GET WELL NATURALLY

LINDA CLARK

AN ARC BOOK   **ARCO PUBLISHING COMPANY, INC.**
219 Park Avenue South, New York, N.Y. 10003

An ARC Book
Published by Arco Publishing Company, Inc.
219 Park Avenue South, New York, N. Y. 10003
by arrangement with The Devin-Adair Company, New York.

Eighth Printing, 1974

Library of Congress Catalog Card Number 65-18927
ISBN 0-668-01762-7

Printed in the United States of America

Foreword

Get Well Naturally is like a well-organized menu. There is something here for every taste. Linda Clark will undoubtedly be taken to task for her boldness in including certain highly controversial approaches to disease. That is to say, they have not yet been accepted by orthodox medicine. But most discoveries are made long before science can explain them, and facts have a way of appearing to be what they are—true, despite all claims to the contrary. So, instead of heeding various critics and removing first this then that item, the author has wisely remembered Aesop's fable of the man with two lady loves: one pulled out his black hairs, one his gray hairs, and soon he was bald.

In these pages are accounts of human experience. I am sure that anyone who reads the book will find suggestions for improving his health and saving his money. Ill health is about the most expensive of all the various fruits of human folly. It is said that the average successful American business executive spends $2,000 to $3,000 per year on medical bills. If he were to concentrate on health-building foods those medical bills would in most cases disappear. But he never gets the tip-off from the usual publicity sources. It must reach him by word of mouth. If this book helps to create such a word-of-mouth campaign it will have fulfilled its purpose admirably.

ROYAL LEE

Lee Foundation for Nutritional Research
Milwaukee 3, Wisconsin

The author explains

As I have stressed in my previous book, *Stay Young Longer*, I do not prescribe and I do not take responsibility for the remedies included here. As a reporter I merely pass on to you what others have already learned. You will find a mixture of orthodox, unorthodox, and folk remedies. I have given sources where feasible, but folklore and home remedies are often handed down through generations; thus they cannot be documented. What sources are available appear in the Bibliography.

In writing *Stay Young Longer* the question, "Is it scientific?" was constantly in mind. On the other hand, *Get Well Naturally* serves an entirely different purpose. My motivation here is "Is it helpful?" If a remedy has already helped—or offers a glimmer of hope—to even one individual, I have included it, orthodox or not. Don't forget that what may be considered unorthodox today might become orthodox tomorrow. I hope you will join me in keeping an open mind in the scrutiny of healing methods which many people have not yet heard of, let alone accepted.

The time has come when human suffering—and its relief—should be put first; whether a remedy is "unorthodox," "unheard of," or "questionable" should be secondary. Obviously, if I had considered any of this information harmful, I would not have included it. Granted, not everything will work for everyone, but if even a small percentage of the remedies help even a few people to feel better, the effort of bringing them out of obscurity and reporting them to you will have been worthwhile.

I hope that doctors, too, will explore and use some of these natural remedies for their patients.

LINDA CLARK

Carmel Valley, California

Contents

PART ONE

SOME UNUSUAL TREATMENTS

1 Believe it or not

In the process of doing research for my first book, *Stay Young Longer*, I came across some surprising information. Some of it—but not all—could be classed as folk medicine. Occasionally an experimenter without funds or expensive laboratories, except his own kitchen or woodshed or basement, would follow a clue, a hunch, a printed sentence, or a sudden chance finding and pursue it relentlessly in order to discover a possible health value. Lacking degrees or funds or commercial backing he tested the results as best he could in limited circumstances. In this section I am reporting on some of these experiments, many of them unusual, to say the least. I am not recommending them.

I do not prescribe and I do not advise. What may be helpful to one person may have no effect whatever on the next, although there are some basic laws which affect all of us. Meanwhile, the experiments are so fascinating that, in my opinion, they should not be overlooked. The solution to a health problem for you may possibly be lurking in one of them.

Many discoveries in the field of health are not accepted today by professional experts. We will examine some of the reasons later. Meanwhile, this should not influence us against experimenting. It behooves us all to keep an open mind about everything having to do with health. History shows that in many fields of science some of the most laughed-at theories later became the pillars of respectable scientific knowledge. For example, the following geniuses were considered "quacks"—or fakers—when they first announced their discoveries:

Samuel F. B. Morse— For his invention of the electric telegraph. He spent his fortune and four heart-breaking years before his invention was accepted.

Thomas A. Edison—	It took him 15 years to overcome prejudice against installing electric lights.
William Roentgen—	The discoverer of X-rays, was accused of being not only a quack, but was criticized for fear his "ray" might invade the privacy of the bedroom.
Charles Goodyear—	Invented vulcanized rubber, yet was called a fool and an imbecile. Without funds, he nearly starved while he was searching for better rubber. Many of his experiments were conducted in prison.
The Wright Brothers—	Were regarded as "cranks" for thinking a machine could fly.

It is an art these days to be yourself. So many people are sheep. They conform to the rule of the majority, no matter how senseless that rule may be. Most of us, for example, read the same books (because they are best sellers and others are reading them), drive the same model cars, follow the clothes trend of the moment, and decorate our homes much in the same manner as our friends and neighbors. Blind acceptance of certain types of health treatments, right or wrong, has been a habit of mankind through history, and many a researcher, belonging to the minority and refusing to be a slave to a pattern set by someone else, has been mercilessly persecuted.

Galen, a physician born around A.D., 130, followed the precepts of his predecessor, Hippocrates, and used diet, massage, and gentle exercise in treating the sick. He was famous and popular. But when he announced his theories of anatomy, which were sketchy but still ahead of the times, he was forced to leave Rome in haste after hiding in dark alleys to avoid the fury of the mob. His views, of course, were later accepted.

Vesalius, a sixteenth-century physician, a teacher of anatomy and surgery at the University of Padua, wrote a book in 1543 announcing new discoveries in human anatomy based on dissection. But because the information differed from the older views of Galen, Vesalius was denounced as an impostor and a heretic. Vituperation was heaped upon his head until he was forced to flee from Italy. Not until after he died were his discoveries accepted.

In the 1600's William Harvey, another physician, discovered what is now considered the most momentous single achievement in the history of medicine: the circulation of the blood. But because it was "different" from the current thinking, he was subjected to ridicule and a storm of abuse. He stood his ground, however, refusing to waver in his beliefs, and his discovery was finally and universally accepted—fortunately while he was still living.

Today there is a tendency to suspect discoveries from anyone who is not a "scientist" or who hasn't a list of degrees after his name. A layman is not supposed to be a "reliable" source of information. So it is not surprising that whenever a layman has made a momentous discovery, he has usually been ignored or ridiculed. For instance, a layman, named Ronssius, discovered that lemon juice was a cure for scurvy 231 years before the British Navy finally accepted the idea! And it took 69 more years before the discovery was put to practical use as a preventive measure in the English Merchant Marine.

Another example of hard-headed resistance concerns beriberi, the disease we now know to be due to lack of vitamin B complex. It was credited to 14 different causes before the truth came home. At one point the accepted scientific conclusion was, "there is no evidence to incriminate any definite food, drink or intermediate host. The host is almost certainly an extra-corporeal or vegetable parasite." The conclusion couldn't have been more wrong. The cause of beriberi was later found in vitamin deficient polished rice, the result of a process which denudes it of B vitamins. When the B vitamins were replaced in the diet, rapid recovery took place in both animals and humans afflicted by it.

Similar persecutions of those who are seeking uncharted avenues to health are taking place today. (Some I shall mention later.) But our modern world of radio, television, air and space travel is so complex and marvelous that nearly anything is possible. What is today's biggest question mark may turn out to be tomorrow's greatest invention. As you read of these unorthodox treatments, at least join me in refusing to pass judgment one way or the other until orthodox science has had a chance to catch up with and either prove or disprove them. If some of these investigators turn out to be ahead of their time, you will have been so informed. If they turn out, on the other hand, to be on the wrong track, at least you will have enjoyed searching in unusual areas. Should you wish to explore further into any of these fields, you will find the sources listed in the back of the book.

2 How to be healthy

We need not be sick. In each of us is a vital force which keeps us living. It also tries to keep us well. An honest physician admits with Hippocrates, the father of medicine, that "Nature cures, not the physician." In fact, the word *physician* is derived from the Greek word *physis*, which means nature.

Professor A. H. Stevens has said, "The older physicians grow, the more skeptical they become of the virtues of medicine, and the more disposed to trust to the powers of nature."

R. Swinburne Clymer, M.D., agrees: "Personally, I do not profess to cure disease. In fact, no man, whatever his system, can do that. Nature alone is capable of curing (eliminating) disease. . . ."

William Gutman, M.D., explains it this way: "Without this healing power of nature, no healing takes place, no cure is possible. . . . If born with a healthy organism, the vital force when not interfered with is capable of carrying us through life free from disease."

This vital, or life, force is the battery within us which keeps us going. It keeps our hearts beating; it exists in every cell, every organ. To achieve health or to maintain it, it must be sustained. If we desire health, we should do everything possible to cooperate with it. Children have a tremendously high voltage of the life force. Old, feeble people have very little. The rest of us are somewhere in between. And when it finally ebbs away, we die. Happily there are ways of charging it while we live.

The human being is incredibly intricate. Earl L. Shaub, an editor and advertising director, gives us a humorous but apt description of our own bodies. "It is staggering to contemplate what our bodies include: camera eyes, radio ears, valves, tubes, pulleys, hinges, arches, temperature control, chemical laboratories, a constant repair system, a telegraphic nervous system, a structural frame, storage space, sewage disposal, pipe lines and a pump. Such is the mechanism of the body, and—what is more—it works!"

Try to visualize the microscopic size of the heart, liver, lungs, eyes, ears, and flying equipment of a mosquito or even a gnat. The human eye cannot even perceive these marvelous little organs, yet they, too, work.

Science must play second fiddle to nature. Dr. Otto Mauset tells us, "Chemistry of today has accomplished wonderful results in many ways, but all the laboratories in the world will never be able to supplant the remarkably fine process which takes place in the living cell. They will never successfully imitate the wonderful methods that nature uses in performing its work in the plant, as well as the human body. Our late American wizard, Thomas A. Edison, expressed himself on the subject as follows: 'Until man duplicates a blade of grass, nature can laugh at his so-called scientific knowledge!' "

How can we cooperate with the natural life force within us, which is trying to keep us well? Dr. Gutman explains that this vital force, though common to us all, differs in each of us. We each have our own special weak spots which flare when we are exposed to a germ, virus, sudden chill, or stress. The life force immediately springs to our defense and tries to begin the healing process. As Dr. Gutman says, "The aim of the treatment is liberation, support and stimulation of the vital force which alone accomplishes the restoration of health."

There are various ways to support this vital force in order to encourage it to take over and begin healing. One method is to let well enough alone. Here are two examples:

A little girl, just four years old, fell and cut her chin. Tearfully, she asked her mother for a band-aid. But her mother advised, "Since the cut is on your chin and can't get very dirty, let it alone. A scab will form instead." The child considered this for a moment, then she answered, "I guess you're right. Maybe a scab is God's band-aid." And maybe it is.

William Fabry, a physician who lived in the seventeenth century, was considered the real father of German surgery. Though a bold and skillful surgeon, he was conservative in his beliefs. In those days of swords and daggers, he devised the "weapon salve treatment" as an alternative to surgery. When a patient appeared with a dagger or sword wound, Dr. Fabry demanded the weapon which had inflicted the wound. Then he carefully and solemnly applied a salve and bandage, not to the *patient*, but to the *weapon!* The patient was advised to go home and return in two or three days, at which time the salve-and-bandage treatment—for the weapon—was repeated. Thus, all attention was concentrated on the weapon, while the actual human wound itself was merely covered with a clean cloth and forgotten. Healing was so successful with this natural, let-alone, healing technique, that "weapon-salve treatment" was used for over a hundred years.

Obviously there are some forms of disease which may not be ignored. In his book, *Prolongation of Life* (see Bibliography), Dr. William Gutman explains how some of them appear, and how to handle them. Dr. Gutman is a staff member of New York Medical College-Flower Fifth Avenue Hospital, New York City:

"The signs of reaction of the vital force in disease we call the symptoms of disease. They signify either successful defense and recovering of the disturbed balance of the organism, or a failing effort.

"Pain and fever are such signs of self-defense; pain enforces rest, the preliminary condition of recovery, and directs attention to the disturbed organ, so that it can properly be cared for; fever and inflammation are the expression of the defense of the organism against infection and toxins, indicating the formation and mobilization of immune bodies and white blood cells, the main fighters against infection. . . .

"The vital force is usually successful, if obstacles to its action are removed in time. If, however, these obstacles . . . continue to operate for a prolonged period, deflection, weakening and finally failure of the vital force result. To the extent that the vital force weakens, degenerative processes take place in the diseased organs and system. . . .

"The logical first step of treatment is removal of the obstacles. . . . the other part of the treatment is the direct support of the vital force, the field of medicine proper. . . . [Still another part of the treatment is] the method of substitution. The use of vitamins and hormones belongs in this field; insulin in the treatment of diabetes is an outstanding example of this practice. The method of substitution is of great importance, for it gives the organism what it lacks or cannot produce in sufficient quantities for some reason. . . . The vital force is assisted in a task which it cannot perform adequately and is thus strengthened in an indirect way."

R. Swinburne Clymer, M.D., in his book, *Medicines of Nature* (see Bibliography) adds, "All that I, or any other man, however great he may be, can do, is to seek the cause of the weakness, learn what the deficiences are that brought it about, then proceed to supply the essential substances. Nature can then do the rebuilding—the reconstructing. . . .

"Drugs, those [synthetic] substances so consistently prescribed, cannot be digested or assimilated. They may be absorbed by the cells just as dyes are absorbed by cotton, woolen or silk goods, but assimilation is not possible. . . ."

Dr. Clymer continues, "[When drugs are given] the hungry cells are not supplied with the foods for which they are crying. Such agents are of no actual value, except in rare instances where they stimulate weakened (hungry and starved) cells to make a greater effort to establish their lost balance.

"The *Natural* physician does *not* attempt to cure, he merely supplies the cells with the *food* (vegetables, herbs, cereals, legumes and fruits, *i.e.* their vital mineral content) which they need. By this he attempts to eradicate disease (cell weakness or cell congestion) and to establish a state of well being. This is my plan of operation and the system I personally advocate."

Dr. Gutman agrees. Drugs, in his opinion, act upon the vital force in a way similar to whipping a tired horse. Far better, he says, to support the vital force with natural foods, vitamins, and minerals. These give the body what it lacks or cannot produce in sufficient quantities, thus assisting and strengthening the life force indirectly through a maintenance program.

This method encompasses prevention as well as cure. H. P. Pickerill, M.D., says, "There is but one rational way of treating disease on a large scale—that is by building up the resistance, active and passive, of the individual to the disease."

His statement may well turn out to be one of the most important in the history of health!

In case you consider the "life force" a mere figment of the imagination, its existence has been proved in the laboratory. Dr. Hans Selye, Director of Experimental Medicine and Surgery at the University of Montreal, has established the actuality of the life force, which he has named "Adaptation Energy," and which reacts to physical, chemical and psychological stresses in maintaining health and resisting disease. Before we discuss methods in which the life force can be charged, let us look at one of the insidious ways in which it can be weakened.

3 Why drugs?

I recently learned the story of a business man who had had an electrifying experience. John, his wife Amy explained to me, had a history of allergy to green onions. It was not a psychosomatic allergy, because he reacted violently to them even when they had been disguised in a salad, and when he was unaware that he had eaten them. His symptoms included severe indigestion and nausea. Amy had learned how to cope with this allergy in a simple, natural way. She merely gave him an emetic, he got rid of the cause of the disturbance, and that was that. The symptoms promptly subsided.

One day, however, when Amy was visiting friends in a nearby town, John, again unknowingly, ate green onions and responded in his characteristic manner. Since Amy was gone, an alarmed friend called a doctor, who, himself, had recently recovered from a heart attack. Noting John's symptoms, which were not unlike those of a heart disturbance, the physician prescribed a round of quinidine, a drug which is an anticoagulant and used in treating heart irregularities.

John grew steadily worse. Amy was hastily summoned, and while the quinidine was being continued, a heart specialist was also called. John at this point developed blood blisters, first on his tongue, then on his face, arms, and even on his eyes. Then, both externally and internally, he began to bleed profusely. He was rushed to the hospital, given transfusions, tests, and various types of medications. Amy was told that there was little hope.

Meanwhile, the quinidine had been laid aside in favor of other drugs, and while his wife and doctors were expecting the worst, to the astonishment of everyone, John began to improve. He continued to get better until one week later he was dismissed from the hospital.

The doctors, who by this time had established by electrocardiogram the fact that John's heart was normal, admitted that quinidine appeared to be the cause of the bleeding. When John asked if it had caused bleeding in others, he was told, cautiously, "Yes, in some cases."

Dr. James A. L. Roth, professor at the University of Pennsylvania Graduate School of Medicine, is an internationally known expert on the effects of drugs on the digestive system. He warns that aspirin can also trigger internal bleeding and may cause low-grade anemia. He adds, "60 to 70 per cent of all people who take aspirin in almost any form will bleed internally in small amounts."

The amount of aspirin that causes trouble is apparently not what one would occasionally use for a simple headache. Dr. Francis

X. Fellers and Dr. John Craig, both of Boston, declare that it is the massive doses, as taken for rheumatoid arthritis or rheumatic fever, which can cause renal pillary necrosis, the illness in which kidney tissue is killed. Drs. Benedict R. Harrow and Jack A. Sloane reported kidney damage from phenacetin, a common ingredient of many pain-killers. As a result of the danger of aspirin and phenacetin, these four physicians believe that both drugs should carry the label: *Danger from prolonged daily use.*

Yet, on the radio, I have heard this commercial: "If you feel hot and headachy this summer, stop and take two aspirins and you will feel better fast. It will just take two minutes to take two tablets. They may be the most important minutes of your day."

We live in an "instant" civilization. We demand instant service, instant food, instant transportation, and instant results. So, since everything else must be instant, we insist on instant relief from sickness or pain. If a person is depressed, he wants an instant lift (pep pill). If he is tired, he wants instant rest (a tranquilizer or sleeping pill). If he has a chill or fever or virus, he wants an instant cure (an antibiotic). The current slogan is: *Do Something Now.* The drug industry knows this and as a result is making hay.

No one enjoys suffering. Although an antibiotic may save a life, it may also produce adverse side effects or even death. Several months ago a young mother took her child to the family physician for a check-up. When this was finished, she said, "Incidentally, I think I am coming down with a virus or the flu. How about an antibiotic, doctor?" The doctor consented, and gave her a shot of penicillin without testing to see if she was allergic. Five minutes later she was dead. John, my friend who took quinidine, was one of the lucky ones.

Lawrence Galton, in an article "A Pill for Every Purpose," wrote, "Medicine is often used to push nature out of the way, not to help nature when help is needed. We rush to stop a cough. But coughing, so long as it is not excessive, is useful; it is nature's defense system.

"We view any fever with alarm. But fever must go very high to be dangerous in itself. And many doctors now prefer to let a fever run unchecked as long as it doesn't become excessive, for they believe that body defenses increase at high temperature."

Are quinidine, penicillin, aspirin, and of course, thalidomide, the only potentially dangerous drugs? No. The reports are endless. The American Medical Association has warned against at least 72 of them, including quinidine, which may cause from mild to serious blood disorders. They cite one of the most popular antibiotics, one of the best-selling tranquilizers, and two widely used anti-diabetes pills. The entire list includes: antibiotics, tranquilizers, sleeping pills, anti-arthritis and anti-gout drugs, pain-killers, anti-diabetes pills, kidney stimulants, anti-coagulants, heart soothers, anti-epileptic drugs, thyroid drugs, sulfa drugs.

Sidney Katz, a reporter, writes on overmedication in two articles in *Maclean's* magazine, "Your Health and the Almighty Pill" and "The Criminal Record of the Miracle Drugs": "A more potent but less frequently prescribed group of drugs are the steroids, which are hormonal compounds. They were hailed with great enthusiasm in 1948 when a Mayo Clinic physician first demonstrated the miraculous way in which cortisone banished the symptoms of rheumatoid arthritis. It was soon learned that the side effects could be devastating. Steroids ignite peptic ulcers; reactivate tuberculosis; kindle diabetes in the susceptible, cause a form of psychosis in the emotionally unstable person. Arthritic children, carelessly treated with steroids, may end up with bones so deficient in calcium that they suffer from merely walking. Some steroids, the sex hormones, can do great harm. Men dosed with them have developed large breasts; women have grown beards. . . . Pregnant women, treated with them for abortion, have given birth to female infants with male genitalia. These have to be removed by surgery. . . . Cortisone has also caused cataracts."

Mr. Katz, in gathering material for his articles, questioned physicians, pharmacologists, hospital clinicians, scientific researchers, and others about the drug problem. His conclusion is that "unless we quickly mend our ways, we are on our way to creating a nightmare of drug-induced heart and blood disease; damaged livers and kidneys; impaired hearing, sight and sexual powers; and the birth of an increasing number of severely deformed babies.

"There are so many drugs on the market that nobody can even count them accurately. Most of them serve no useful purpose; they confuse and bewilder laymen and doctors. . . ."

Antibiotics, according to his findings, may have saved many lives, but they are also doing incalculable harm. One doctor pointed out that a drug potent enough to poison a germ could also poison a person.

Some doctors, when not successful with one antibiotic, try a second and even a third. Worst of all are the effects of some of these drugs in combination.

The death of Alan Ladd, the Hollywood film star, according to Coroner James T. Bird, was due to a combination of a high level of alcohol and three drugs which acted upon his nervous system. The drugs were identified as two types of tranquilizers and one barbiturate.

According to Morton M. Hunt, a reporter and author of an article, "Side-Effects: A New Worry for Doctors" (in *Look*, December 31, 1963), "A twenty-four-year-old soldier with a sore throat reported to sick bay at an Army base not long ago. The medical officer prescribed a gargle and some antibiotic lozenges. The soldier went to the dispensary and got his prescription, then put a lozenge in his mouth and walked two blocks to his barracks. There, he fell down in convulsions, bloody froth coming from his mouth. In a few minutes he was dead from 'anaphylactic shock'—and a systemic overreaction due to his individual hypersensitivity to the antibiotic."

Tranquilizers, originally intended for mental hospitals, are now anybody's game. Sidney Katz thus concludes his article on the subject: "Obviously there are ordinary, usual situations which every normal human being must be prepared to face without leaning on a drug. [Yet] manufacturers, in their advertisements, have recommended tranquilizers for . . . homesickness, restlessness in children, fear, fatigue, itching, working in a noisy place, going to weddings and funerals, giving a speech, having differences of opinion with somebody. One advertiser boasted in print that his product so alleviated 'hostilities' that the average patient wouldn't even be able to start an argument after one dose."

Who is to blame for this hurricane of drugs sweeping the world? Is it our doctors, the drug industry, or the people themselves? I have spent several years trying to solve the mystery. By picking up a clue here and there from guarded statements of professionals who know the inside story, I finally learned the truthful solution. To call it shocking is an understatement.

4 Who is to blame?

In trying to unravel the mystery of who is to blame for the avalanche of drugs being foisted upon us, I began to feel like a second Erle Stanley Gardner. People who should—and did—know about such things were very cautious for fear of being quoted and of consequent persecution. So, in order to protect them, I cannot give their names. A few courageous people who have already spoken out in other publications can be mentioned.

I began by questioning an internationally famous anthropologist. "What," I asked, "causes out-and-out lies to be fed to the public?" I was thinking about the radio commercials praising aspirin, and ads in the medical journals extolling the virtues of specific drugs as "safe," "harmless," and "with little or no side effects," when tests have proved otherwise! The anthropologist gave me a simple answer. "Money," he said. "Everybody wants to make money. This is more important to some manufacturers than integrity or honesty."

The Nation (September 21, 1964) states: "The ethical drug business has an advertising/sales business of 10.5 per cent, only the fourth highest in American industry, but fantastic in terms of expenditure per prospect. About $750 million is spent every year to persuade 180,000 physicians to prescribe the products of some sixty drug companies. Every possible dodge is used, from seductive advertising in medical journals to free cocktail parties and including, of course, the visits of detail men. As the late Pierre R. Garai put it . . . , 'perhaps no other group in this country is so insistently sought after, chased, wooed, pressured and downright importuned as this small group of doctors who are the *de facto* wholesalers of the ethical drug business. . . .'"

American Druggist rejoices that the doctor's pen is flowing more freely than ever, and new prescriptions and refills are booming. Some of these drugs are life savers, but many are worthless, not a few are actually harmful, and occasionally one is dangerous. Dr. Dale G. Friend, professor of medicine at Harvard and head of clinical pharmacology at Peter Bent Brigham Hospital in Boston, says flatly that there is no such thing as a safe drug.

I asked the anthropologist, a pioneer in the study of people who lived many years ago under natural conditions and enjoyed abundant health, why herbs and roots are no longer used today as medicines. He answered, "Because they don't make as much money for the processors as drugs. Also, the natural cure is apt to be longer-lasting. There is no money in prevention." In other words, *there is money in them thar' ills!*

One physician told me that every morning he opens his post office box to find it loaded with drug samples. A legal authority added that one drug company tried to lure the physicians to use these drug samples on their patients by baiting the physicians with such rewards as points toward a tape recorder, or butterflies for a butterfly collection!

The drug industry, another retired physician told me, is giving huge grants to medical schools. Professors are paid to "teach" young medical students about the "new" and "wonderful" drugs. When this physician cautioned his two young nephew medical students about using untested drugs, their retort was, "Oh, Uncle, you are so old-fashioned! These drugs are the *newest* things!"

Dr. Harry Lillie, a London physician, considers modern drugs "99 per cent useless." In an interview published in the *Winnipeg Free Press* (Canada), September 5, 1961, he said, "Drugs patch up the symptoms, not the causes. When I first qualified, I thought the use of drugs was just the thing. But I'd never go back to that now.

"The medical profession on both sides of the Atlantic is being run and dictated to by the pharmaceutical houses."

Dr. Lillie also disputes claims that diptheria and smallpox have been wiped out by inoculation and vaccination. He says, "The advances made in this field are largely advances in sanitation engineering."

Senator Ernest Gruening of Alaska, himself an M.D. and a Harvard graduate, told the Senate Government Operations Committee, investigating the Food and Drug Administration (F.D.A.), "For twenty-five years the A.M.A. has been silent in face of the fact that the Food and Drug Administration has 'buried' scientific data within the 13,000 new drug applications on file. No medical scientist can obtain purely medical information which F.D.A.—by administrative decision, not by law—labels 'secret.' "

Dr. William Gutman, on the subject of drugs, cautions, "This method [the use of drugs] treats each symptom or complaint separately, and by its opposite; for instance . . . pain by giving a pain-relieving drug or narcotic; fever by temperature-depressing drugs; constipation by giving a laxative, etc. . . . Such treatment considers neither the disease nor the patient as a whole. It has only a very limited place as a momentary measure to give the organism some rest, a night's sleep, or a pain-free interval so that the vital or life force can recover more quickly, and it is applicable in the final stages of incurable conditions where relief only is possible.

"Treating only a symptom, one loses sight of the disease process. . . . Catering to the patient's complaints one is apt to lose sight of the cure in concentrating more and more on relieving unpleasant subjective symptoms. The dangerous consequence is suppression of the disease process. This leads to new complications through deflecting the vital force which produces new symptoms in another organ.

"Finally, treating single symptoms needs large doses of a drug, and this in itself has a great disadvantage. First of all, large doses 'backfire' mostly; that means that their desired effect is followed by the opposite effect; a laxative leaves the intestines more sluggish and constipated than before; an anti-acid for the stomach produces in its secondary effect higher stomach acidity; a narcotic, in its after-effect, a state of greater sensitivity and irritability; therefore, new and often large doses are required constantly to relieve the isolated symptom. If recovery takes place, then it does so not because, but in spite of, such treatment. In addition, the large dose or repeated larger doses of drugs have toxic side effects."

Dr. A. Dale Console, a former medical director of a major drug concern (according to a *New York Times* report) told Senate anti-trust investigators: "Doctors and the public are subjected to a constant 'barrage' of new drugs, some worthless, and others with a 'greater potential for harm than good. . . . since so much depends on novelty, drugs change like women's hemlines.'

"More than half the research of drug companies is directed toward projects that are really not worth-while, but are purchased simply because there is profit in it.

"The drug industry has high-pressure sales techniques based on the maxim, 'If you can't convince them, confuse them.'

"Most medical leaders and educators 'face the problem with denial, complacency or futility' because the industry is unique in that it can make exploitation appear a noble purpose."

Dr. Wendell Macleod, dean of medicine at the University of Saskatchewan, Canada, urges us to get back to nature. "Confidence in the healing power of nature," he says, "has been displaced by undue dependence upon the popular drugs of the moment. . . ."

In September, 1963, the F.D.A. announced that the birth-control pill, Enovid, had mistakenly been declared dangerous. When investigators rechecked their figures they found, ". . . that they had used the wrong set of statistics for the normal death rate of women over 35. It is a horribly embarrassing mistake," they said. But the go-ahead on sales of Enovid, which the F.D.A. finally permitted without a warning label that it can lead to dangerous blood clots, is a serious error according to Dr. Louis Lasagna, associate professor of medicine, pharmacological and experimental therapeutics, at Johns Hopkins University. He still believes that Enovid can "lead to thrombo-embolic disease and death." He states that he has met a number of other doctors who agree. One doctor told him, "I wouldn't give Enovid to my own wife, so I wouldn't prescribe it for anyone else's wife." (*Health Bulletin*, October 26, 1963). Enovid is only one trade name for "the pill"; there are others. Before using any of them consult your doctor!

Dr. Herbert Ratner, director of public health, Oak Park, Illinois, has predicted that birth-control pills may be removed from the market because of the role they play in cancer. Researchers at the University of Oregon found that Enovid "markedly accelerated both the development and growth of all tumors" of the breast in mice. (*Health Bulletin*, June 6, 1964.)

Four Detroit doctors, at Henry Ford Hospital, emphasize the danger of blood clots from taking Enovid. One woman, age 39, suffered from a blood clot below the knee requiring a leg amputation. (*Journal of the American Medical Association*, May 4, 1964.)

The use of Enovid is apparently also suspect for older women. Dr. Barnet M. Hershfield, writing in the *New York State Journal of Medicine*, mentions the fact that Enovid is often prescribed for menstrual disfunctions in older women and may be dangerous for them, too.

Many drug firms are on the bandwagon with new brands of oral contraceptives all spoken of collectively as "the pill."

Dr. Herbert Ratner charges, as quoted by *Health Bulletin*, "One of the difficulties in this field is that there is a reluctance to publish anything critical about the pill because it is so popular and so lucrative to drug companies."

Elise Jerard, reporting in *Modern Nutrition* (October and November, 1963), adds, "In short, it is reasonably clear that products are being protected rather than people. There is a growing rebellion among informed physicians and consumers against such a philosophy and such practices."

How about the doctors? Are they to blame? For the most part, no. They are caught between the pressures of the drug industry, which wants to sell more drugs, and their patients, who, motivated by advertising, want to take more drugs.

Morton M. Hunt explains the plight of the doctor. "Ninety per cent of the prescription drugs now in use did not exist twenty years ago. Virtually all the antibiotics, steroids, histamines and tranquilizers have been developed since the average forty-five-year-old doctor left medical school . . . adding new data at a rate he cannot possibly absorb while practicing his profession. . . .

"Even with large-scale testing on human beings, there is no certainty that drugs which seem to work out all right now won't later prove terribly harmful. In complete despair, most doctors look for short cuts; they learn about the drugs from the 'detail man,' the advance runner of the drug companies or from drug-company advertising and direct mail brochures. None of these could, by the wildest stretch of the imagination, be considered impartial and scrupulously accurate sources. . . ."

It is common knowledge that the busy doctor gets much of his information about drugs from drug salesmen. An article on the American doctor, which appeared in the *Saturday Evening Post* reports that a doctor simply hasn't enough time to read. "In the unlikely event that some patients miss appointments, he [the doctor] can work over the approximately fifty pieces of mail that arrive daily. These include drug literature . . . and forms for insurance companies. Or he can read the medical journals that, 'I never seem to catch up with.' Or he listens to the economic-scientific intrusion of the drug salesmen."

To complicate the doctors' crowded schedules and pressure from the drug industry, patients seem, somehow, to believe that health, like many other things, can be bought. They often demand a drug, either because of the influence of advertising or because a friend has recommended it. They forget that although new drugs have seemingly produced miracles, they also—on prolonged use—have often led to disaster. This disaster, as in the case of untested penicillin mentioned before, has caused death in a single dose.

SOME WAYS TO PROTECT YOURSELF

I asked a physician if there were a test to determine the allergic effect of penicillin on a patient. He told me there was a simple test—involving a drop of blood—a procedure which took about ten minutes, but that few doctors use it. He said, "I hate to admit that in giving drugs, many of my own profession are delinquent."

Unfortunately this test is not always reliable. But it is better to take it than not. As an added precaution, if the doctor *has* administered an injection of penicillin, the patient should remain in his office for a short while afterward. If serious allergic symptoms do appear, the physician can provide prompt treatment in case it is needed. One method is to administer penicillinase, an enzyme which acts as an antidote to penicillin. Other first-aid measures are available, and may help if given immediately.

Do not accept medication from your relatives, friends, or neighbors. A physician told me that one of his patients developed some mysterious and distressing symptoms. Quick detective work on his part led to an antibiotic tablet labeled only with a trade name. A neighbor had generously given it to her friend because the tablet had helped her! An analysis revealed that the "antibiotic tablet" contained a form of penicillin, a fact of which neither the patient nor the neighbor was aware.

Sometimes the source is harder to pinpoint. For example, cows are often given penicillin, which appears in their milk and is in turn passed on to people.

The *New England Medical Journal* (December 12, 1963), suggests that if an individual disturbance is known to exist, such as epilepsy or diabetes, that person should wear a "dog tag" stating the precautions and treatment in case the patient goes into shock. It would be equally helpful to have penicillin or other antibiotic allergies mentioned on an identification tag.

I was told by a spokesman who did not wish to be quoted that the demand for penicillin became so great that the massive amounts needed could not be grown fast enough by the natural process. Hence the drug began to be synthesized. At this point, said my informant, the disturbing penicillin reactions became widespread. Whether a cause and effect relationship exists is an interesting speculation.

For a long time I could find no supporting evidence for this information. Recently, what appears to be confirmation, came from the *New England Medical Journal* (November 21, 1963), which reports, "As early as 1960, it was estimated that more than 500 new penicillins had been prepared that could not have been made by fermentation technics alone. . . . Careful study of larger numbers of patients treated under controlled conditions will be needed to determine the full potential and comparative value of the various new derivatives already available or soon to be released for general use."

Another reason some doctors yield to the demands of their patients for a specific drug is that if they don't prescribe it the patient will go to a doctor who does!

Many doctors will testify that the average patient doesn't want to improve his living habits to improve his health. Patients would rather break every known health rule, then seek absolution in a pill. According to Alexander Bryce, M.D., "They don't want to be cured. They are content to be patched up sufficiently to continue their practice of self-indulgence in various forms."

Dr. Herbert Ratner, former professor of preventive medicine at Loyola University, Chicago, who was mentioned in the Katz report, says, " 'We are too impatient to give nature a chance. At the first sign of a minor or even trivial illness we impose drastic drugs and techniques intended for serious conditions. Many of the illnesses are self-limiting—they would do better without interference from a physician. America is the most over-medicated, the most over-operated, the most over-inoculated country in the world.' "

In the same report Dr. Alton Goldbloom says, " 'I have cured more people by taking away drugs than by giving them.' "

So the mystery is solved. The finger of suspicion does not point to the physician, but to the pressure put upon him.

In every profession there are good and bad examples. One cannot make a generalization that most doctors are ruthless, money-mad, given to unnecessary surgery, or abnormal use of drugs. I know many fine physicians who are dedicated to getting and keeping their patients well, at the same time trying to keep themselves free from the entangling web of drug-industry or patient pressure. If you locate this type of doctor, you have discovered a gem. By all means, cooperate with him.

WHAT HAPPENS BEHIND SCENES

Richard Harris, in three articles in the *New Yorker* (March 14, 21, and 28, 1964) brings to light facts which were discovered by

Senator Estes Kefauver in his long attempt to safeguard people from dangerous and overpriced drugs. These articles now appear in Mr. Harris's book, *The Real Voice* (Macmillan, 1964).

Kefauver learned that the drug industry was making huge profits on "wonder drugs." For example, 1,118 per cent profit, and 7,079 per cent profit were made on just two drugs alone.

John Lear, science editor of the *Saturday Review* flushed out the information that one large drug company had extolled an antibiotic, which, said the company, was endorsed by eight doctors. The names, addresses, telephone numbers, and office hours were listed. When John Lear wrote to these doctors for verification, the letters were returned. When he telegraphed them, he was told there were no such addresses. And when he telephoned, he found that no such numbers existed.

Meanwhile Senator Kefauver learned that physicians, themselves, were being fooled: One instructor, an M.D., testified, "The average practicing physician—and I have helped train hundreds of them—just does not have the time, the facilities, the skill nor the training to be an expert in the determination of drug efficacy."

Dr. Solomon Garb, of the Albany Medical College, added, "The majority of the mailed ads are unreliable, to the extent that a trusting physician could be seriously misled."

Dr. J. Murray Steele, professor of medicine at New York University, called attention to "the extravagant and distorted literature which some of the drug houses are distributing to the medical profession. . . . it may recommend a product in such a way as to lead to, if not encourage its indiscriminate use . . . with little or no mention of side effects. . . ."

The hearings revealed that nearly every drug produced adverse side effects on certain people under certain conditions, yet few drug manufacturers had issued such warnings.

Senator Kefauver learned that generic names are seldom used. Trade names are handier and easier to remember and to prescribe.

Dr. Console said, "By the time the doctor learns what the company knew at the beginning, it has two new products to take the place of the old one."

Sometimes the same drug has different names. Dr. Walter Modell, associate professor of pharmacology at Cornell University

Medical College and editor of *Drugs of Choice*, reported that one drug with which he was acquainted had as many as 25 names. He testified, "No practicing physician can possibly deal with this Hydra-headed monster of terminology. . . . if a patient is allergic to a drug under one trade name, and if the doctor, in trying to avoid it, gives him the same drug under another trademark because he doesn't know the two are identical, he can cause a catastrophe."

The Senator learned that advertising practices were voluminous and unscrupulous.

As for advertising reliability, Harris reports the policy of the *Journal of the American Medical Association*, which proclaims, "Every statement which appears in A.M.A. publication ads must be backed by substantiated facts . . . or we won't run it! This is why you can rely on what you read about products which are advertised in the pages of the A.M.A. scientific journals."

Yet in two issues of the *Journal* a week apart, appeared two ads. One, for Equanil, warned of dangers from its indiscriminate use. The other ad was for Miltown, which, in part encouraged its use with assurance of ". . . no cumulative effects . . . does not impair mental efficiency or normal behavior." Yet Equanil and Miltown are different names *for the same drug!*

Mr. Harris quoted Paul Dixon, a lawyer, one of Kefauver's assistants, who said, "These drug fellows pay for a lobby which makes the steel boys look like popcorn vendors. In the end, they mounted against Estes the most intense attack I've seen in a quarter of a century in Washington. Anybody who dares seek the truth will be accused of being a persecutor. Estes was certainly accused of that and much more."

Some physicians have given up the use of drugs entirely. Others have testified that they could manage to keep patients well with about 20 drugs, instead of the thousands which are now on the market.

H. G. Cox, M.D., formerly of the College of Physicians and Surgeons (New York), remarked, "The fewer remedies you employ in any disease, the better for your patients."

Drugs are not the only menace. Some cosmetics have been proved dangerous to those who use them. One woman, whose doctor diagnosed a large swelling under her armpit as due to her reaction to the use of a deodorant made by a well-known cosmetic company, was told by the firm that if she pressed charges, she would be sued in return for an exorbitant amount.

Several medical tests have ascertained that certain hair sprays have caused lung tumors in women who inhaled the spray. When the spray was discontinued, the tumors disappeared. An acquaintance recently told me that her face had swelled after using a well-known hair spray.

Dr. Kenneth G. Baker, a dermatologist, reported that hair sprays are definitely related to some acnes in teen-age girls. The acne appears on forehead, face, and neck. Dr. John M. Gowdy, of the F.D.A. agrees. He cites the reports of other clinicians who suspect that sprays, hair dye, and home-permanent solutions can cause skin disturbance. (*Health Bulletin*, May 23, 1964.)

There are safe, organic cosmetics, deodorants, and even a safe, organic hair spray available at health food stores.

WHAT CAN YOU DO?

How can we defend ourselves these days in this high-pressure era in which we live? One way is to refuse to be dominated or hoodwinked into accepting what you do not want to accept. Become an intelligent consumer. An aroused and educated public can turn the tide in the opposite direction. Manufacturers, who admittedly must make a living, can be made to manufacture harmless products instead of harmful ones, providing the demand is great enough. There is no need for any of us to be a puppet of the advertising industry.

One example of the think-for-yourself attitude came from a young mother who told me, "I didn't take a single drug during my pregnancy." And her own radiant health and beautiful, perfect baby bore testimony to her intelligent program.

Pauline Beregoff-Gillow, M.D., feels that while bigger and better hospitals are being feverishly built, progress in health should mean, instead, eliminating disease and closing hospitals. Her suggestion is to substitute "Preventoriums" for hospitals.

There are two ways out of the drug dilemma—if you want to get well and stay well. One is to *prevent* chronic poor health; the other is to get well via the natural, drugless way.

There are natural techniques (usually hidden or belittled to prevent public acceptance) which can often relieve pain and eliminate disease as effectively as drugs, without dangerous side effects. There are also ways to immunize your body from various threats through herbs and natural foods. These techniques have brought me—and scores of others whom I know personally—safely from poor health to good health, so I *know* it can be done. Many of these remedies and techniques appear in this book.

5 Is it safe to do it yourself?

Prevention is easier and cheaper than cure. But if you have passed that point, need help, and have some remedies at your disposal, is it wise to use them instead of relying on a doctor?

In *This Week* magazine (December 18, 1960), D. Vincent Askey, M.D., a past president of the American Medical Association, reported his opinion of self-help: "Home remedies always will have a place in the treatment of mankind's aches and pains. Physicians do not expect and do not desire that patients shall dash to the doctor with every minor discomfort, every trifling injury, every small ache and pain. It is sensible to care for such things by simple, safe home means."

But Dr. Askey feels that folk medicine has potentialities for great harm in that some serious illnesses have small beginnings, and that it is important to know when *not* to rely upon traditional home remedies. He warns, "The use of home remedies must be tempered with judgment, and in case of doubt, prompt resort to modern scientific care is the course of wisdom."

Dr. Askey's rule of thumb is this: Whenever any pain persists, returns again and again; when any inflammation, lump, or growing mass is obviously not temporary, the time for home medication has passed.

Mildred W. McKie, M.D., a physician who has worked for many years in India, is the author of an excellent booklet, *Natural Aids for Common Ills*. She points out that long ago early man lived close to nature. She considers it a pity that much of his knowledge has been lost or forgotten.

She writes, "One should *never underestimate* the healing forces of nature for they are a vital aid to the body. . . . Ancient people knew their value and worked out various methods to utilize their healing and health-giving power. These simple [nature] methods can easily be learned by all and should be reinstated. Not only are they used for treating illness but more largely for building strong healthy bodies."

Dr. McKie adds, "We need to know the Laws of Nature which control our health and life, so that we may live according to them, as our ancestors did. Somehow or other, by trial and error, or by a higher science than we now possess, they worked out a system of healthful living. These same fundamental principles hold true today. Science is now gradually proving that their 'old empirical knowledge' was and still is sound, that the natural methods they evolved are scientifically correct and the 'ancient way of life' is still the best. It is up to the present generation to discover that way of life and health, to understand and recognize its value in order to make a modern application of those ancient principles to meet the needs of today."

In an address in defense of the right to self-medication, Clinton Robb, an attorney of Washington, D.C., stated, "The privilege of choosing one's own remedies for one's own ills has been regarded, from time immemorial, as one of those natural or inherent rights which are the heritage of all those worthy of the name of freedom.

It belongs to that group of intimate personal privileges and liberties that countless generations of men have struggled to establish and maintain.

"In primitive times, of course, self-diagnosis and self-medication were absolute essentials of existence and the privilege of practicing such self-treatment went unchallenged. As society developed and the rights of the individual gradually became more interwoven with those of the general public, some limitations and qualifications of that right became necessary for the common good. But it is to be clearly noted that in the United States of America at least, the broad and general right of the individual to attempt to diagnose his own ailments and attempt their relief through remedies of his own choosing never has been denied by our courts. Indeed, there are affirmative rulings in many adjudged cases to the effect that, with certain well-defined exceptions, the rights of self-diagnosis and self-treatment belong to every individual of proper age and sound mind. One court has expressed the general or basic principle thus: 'Every human being of adult years and sound mind has a right to determine what shall be done with his own body.' "

6 Who can help you?

A woman came up to me one evening after I had finished a lecture and asked in a self-conscious stage whisper, "What do you think of chiropractors?"

I answered her, definitely not in a stage whisper, but in full voice, "I feel the same way about them as I do about other physicians. If you find one who is being truly helpful, consider him one of your treasures."

She looked vastly relieved and said, "Oh, I am so glad you said that! I have a wonderful one, but some people make fun of me for going to him."

If we are trying to put down discrimination among races in this country, it is high time we put down discrimination among health practitioners, whether it be a doctor of medicine, a doctor of chiropractic, a doctor of osteopathy, a doctor of naturopathy, or a spiritual healer. In building a house, many artisans are needed: architect, carpenter, electrician, plumber, painter, and perhaps a landscape gardener. The work of each does not duplicate; it complements, and together they complete the structure.

People who are afraid to accept a certain type of treatment because it is unusual or unfashionable are entitled to their opinions, of course. On the other hand, those who are independent thinkers should be allowed to choose whatever professional assistance they wish, if they feel they will derive help from it, without being made to feel guilty or peculiar just because it is "different."

I asked a friend, an M.D., what he, personally, thought of these various professions.

He replied, "I think each group, whether it is chiropractic, osteopathic, naturopathic, or homeopathic has something to contribute. It is my opinion that no one of us has the *only* right method; a patient should be entitled to help from all methods, according to his need."

Three of the most successful M.D.'s I know (I am measuring success in the ability to achieve health for patients, not to make money from them) have studied all of these forms of treatment and use whatever is necessary to keep their patients well.

Each philosophy is consistent with its own objectives, although in many cases some of the treatments of each of the following groups (listed alphabetically) overlap, as you will see. Please maintain an open mind until you have read *all* of the facts.

Separate chapters are devoted to homeopathy and other therapies less well known than the four which follow.

CHIROPRACTIC

David Daniel Palmer, rediscoverer of the principles on which chiropractic is based, states: "Chiropractic is founded on the relationship of bones, nerves, and muscles. Displacement of any part of the skeletal frame may press against the nerves . . . leading to possible disturbance or disease.

"Chiropractors adjust, by hand, all displacements of the 200 bones, more especially those of the vertebral column, for the purpose of removing nerve impingements which are the cause of deranged functions. . . ."

Dr. Palmer adds, "I think there is some good in all methods; but when the chiropractor adjusts the bony framework to its normal position, all pliable tissue will respond and resume its proper position and consequently the usual functions—health being the result.

"I have never felt it beneath my dignity to do anything to relieve human suffering."

Professor Bircher-Benner stated, "Up to now I have not met one M.D. who could judge the spinal column half as well as a competent chiropractor."

Chiropractic is not new. It probably originated with the ancient Greeks. Hippocrates warned, "One or more vertebrae of the spine may or may not go out of place. They might give way very little and, if they do, they are likely to produce serious complications and even death, if not properly adjusted."

Charles Greenbert, M.D., a modern physician, in a recent study, "Report on Spinal Adjustment and its Relation to Health and Disease" concludes, "Time and again this theory [the chiropractic theory of spinal adjustment] has been confirmed not only by chiropractors but by eminent leaders of medical science.

"The following conditions are the ones which respond successfully and quickly to spinal adjustments:

"Sacroiliac strain, neuralgia of arms, legs, back and face.

"Neuritis and sciatica.

"Asthma.

"Migraine, and all other types of severe headaches; dizziness, nervous tension.

"Lumbago, and all other back pains.

"The above respond with dramatic results with as few as three to four treatments.

"Many other conditions, too numerous to mention, are also greatly helped when other types of medical treatments fail.

"Many members of the medical profession have spoken up vigorously at one time or another in support of the principles of chiropractic. Sometimes it is because they have observed the remarkable results achieved by chiropractic after medical methods have failed. At other times, results from scientific investigations reveal that chiropractic has indeed something to offer those seeking health."

Thorp McClusky, author of a book about chiropractic, points out that since the preceding report is by a medical man who prepared it for the medical profession, it cannot be considered as biased in favor of chiropractic. McClusky concludes, "Chiropractic is the process of restoring the body to a well-functioning state. . . . The net result will be that the person will have a better functioning nervous system and an improvement in structural balance. This, combined with sound hygienic habits and good nutrition, will lead to greater efficiency and better health. In this sense, the chiropractor is a 'doctor of health' rather than a 'disease treater.' He serves a most important function in this modern world where the hazards of daily living put strains on us that make the preservation of health more important than ever before."

NATUROPATHY

The U.S. Department of Labor's *Dictionary of Occupational Titles* gives the following definition of "Doctor, Naturopathic": "A healer: Diagnoses and treats patients to stimulate and restore naturally bodily process and functioning; a system of practice that employs physical, mechanical, chemical and psychological method: utilizes dietetics, exercise, manipulation, chemical substances naturally found in or produced by living bodies, and healing properties of air, light, water, heat, and electricity.

"Provides for care of bodily functions, processes, or traumas, and treats nervous or muscular tension, abnormalities of tissues, organs, muscles, joints, bones and skin; pressure on nerves, blood vessels, and lymphatics; and assists patients in making adjustment of a mental and emotional nature.

"Naturopathy excludes the use of major surgery, X ray and radium for therapeutic purposes, and use of drugs with the exception of those substances which are assimilable, contain elements or compounds which are components of bodily tissues, and are usable by body processes for maintenance of life."

Dr. John W. Noble, President of the National Association of Naturopathic Physicians adds that the men and women who practice naturopathic medicine are adequately trained to diagnose and treat any and all disease because of the strict academic program followed in naturopathic colleges.

Before a person can be admitted to any accredited college of naturopathic medicine he must submit satisfactory evidence of having completed two years in any college accredited by any state board of higher education where he must maintain a grade point average of 2 or better.

Before being admitted to licensure he must submit satisfactory evidence of having attended a recognized college of naturopathic medicine for a period of four years of nine months each, with a total of not less than four thousand seven hundred hours in class attendance.

Naturopathic medicine has steadfastly maintained that nature's agents, forces, processes and products are the remedies of choice in the treatment of disease and that the use of these agencies is on the increase is evidenced by the worldwide search for new remedies from natural sources.

Indeed, many of the old remedies that have been so blithely dismissed as "old wives' tales" or mythical folklore, are now being tested and *proven* to be of great benefit as bactericides and antibiotics, as well as having other properties of proven benefit to mankind.

Naturopathic physicians no longer employ the term "drugless" be entirely non-drug. This has been particularly true since 1938 as the term "drugless" is incongruous since no true physician can when the United States Pure Food & Drug act was broadened to read "The word or term DRUG as used in this Act shall include ALL medicines and preparations recognized in the United States Pharmacopoea or National Formulary for internal or external use and any substance or mixture of substances intended to be used for the cure, mitigation or prevention of disease either of man or animal."

As a result of this broad definition, the term "drugless" became obsolete and because naturopathic physicians do prescribe natural substances as remedial agents, they must therefore be considered in the category of a system of medicine.

Quite often naturopathic physicians are confused with so-called "Nature Curists." While the basic philosophy of each is similar, the "Nature Curist" has a very narrow, self-limited scope of practice while the naturopathic physician's scope of therapy, as can be seen in the definition contained above, is very broad.

While the naturopathic physician uses minor surgery when necessary, he believes that major surgery is a highly specialized limited field in medicine and should serve all systems of medicine and their respective branches, therefore they do not include it in their practice.

OSTEOPATHY*

Osteopathy is a school of medicine and surgery. The most distinctive aspect of osteopathy has been and is the continuous development of technics for releasing man's natural abilities to combat strains and stresses which may result in disease. Osteopathic physicians and surgeons integrate all accepted methods of treatment of disease and injury, including manipulation, drugs, operative surgery, and physical therapy, as dictated by diagnosis of the individual patient.

Health is held to be a total condition of the entire body; moreover, the focus of osteopathy is upon treating the man, not just his disease. Osteopathic physicians favor those treatments which

* This description is based on information supplied by the American Osteopathic Association, Chicago.

stimulate or assist man's natural abilities to maintain or return to a state of health.

There are two categories of osteopaths: osteopathic physicians, who employ manipulations and in some states prescribe drugs (only a few of these remain); and osteopathic physician-surgeons, who employ manipulations, prescribe drugs, and perform surgery. Like M.D.'s, these practitioners are well trained with three years of premedical training, four years medical and osteopathic training, and one year internship.

California has outlawed osteopaths as such by absorbing those with proper training who elected to change their licensure from D.O. to M.D. Approximately 300 California D.O.'s refused to make the change. Those who did change can no longer be distinguished in the yellow pages of the phone book from other M.D.'s. For California D.O.'s-become-M.D.'s, now to use the title of D.O. is considered a misdemeanor.

When the new law went into effect, the one osteopathic college in California was renamed "The California College of Medicine," and its D.O. faculty members were granted M.D. degrees. It can no longer graduate D.O.'s.

This merger has produced unexpected complications, according to David Dobreer, D.O. president, Osteopathic Physicians and Surgeons of California. He says, "None of the new M.D.'s has been allowed to join the medical society in the county in which he practices. He can belong to the state medical association only as a member of this special ghetto or concentration camp for former D.O.'s.

"Eight men who originally elected to join the merger and practice as M.D.'s have already come back into our profession, and others are taking steps to follow. Our court case challenging the legality of the merger and its implementing legislation is proceeding at the appellate level.

"California was chosen as the first point of attack for several reasons: It was the largest osteopathic state in the country . . . and it was felt that if the osteopathic profession in California was wiped out, the other states would rapidly be brought down by the same process. . . . Another merger is under way, this one in Washington State." Others in various states are expected. In the meantime the five osteopathic colleges in the United States are expanding their facilities and will continue to graduate physicians and surgeons, D.O. Today there are 387 osteopathic hospitals in the United States and 12,000 members of the osteopathic profession.

Elsewhere, new multimillion-dollar osteopathic hospitals or colleges are planned in Michigan, Kansas, and Pennsylvania. The Chicago College of Osteopathy recently opened its new $1,800,-000 hospital wing.

Unfortunately, while there is often rivalry among some of the healing professions, there is also a tendency for some of them to belittle other healing methods which they consider useless or less "respectable." As I have already pointed out, each would seem to have a contribution to make and all should work together for the common goal of health for suffering humanity. The discrimination not only applies to patient referral, but it is almost unheard of for an M.D., for example, to seek treatment, himself, from a chiropractor or osteopath.

I have heard of one amusing case, however. A patient was receiving help from an M.D. for a back ailment, without noticeable improvement. His nagging pain was so uncomfortable that after several months he yielded to urges of friends to seek help from a well-known osteopath in the area. This osteopath (whom I know and respect) has relieved hundreds of back problems, and he is beloved by all who know him. He resides in a state where D.O.'s and M.D.'s have not merged.

When the patient announced his decision to go to the osteopath, the physician appeared horrified and warned him that he would not assume responsibility for what might happen. But the osteopath relieved the man's suffering, and when his pain finally disappeared, the patient joyously reported his recovery to the physician.

Several months later, the osteopath received a mysterious call from the physician, who whispered over the phone that he, too, had a back ailment; could the osteopath help him? Then he asked, "Is it all right for me to park around the corner so no one will recognize my car sitting in front of your office?"

There is no reason why a physician should not be helped by an osteopath or a chiropractor, or vice versa.

In general, as I see it, the natural-health professions attempt to strengthen the vital force of the body in some way, or to remove obstructions (such as nerve impingements and pressures) so that the body can heal itself.

It is my own opinion, after talking with many fine medical men, that, left to themselves, they would be more than willing to give the drugless "doctors" their due. But fear prevents such action.

SPIRITUAL HEALERS

Spiritual healers also have a contribution to make. Through prayer they help to stimulate the vital force via the source from which the vital force originated. If you believe in God, you believe in nature; for God created nature in the first place. Hence, applying the original source of power to the human body, as proved from biblical examples down to the present day, can and has stimulated the vital force to heal, often miraculously. Nobel prize-winner Alexis Carrel wrote as early as 1935 in *Man the Unknown*, "The miracle is chiefly characterized by an acceleration of the processes of organic repair. . . . Miraculous cures seldom occur. Despite their small number, they prove the existence of organic and mental processes we do not know. They show that certain mystic states, such as that of prayer, have definite effects. . . . There is a slowly growing literature about miraculous healing.* Physicians are becoming more interested in these extraordinary facts. Several cases have been reported at the Medical Society of Bordeaux by professors of the medical school of the university and other eminent physicians. . . . The only condition indispensable to the occurrence of the phenomenon is prayer."

Still another mystery is the effect of prayer on plants, already covered in my book *Stay Young Longer*. Spiritual healing of people, even in orthodox churches, by the orthodox clergy, has passed the point of conjecture. Though the laws of spiritual healing are not yet completely understood or successful in all cases, the fact remains that some people have been healed by such means. Often a physician who made the original diagnosis will not admit that

* Spiritual healing is discussed in *Stay Young Longer*, with a review of recent literature on the subject.

the healing was due to religious intercession or prayer. His usual response: "Wrong diagnosis!" Yet I know a reputable physician, an M.D., who found that he could heal some of his own patients by prayer. His colleagues in his community were so derisive, telling him that it "was all in the mind," that he finally closed his office, sold his house, and is now studying for a degree in psychiatry so that he can answer his critics with authority. I have even known some people who, through prayer, have cured themselves. (Further information appears in *Stay Young Longer*.)

COOPERATION IS NEEDED

James W. Bishop, D.C., and A. Mercer Parker, D.C., sum up what *ought* to be the attitude of all the healing professions: "The physician does not cure, be he a natural, medical, or a drug-and-surgical practitioner [or a spiritual healer]. Activation of the patient's inherent powers of recovery by natural means can best restore normal functions.

". . . Natural healing practitioners, in the eyes of the law and the courts, are practicing medicine and are medical doctors, practitioners and physicians, regardless of the branch, system and method they are licensed to practice. . . .

"Therefore, all medical practitioners should pool their intellectual efforts and financial resources and cooperate enthusiastically in an educational and legislative program for the greatest good for the greatest number, with equal rights and liberties of all lay individuals and groups to make a choice. . . ."

In my own opinion, it is more important for people to get well and stay well than to quibble over who is best qualified to give help. We need every shred of information to ensure health, no matter who contributes that help, or where it comes from, as long as it is not harmful. And we should not even be too quick to accept the judgment of what someone else considers harmful.

The choice of all branches of healing, and of any substances, whether vitamins, herbs, or food, should lie in the hands of the people as their God-given right to treat their own bodies as they see fit.

7 Homeopathy

When I first heard of homeopathy, I shrugged it off as another foolish idea. But I had a startled awakening. At a time when I was suffering from a disturbance which refused to yield to any other treatment, a physician prescribed a homeopathic remedy. To my amazement the disturbance disappeared not only miraculously and rapidly, but with no side effects. It has never returned. Thus encouraged, I decided to try again. So, when a minor ailment made its appearance, I promptly took, on my own, a remedy which had helped a friend with similar symptoms. Results: none. Still persistent, I tried another remedy (as one would a drug or even a vitamin). I received absolutely no help from that remedy, either. Swallowing my pride, I asked the physician why these remedies hadn't worked.

He explained that homeopathy never works like allopathy (drugs). He pointed out that a trained expert treats the *person*, not the symptom; and what will cure one person will not cure another, even though the symptoms may appear to be identical. As for the second remedy taken indefinitely, he said, "You were on the right track with the right remedy, but you took too much too long. If you had stopped the minute your symptoms lessened, you would probably have had good results. In homeopathy, if a little is good, more is *not* better."

Since the public has been urged not to treat itself, you are no doubt surprised that I should have tried this self-help in the first place. Let me assure you, as the physician assured me, that homeopathic substances are not considered harmful. So I have continued to experiment until I finally have discovered that used correctly, they are often near magic.

In order to learn more about the subject, I studied every book I could find on the subject. One of these, by Alonzo J. Shadman, M.D., *Who is Your Doctor and Why*, marked one of the turning points in my life.

Dr. Shadman says, "I suggest that a family have a case of homeopathic medicine. Owing to the fact that the indications for the prescribing of homeopathic remedies never change, people of average intelligence may learn how to prescribe for their own *simple* ailments. . . . I know of many families who have not had a doctor for years because of this advice." He adds, "Before that their apprehension and fear of sickness cost them hundreds of dollars each year for doctors and drugs."

After studying several repertories (the name given to symptoms with their corresponding remedies) I made a list of the most commonly used remedies, took it to a homeopathic pharmacy and laid in a supply. Since each remedy costs less than a dollar, the financial outlay was not great.

Several physicians whom I know who now use homeopathy for their patients were not only skeptical at first, but even violently antagonistic. After being converted by another physician, and noting almost miraculous results in many, many cases, they eventually became as enthusiastic as their converters. But why? How does homeopathy work?

The credit for discovering homeopathy goes to a physician, Samuel Hahnemann, originally trained in 1790 to respect drugs. After noting their disturbing side effects, he began to rebel against them, particularly when used in large doses. He wrote, "I set out to discover if God had not indeed given some law whereby the diseases of mankind could be cured. . . . Infinite wisdom should be able to create the means of assuaging the sufferings of His creatures."

Dr. Hahnemann first experimented on himself. While he was well, he discovered that if he took Peruvian bark (source of quinine) in the usual doses, he developed all the symptoms of malaria. In minute doses, however, it cured the disease.

Later, his students continued the testing of other drugs, which was called "proving." Together they eventually proved that 3,000 remedies repeated the principle of the quinine-malaria discovery and its reverse; that *what disease symptoms a drug can cause, those symptoms can it cure*. In other words, based on the principle of similars, *like cures like*. This marked a new approach to treating disease.

Meanwhile, contrary to orthodox medicine which was apt to use the largest drug dose that could be tolerated by the body, Hahnemann kept diluting his doses until he discovered that a tiny, *minimum* dose was more effective than a large one. You must bear in mind, too, that the word "drug" in 1790 had a different meaning from its present one. In those days drugs were derived largely from roots and herbs. Thus, Dr. Hahnemann used only natural substances. He also limited his drugs during treatment to one at a time.

Dr. Hahnemann was so successful with this new method, which he named "Homeopathy," that in one epidemic he cured 72 out of 73 patients. Dr. Shadman, in his book, reports that the system still works successfully today. He has seen cases of malaria cured by an almost infinitesimal dose of quinine, whereas large doses sometimes failed. He has seen cases of typhoid cured with unbelievably small doses of a suitable remedy when the usual treatment of strong drugs has led to death. He has seen cases of cerebro-spinal meningitis cured by the homeopathic method, when others died from the current orthodox treatment. Dr. Shadman says that he has never lost a case of pneumonia in his entire half century of practice, and he has never used anything but homeopathic remedies. In his opinion, "It always helps; it never interferes."

WHY IS HOMEOPATHY SUCCESSFUL?

Why does this system produce such good results? According to those who use it, it is because:

Homeopathic drugs are drawn exclusively from natural substances —animal, vegetable, and mineral.

They are used to stimulate or "charge" the vital force into bringing about a natural healing of the body.

The patient is considered as a whole: his mental and emotional states as well as his physical condition.

Doses are microscopic because the small dose challenges or gives the vital force a gentle nudge instead of "whipping" it. A diseased body is far more sensitive to a drug than a well body. There is proof, for example, that a gouty person is 250,000 times more susceptible to formic acid than a well body.

Homeopathic drugs are prescribed for the symptoms which they produce when given to healthy human volunteers. Tests on animals are not used because only humans can report the sensations produced by a drug.

Homeopathy is based on the principle of individual differences. People with the same symptoms do not necessarily react to identical homeopathic remedies.

All methods at variance with homeopathy must be avoided. This means no laxatives, salves, mouth washes, or other drugs are to be used simultaneously.

Homeopathic remedies usually come in very tiny pellets or tablets, diluted with milk sugar so that they are sweet to taste. The potencies are microscopic, starting with one part of the mother remedy to nine of the diluting (milk sugar) substance. This dilution sometimes goes as high as 1/1000 or even more. The potencies are accordingly labeled 3x, 6x, 12x, etc. For home use Dr. Shadman suggests the 6x potency. Some people might conclude that a minute dose is useless, but homeopathy proves otherwise. Nearly everyone knows that a large dose of iodine can be poisonous, whereas a minute or "trace" amount of iodine is an absolute necessity for health. A solution of adrenalin, 1 part to 1,000, has been found to constrict a blood vessel, while 1 part to 1,000,000 of the same drug produces the opposite effect: it expands a blood vessel.

Dr. Melvin E. Page, of the Page Biochemical Foundation, St. Petersburg, Florida, told me a story which illustrates the effects of the minimum dose. In his rehabilitation of patients through nutrition and related techniques, he helps to achieve balance in sluggish glands by the use of certain glandular substances. But he uses these substances not in the large, orthodox dose usually prescribed, but in tiny doses, often 1/1000 of the usual amount. He has found that this "charges" or "stimulates" the gland into manufacturing its own secretions, at which time he may withdraw the dose entirely.

A physician, reading about Dr. Page's method, decided to try a specific glandular substance on himself. Since he did not accept the fact that a tiny dose would be effective, he used the usual large dose he was accustomed to prescribing for his patients. He then wrote to Dr. Page complaining that he had achieved none of the results Dr. Page had promised. Dr. Page promptly answered suggesting that the physician stick to the microscopic dose. The doctor tried again and responded that, to his surprise, the small dose had worked where the large dose had not.

HOMEOPATHIC PHYSICIANS

How do physicians receive homeopathic training? Homeopathy is a postgraduate course, which may be elected after receiving an M.D. degree. At present I believe there is only one school in the U.S. which provides this training. It is the American Institute of Homeopathy, 1011 Arch Street, Philadelphia 3, Pennsylvania. You will not be surprised to learn that because homeopathy so often eliminates the need for tests, drugs, and surgery, and is simple, painless and inexpensive for the patient, it does not carry the approval of giant organizations to whom the method is a threat of competition. Perhaps for this reason homeopathy has been ignored, ridiculed, even persecuted.

In times past such well-known people as Nathaniel Hawthorne, Henry Wadsworth Longfellow, Wendell Phillips, Julia Ward Howe, Louisa May Alcott, Thomas Bailey Aldrich, and Mark Twain adopted homeopathy and were said to have achieved amazing curative results.

To find a homepathic physician near you, write to the American Foundation of Homeopathy, 2726 Quebec St. N.W., Washington, D.C. (Homeopathic pharmacies are listed in the bibliography, p. 378).

Dr. Shadman says, "The usual method of giving the medicine is in doses of one or two or three hours, dry on the tongue, to be dissolved in the mouth. (It is not washed down with water). The medicine is to be discontinued as soon as improvement is apparent. Doses repeated too often may be harmful. The rule is the single remedy, the minimum dose, and only as often as is absolutely necessary—which is best learned by experience."

A repertory of symptoms and the corresponding remedies appears in Dr. Shadman's book. Since this book—*Who is Your Doctor and Why?*—explaining the use and good results of homeopathy, was a turning point in my life, I hope it may also be in yours, because homeopathy, tested for nearly 200 years, provides a safe and simple means of getting well naturally. For proof of this, read Dr. Shadman's book. It is available from the Lee Foundation For Nutritional Research, Milwaukee 3, Wisconsin.

8 The biochemical cell-salts —flower remedies

Biochemistry may be applied in maintaining health in the living tissues of the body. Biologists usually endeavor to supply the necessary elements to the body for its own self-repair and maintenance. If a plant is ailing, the botanist may decide that the plant is suffering from a deficiency and in such cases supply specific nutrients and restore the plant to health. The same method is used with prized animals—show dogs, race horses, and zoo animals. In animal husbandry body disturbances are almost always corrected by supplying the missing elements through correct nutrition. Only in emergencies are animals given drugs.

Humans can be and should be treated in the same way. Many people have already discovered that correcting nutritional deficiencies has vastly improved their health and consequently they have become enthusiastic about the nutritional (biochemical) approach to living.

Plants take up their nutrients in microscopic amounts via the soil. In people the blood stream picks up the nutrients after digestion and processing and delivers them to every organ and cell. If the proper nutrients are lacking in food, there is little or nothing of value to deliver and, like the ailing plant, the body first becomes impoverished, then begins to degenerate. Although degenerative diseases differ from infectious or contagious diseases caused by a virus or a germ, there is much evidence to show that a body abundantly supplied with the proper nutrients resists degenerative diseases, and, to a large degree, infectious diseases as well. This further explains the fallacy of trying to treat a degenerative disease with a drug, which provides only temporary stimulation. Since nutrition is a slower way, and since these days people are in a hurry about everything, countless patients turn to drugs. Instead of being called *patients*, these people should be called *impatients*.

One method, considered quicker in some instances than nutrition-through-food, can be used in conjunction with a correct nutrition program. It provides necessary elements to cells and organs quickly, bypassing the slower process of digestion. This method is known as the "Twelve Schuessler Biochemic Cell-Salts," related to nutrition.

As early as 1873, W. H. Schuessler, M.D., wrote, "About a year ago I intended to find out by experiments on the sick if it were not possible to heal them, provided their diseases were curable at all, with some substances that are natural. . . ."

Dr. Schuessler analyzed human blood and isolated 12 minerals or cell-salts which he found were constantly needed and being built into the human structure. He considered these 12 mineral salts essential to proper growth and maintenance of health. A book, *Dr. Schuessler's Biochemistry*, by J. B. Chapman, M.D., explains, "Should a deficiency occur in one or more of these cell-salts, some abnormal or 'diseased' conditions arise, and according as they manifest themselves in different ways and in different parts of the body, they have been given various names. Every disease which afflicts humanity reveals a lack of one or more of these inorganic cell-salts. Health and strength can be maintained only as long as the system is properly supplied with these cell-workers or tissue builders."

Dr. Schuessler adds, "The inorganic (mineral) substances in the blood and tissues are sufficient to heal all diseases which are curable at all. If the remedies are used according to the symptoms, the desired end will be gained by means of the application of natural laws."

Dr. Schuessler's biochemic method is to ascertain which cell-salts are lacking and supply them in the form needed. He feels that a symptom is merely a distress signal, warning that an element is lacking. When it is restored (if the disturbance is curable at all) a normal condition follows.

The twelve Schuessler salts are:

CALCAREA FLUOR. (Fluoride of Lime)	KALI SULPH. (Sulphate of Potash)
CALCAREA PHOS. (Phosphate of Lime)	MAGNESIA PHOS. (Phosphate of Magnesia)
CALCAREA SULPH. (Sulphate of Lime)	NATRUM MUR. (Sodium Chloride)
FERRUM PHOS. (Phosphate of Iron)	NATRUM PHOS. (Phosphate of Soda)
KALI MUR. (Chloride of Potash)	NATRUM SULPH. (Sulphate of Soda)
KALI PHOS. (Phosphate of Potash)	SILICEA (Silica)

Mira Louise, of Australia, in a booklet, *More about Biochemistry*, says, "Although the twelve Schuessler cell-salts are usually sufficient to bring about a restoration of health and vitality, there are occasions when some of the newer cell-salts introduced by Dr. Eric Graf von der Goltz will be found of great assistance, especially for chronic sickness. Indeed, the action of these cell-salts, if wisely administered, is very little short of miraculous. As they are trace elements, only very small doses are required."

These additional salts are:

BARYTA CARB.	PLUMBUM
(Carbonate of Barium)	(Lead)
CALCIUM IODIDE	STANNUM
(Calcium Iodide)	(Tin)
CUPRUM	ZINCUM
(Copper)	(Zinc)

Mira Louise's booklet contains descriptions of some symptoms of deficiencies that may be regulated by the cell-salts, with rules on how to take them. *Dr. Schuessler's Biochemistry* is a more complete document, discussing complete deficiency symptoms of the 12 Schuessler cell-salts. Together, the two books provide excellent guides to the treatment of practically every disease. These salts are similar in appearance and taste to homeopathic remedies and are available from most of the homeopathic pharmacies. They are also dissolved dry on the tongue to facilitate rapid assimilation. For severe cases, according to Dr. Chapman, they work better and quicker in hot water. Like homeopathic remedies, they too are used singly. If more than one remedy is needed, they are alternated. Dr. Chapman concludes, "They are perfectly safe for adults and children." They are also inexpensive. (See bibliography for sources.)

THE FLOWER REMEDIES

A sort of hybrid of the Schuessler, homeopathic, and herbal remedies are the flower remedies. These were developed in England by Dr. Edward Bach, a scientist, bacteriologist, and practicing physician who died in 1936. They are made from the essences of certain flowers and aimed primarily at relieving mental states. However, as the mental states improved, Dr. Bach noticed that physical symptoms seemed to disappear too. The 38 remedies he produced were designed to eliminate fear, uncertainty, insufficient interest in present circumstances, and loneliness, and to help those people oversensitive to influences and ideas, or tending to despondency and despair, and overconcern for the welfare of others.

A combination of several of the flower essences is called the "Rescue Remedy." Marcus Bach a present-day writer, apparently no relation to Dr. Edward Bach, in an article "Let the Flowers Heal You," cites an example of a man shipwrecked in 1931 off the north coast of England. He was picked up unconscious. A few drops of Rescue Remedy applied to his lips helped him to regain consciousness in a few minutes and to recover fully. Another man, injured in a car crash in Australia, was found bleeding and in deep shock. After receiving three doses of the Rescue Remedy he was sufficiently fit within 12 hours to travel to his home 1,000 miles by train.

As for using the individual flower remedies, Marcus Bach suggests this, "You are the uncertain type and need four drops of Clematis, three times a day." Or one could say, "I am afraid, I will take Mimulus," or, "I am irritable, I will take Impatiens."

Aubrey T. Westlake, M.D. of England, in his book, *The Pattern of Health,* admits he found the reports of miraculous cures by Dr. Edward Bach hard to accept. He knew Dr. Edward Bach was a highly esteemed practicing physician and that no one could understand why he suddenly gave up his career to pursue and develop the flower remedies. "As with all pioneers, his path was by no means easy. His medical colleagues thought he was slightly mad, and his friends were filled with regrets for what they felt was a sheer waste of his brilliant talents."

But Dr. Westlake was still curious about the reports of cures achieved by the Bach method. He says, "So I proceeded to try the remedies. To make a test as conclusive as possible, I eliminated all other therapeutic factors so that only one factor was operating— the Bach remedy—if anything happened it would presumably be due to the remedy and to nothing else. I treated a variety of conditions in this way, and much to my surprise I became completely convinced that the remedies acted as Dr. Bach claimed; anyhow in acute conditions. . . . As a user of these remedies for twenty years I can affirm that, generally speaking, it is just as simple and just as sure as that, surprising as it may sound."

Since Dr. Edward Bach's death, his work is being carried on by

Miss Nora Weeks at the Bach Healing Centre, Sotwell, Wallingford, Berks., England. Testimonials of healing, fully certified, are on file there. Practitioners are trained at this center or by correspondence. Medical doctors, osteopaths, chiropractors, herbalists, and spiritual healers are included in a group of 200 practitioners throughout the world who use the flower treatments in conjunction with their own healing methods.

Marcus Bach, the writer, reports a statement by Miss Weeks: "'An intelligent patient can be his own diagnostician, for Dr. Bach taught that we need to take no notice of the disease, but must analyze the outlook on life of the person in distress. Treat the patient, not the disease, is the rule.'"

The 38 Bach remedies come in tiny bottles from England* for a very modest price. One adds a few drops of the remedy indicated to water and takes several drops four times a day, preferably on empty stomach for quick assimilation. Dr. Edward Bach's own explanation of the remedies and how to take them is contained in a small pamphlet, *The Twelve Healers and other Remedies*. Dr. Bach gives assurance that the remedies are pure and harmless.

The publisher describes the booklet this way: "A simple herbal treatment by a late Harley Street Specialist, for the lay healer and the home, capable of healing all types of disease in those who wish to get well . . . with instructions regarding the finding of the herbs, preparing the remedies and doses and administering."

Since the technique is safe, simple, and inexpensive, however, it could be a fascinating experimental project for people who want relief from uncomfortable emotional and mental states without taking tranquilizers.

It should now be evident that there are unpublicized and drugless remedies such as those embraced by Homeopathy, the Schuessler Cell Salts, and the Bach Flower Remedies. They are considered, by those who originated and tested them for years on many individuals, safe and simple. They are also inexpensive. Any intelligent person can study, order and apply them for a variety of ills for which they have been found helpful.

Herbs are another timeless source of help.

* See Bibliography for sources of books and remedies.

9 Do herbs help?

It would have been very thoughtless of nature to create such complex living machines as insects, birds, mammals, or man himself, without at the same time providing fuel to keep them running or remedies to keep them well. Fortunately nature was not thoughtless. She has supplied these resources which are, in their way, as wonderful as the body machines themselves. Wild roots, herbs, berries, grasses, even flowers have been found to contain food or healing elements.

No one teaches the various species of animal life how to use these natural bounties; they know by instinct. Some bears, after winter hibernation, eat ivy and Mandrake leaves before a copious meal to strengthen their depleted forces. At the first hint of spring, honey bees use pollen for an internal cleansing. Animals suffering from fractures crawl into a ditch or low place and remain immobile while healing takes place. Dutch planters have observed that sick monkeys not only ate two kinds of herbs themselves, but carried these same herbs to companions too sick to hunt for themselves. In a short time the entire tribe of monkeys became well. And most amazing of all, certain crows and jackdaws were able to find antidotes after an attempt by townspeople to poison them. They ate sorb berries (which they swallowed to induce vomiting) or large amounts of mistletoe berries and thus survived the poisoning. Wildlife has always instinctively found food and natural remedies. Botanic therapy—the use of naturally grown, sun-dried tonic and cleansing herbs, roots, leaves, and barks—has also played an important role in human health from the beginning of time. There is no good reason why we can't continue to take advantage of it today.

Dr. Walter C. Alvarez says, "Back in 1907, when I started the practice of medicine, I soon discovered that I had better learn something—then show some respect for it—otherwise I could easily outrage the patient's grandmother, and perhaps be dismissed by the family for 'gross ignorance.' Accordingly I started buying and reading many books in several languages on folk medicine. . . . Many people feel sure that an old herb doctor knows some things about medicine that a scientific physician doesn't know.

"In my early years of practice, when I saw sick people in their homes, I always made friends with the grandmother by asking her what she thought would be a good thing to do, and then suggesting that she try it—like putting a piece of flannel dipped in some preparation of an ancient herb around the child's sore throat or aching knee joint. Then when the child got well, the grandmother and I shared the credit. . . .

"For years representatives of our great drug houses have been going all over the world to search through the pouches of old witch doctors and primitive 'medicine men' to see if they could find some new and useful drug."

William Engle, science editor of the *American Weekly* illustrates with this story from the November 15, 1959, issue, which I quote: "Little Pao Ping lay dying of a deadly brain infection. Her doctors, modern men of science at Children's Hospital in Peking, had exhausted all their resources. . . . A call went out to a specialist in herbs and roots, buds, leaves and berries, a healer known as Dr. Chiang Chien-an.

"The child has Encephalitis-B," Dr. Pei Li, head of the hospital's Encephalitis-B ward, told the herbalist. 'We think she can live no more than a day or two.'

"Dr. Chiang examined the small girl gravely.

" 'I can cure,' he said. 'I shall give white tiger soup.'

"He mixed the ingredients of this potion and of others. He put in gypsum, rice powder, dried gold and silver blossoms, wild *shou tan* buds and mulberry leaves to lower temperature; roots of wild herbs, *yuan sheng* and *sheng ti*, to give energy; camphor from Borneo to calm nerves; ginseng roots to build resistance; and *peilan,* a fragrant orchid, to combat infection.

"Nine days later, Pao Ping was discharged as well.

"Mere chance? A one-in-a-million bit of luck?" asked Mr. Engle. "Well, according to an official medical association report, thirty-two other boys and girls in the same hospital, between the ages of one and fourteen, were also saved from an encephalitis death in this seemingly primitive and fantastic way."

Among the ailments the Chinese believe folk medicine can cure are: gallstones, kidney inflammation, whooping cough, scarlet fever, mumps, measles, cirrhosis of the liver, prolapsed uterus, typhoid, meningitis, encephalitis, influenza, pneumonia, tuberculosis, infectious hepatitis, and acute bacillary dysentery.

More than 1,000 herbs are used for curative purposes in Russia, according to a statement describing the collaboration of Soviet scientists and the Medical Academy. These herbal remedies constitute 40 per cent of the curative therapy of the Soviet Union. (*Organic Consumer Report*, Vol. 44, No. 2.)

Elsewhere, on five continents, 750 physicians and medical scientists are collecting plants and folk remedies for experimentation at 170 clinics and hospitals run by the College of Medical Evangelists, in California. These herbal concoctions must be studied and tested, but they hold hope for various disturbances. Dr. Orville H. Miller, professor of pharmacy at the University of Southern California, notes that diseases resembling cancer have been reported cured by Mexican medicine men using wild plants. Dr. Bruce Halstead reports a leafy poultice used with similar success by witch doctors from Nicaragua. There are two types of witch doctors (*bruhos*) according to Saleem A. Farg, Ph.D., of the College of Medical Evangelists' department of bio-toxology. One type deals in magic and invokes spirits, the other in herbal medicine. It is the latter in which the college is interested, for these men may possess priceless keys to human health.

Folklore and kitchen or herbal remedies must have value, or a worldwide revival of their use would not be under way. Natural, herbal remedies have been used everywhere, for centuries, for health.

In this country, Ann Counselor, who has worked with and lived close to the Navajo Indians, has collected some of their natural remedies and made them available for this book. During the many years in which she worked with the Navajos, she did not witness high blood pressure or overweight until the Indians began to eat white man's food. A missionary doctor who worked with these Indians for many years did not report a single case of cancer. Only recently, according to Mrs. Counselor, has one case come to light. Smoking did not seem to be harmful, she adds, for both Indian men and women smoke from early youth. Nor did they have allergies. However she laments their growing addiction to alcohol, which she feels is causing general deterioration.

Here are some natural remedies which Mrs. Counselor has watched the Navajos use with great success.

Headache: Snuff was prepared from the gentian; also used for nose trouble. Blue-eyed grass was also used for nose trouble, as well as aster and milkweed.

Gout: A tonic beverage was made from crushed leaves and branchlets of the *Gaillardia,* (a carduaceous herb) added to lukewarm water and applied internally and externally.

Rheumatic Stiffness: This was cured by a tonic boiled from the leaves and branchlets of the barberry bush.

Birth Medicine: Watercress was used as a tonic after delivery. To aid delivery, greasewood and sage brush.

Insect Stings: Stings were treated by chewing dodge weed or greasewood and placing the pulp on the swelling caused by the sting of ants, wasps, and bees.

Dandruff: Red Juniper and a grass called *te'ole* were rubbed into hair.

Cuts and Wounds: Fresh green camphor leaves were placed on wound; also the pitch from piñon trees.

One remedy which the doctors have been trying to pry out of the Indians, so far without success, according to Mrs. Counselor, is their cure for rabies.

America has her own heritage of folk remedies. There are many of us who still recall a spring "tonic" of sulphur and molasses. Many families depended on flaxseed cough medicine, the traditional mustard plaster, bread-and-milk poultices for skin irritations, or lemon juice and honey in hot water for colds.

The good effects of herbs for health is no surprise to physicians who are old enough to remember them. Doctors formerly used them with respect and success. Today, many medications include, or are derivatives of, herbs.

There is now an explanation why these natural medicines work. Recent scientific analysis has revealed that herbs contain certain vitamins and minerals, unheard of and unidentified in the early days. At that time, no one cared about *why* family remedies were successful. The health of the patient was more important than whether the remedy was "unorthodox" or "unscientific."

For example here is an excerpt from the *Encyclopedia of Health and Home,* by George P. Wood, M.D., and E. H. Ruddock, M.D. (Chicago: M. A. Donahue and Co., 1913):

"Diphtheria—This dangerous disease can be cured with lemon juice. Patients apparently in the last stages have been saved by this remedy. Mrs. Loveland, of Buffalo, N.Y. had a daughter so far gone with diphtheria that the attendant physicians had given up the child to die. After the doctors were gone the family was in despair, a friend suggested a trial of the lemon remedy as found in this book. It was accordingly administered and the patient began to improve almost as soon as the first dose was given. When the doctor returned the next morning expecting to write out the certificate of death he was surprised to find the child well on the road to recovery.

"Asking in surprise if they had given his last remedy, Mrs. Loveland said, 'No, doctor, we did not. You said Clara would not live, and we decided as a final resort to give her the lemon remedy.'

" 'Oh,' " said the doctor, 'I've heard that it is an excellent remedy.'

"When asked why he himself did not administer it, his only reply was that it was not professional."

Drs. Wood and Ruddock supply this diphtheria remedy "to be used as follows: The throat should be gargled with the juice every half hour or two, and at the same time from a half to a teaspoon swallowed. This cuts loose the false membrane in the throat and permits it to come out. In case the clear juice is too strong, it may be diluted with water."

WHY DO HERBS WORK?

What is the "scientific" explanation for this remedy? Lemon juice, as we know today, is rich in vitamin C. German doctors have called diphtheria "Fulminating Scurvy" because its toxin cannot exist in the presence of vitamin C.

American Indians used pine needles for colds. Today, we have learned that pine needles are also rich in vitamin C. Prior to the discovery that limes and lemons—sources of vitamin C—could cure sailors sick with scurvy, the Iroquois Indians provided Cartier's sailors, sick with scurvy, with a "miraculous cure"—an infusion of tea made from hemlock leaves and bark. Hemlock was later identified as an abundant source of vitamin C. Rose hips provide another rich source of vitamin C, and are now used commercially to provide it.

Claudia James writes that parsley, considered an herb, contains 22,500 units per ounce of vitamin A, whereas carrots contain only 1,275. Parsley contains three times as much vitamin C as lemon juice. And parsley contains 5.763 mg. of iron per ounce while spinach contains but 1.2 mg.

Dandelion leaves and root have been long used as a diuretic and blood purifier, according to Ebba Waerland, author of *Rebuilding Health* (Devin-Adair). She writes, "Arabian physicians in the early Middle Ages used the dandelion as an eye remedy. . . . It also encourages the digestion."

Undoubtedly those who prescribed it, or benefited from the use of the dandelion, did not understand why it was helpful. Only in recent times has an analysis become available. Mrs. Waerland reports it: "The percentage of nutritional salts in the dandelion is 1.9, consisting of potassium 38 per cent, calcium 20 per cent, sodium 11 per cent, magnesium 9 per cent, phosphorus 8 per cent, silicium 7 per cent, sulphur and chlorine 3 per cent. The herb is rich in vitamin C, containing the bitter substances saponin and colocynthin, and is stimulating to all the glands of the body. The content of inulin, a carbohydrate allied to starch, in the root may be as much as 40 per cent. It also contains levulin, which corresponds to the dextrine of starch."

For centuries, the Chinese have used toad skins for respiratory ailments. This remedy was considered pure superstition until an analysis reported that the toad skin contains ephedrine. Ma Huang, another Chinese herb containing ephedrine, has been used successfully for 5,000 years.

In India, Dr. S. S. Nehru, president of the Agriculture-in-Indian-Science Congress, and a member of the Imperial Council of Agricultural Research, demonstrated good results in relieving inflammation of the throat and sinus with onion poultices. To learn why the onion, used in this way, was beneficial, Dr. Nehru mashed onions, put them in cellophane or quartz containers so that they could not touch the skin. Even so, the onion still produced good results. But when the onions were placed in glass, lead, iron or aluminum, the good results ceased. On further investigation, Dr. Nehru found that onions radiate an electrical energy which can pass through cellophane or quartz, but not through glass, lead, iron, or aluminum.

Science News Letter (June 12, 1943), noted that penicillin also produced a charged electrical field. We have much to learn about how—and why—natural remedies are effective.

Many home remedies (without side effects) are mentioned in the book, *Kitchen Remedies*, by Ben Charles Harris, Ph.G., R.F. Mr. Harris is no "faddist." He is a registered pharmacist, herbalist, and curator of economic botany of the Museum of Science and Industry, Worcester, Mass. He tells of two men close to 75 who rubbed a thin slice of garlic over their bald spots three times a day, and in a few weeks were rewarded with an abundant crop of hair. He tells of a woman who removed a large and unsightly mole from her nose by alternate applications of castor oil and the juice of fresh, raw cranberries. He also cites the case of a man who, in the process of cleaning out his fireplace, got soot in his eye. He remembered a family remedy and put a whole flax seed in his eye, and the "jelly" from the seed absorbed the soot and removed the irritation.

Professor Heber W. Youngkin, in his *Textbook of Pharmacology*, writes that rutin, which decreases capillary fragility, reduces the incidence of recurring hemorrhage in diabetic retinitis and pulmonary hemorrhages if not caused by tuberculosis. Rutin is found not only in the grains, rye and buckwheat, but in the flowers, rue, hydrangea and forsythia.

The Mayo Clinic reports finding a new substance in yellow clover which may replace heparin or dicoumoral for dissolving blood clots without side effects.

Mr. Harris suggests as substances which will prevent hardening of the arteries: dandelion, spinach, and beet tops (all sources of choline and inositol, B vitamins already shown beneficial in scientific studies). And he recommends burdock as a blood purifier.

A 1960 medical study has reported therapy with mulberries. When given to 18 patients with heart disturbance, all but two improved. Breathlessness and pain were reduced; improvement of heart sounds was noted, and in some patients, swelling of ankles disappeared.

Obviously, there are exceptions to every rule, and nature has her exceptions, too. For instance, there are poisonous plants—poisonous mushrooms, and poison ivy, oak and sumac being the commonest to most of us. No one should indiscriminately chew a leaf or bite a twig without knowing what he is putting into his mouth—or rubbing on his skin. Here are some warnings, contributed by *Good Housekeeping's* "Better Way," of plants to watch out for:

Beans of the castor-oil plant. Eating even two beans has proved fatal.
Wisteria seeds and seed pods. Two seeds have produced poisoning.
Oleander. All parts are dangerous including honey produced from nectar from the blossoms. Children have died from nibbling blossoms, leaves, and twigs. Contact with the bush itself may cause skin irritation and smoke from burning cuttings or leaves is particularly irritating.
Boxwood leaves and twigs are poisonous.
Rhubarb leaf stalk is good food, but according to the Poison Control Center of New York the leaves or the blades of the plant can be poisonous, even fatal, due to the presence of oxalic acid.

A 23-page booklet for quick identification of common poisonous plants of New England (also helpful for other areas) has just been issued by the Public Health Service of the U.S. Department of

Health, Education and Welfare. The booklet, Public Health Service Publication No. 1220 is available for 35 cents from the Superintendent of Documents, U.S. Government Printing Office, Wash. D.C. 20402.

Be sure to identify an herb before taking. Fortunately those which are commercially prepared for human consumption are safe. This warning applies to any plant.

One woman, trained as a physician in Germany, tells me that there is an herb tea for every ailment. She keeps her family in good health through good nutrition and herbal teas. While the rest of us are buying salad greens from the supermarket, this woman is out in the fields, gathering wild greens. She has taught me to look forward to spring and fall, at which time I gather young dandelion leaves before they have developed into "rosettes." The leaves, if they are very young, are not bitter, and added to a salad of other mixed greens, have a delightful flavor.

My German friend and her family are among the healthiest and most energetic individuals I have seen anywhere. Their kitchen cabinets contain a huge supply of herbs, which they use in the form of teas. This woman reminded me, however, that the same herb does not necessarily suit all people; that the practice of herbal medicine is an art, not an exact science, and that wide generalizations are not wise due to individual differences. She relies on herbal and nutritional therapy exclusively to maintain the health of her family. She refuses to use—or prescribe—a single drug.

Mildred McKie, M.D., writes of her use of herb teas for medicinal purposes in India. She says, "Leaves and flowers are best steeped in boiling water to preserve the delicate flavor. Have the water boiling, add them, cover with a lid and set aside for five minutes."

In spite of the intensive search for herbal and other natural remedies, they are not being officially offered to the public in the United States. Herbal and botanical dispensaries are no longer allowed to make claims or print any testimonials for the use of herbs. In fact, there seems to be a trend to discourage us from taking folk or herbal remedies at all! Books on folk medicine, even those written by physicians, have been belittled and openly attacked. So potent are the influences in favor of laboratory or synthetic preparations, that between the years 1900 and 1910, 44 botanical remedies were dropped from the U.S. Pharmacopoeia, and between 1910 and 1920, 35 more were omitted. Today, herbal remedies are largely replaced by synthetic drugs.

But the products of field and forest still possess, in some degree at least, the virtues and remedial possibilities so well known to our forefathers. If botanical and vegetable remedies were good enough for them it is a pity that they are disappearing from the family medicine shelf today.

A certain American Indian herb doctor, in his late 70's, has been permanently curing diseases in scores of people, including white men and women. He uses herbal remedies handed down from his forefathers. More and more people in his community were turning to this successful herb doctor for help and away from conventional doctors in the same community who were treating the same diseases with drugs—unsuccessfully.

Some time ago the Indian suddenly and mysteriously disappeared. His bewildered patients tried to locate him. Finally he was traced to an insane asylum where he had been committed. Through the efforts of a lawyer, engaged by those who knew he was perfectly sane, he was released.

Now he has moved to a new community where he is watched over by the lawyer and where he is practicing his native lore. (Please do not write me for his address. To protect him I have been sworn to secrecy.) Sincere doctors have begged him for his remedies. He refuses to divulge them for fear of further persecution. Can you blame him?

As I write this, a white man, given the name of an herb by another Indian herb doctor, for a disease (cancer) which baffles all mankind, has made this concoction available at a modest sum to those who have requested it. Its good effects have been witnessed by people of integrity and honesty who have vouched for the man and the product. The result? The man is now in prison for three years. Like the Indian, he, too, is being silenced.

So search for and cherish every home, folk, and herbal remedy you can find. While some countries are searching for them, other countries, including ours, are apparently trying to suppress them. Soon, if the campaign continues, folk remedies will die out with those fortunate few who still remember them and will be forgotten or lost forever.

10 Pressure therapy —acupuncture

Have you ever accidentally bumped or pinched yourself and felt an answering twinge in a distant area of your body? William Fitzgerald, M.D., a former physician in Hartford, Connecticut, supplies an explanation: "There are ten invisible electrical currents through the body." These lines of current, according to a chart in Dr. Fitzgerald's book, *Zone Therapy*, travel from each toe, running in parallel directions up the body to the head. (Lines from each finger are also pictured running to the head.) Presumably when a strong pressure is made at a point on one of these lines or zones, there is a reflex response (not always felt) at some other point in the same zone. Dr. Fitzgerald discovered that by applying pressure at one point relief could be obtained in another part of the zone. He named the method "Zone Therapy."

George Starr White, M.D., gives his opinion of it: "Zone Therapy is pressure therapy, and can be used at home by anyone who has studied it. The system is simplicity itself, yet the technique must be carried out in an exact manner. It cannot be done in a haphazard way. . . .

"The first time I ever saw it used was among the American Indians in Connecticut. I was surprised, although I was very young at the time, to see how many troubles were relieved by this pressure treatment. . . .

"You can imagine my surprise, about thirty-two years ago in Carson City, Nevada, when I met Indians who were using pressure therapy for all sorts of aches and pains, and getting fine results.

"Pressure on the feet—for example rolling them on a child's marble, or on a hard ball, is doing wonders for relieving the symptoms of many obscure conditions, when all other known methods have failed."

Since Dr. Fitzgerald and Dr. White initiated the use of pressure therapy, others have expanded the principle and also report excellent results in many types of ailments.

To give you some idea of the wide range of disabilities which these therapists claim can be treated, here is a list from the book, which represents the combined advice of Dr. Fitzgerald, Dr. White, and Dr. Bowers, all M.D.'s. The lists include: Bright's Disease, pneumonia, high and low blood pressure, asthma, sore throat, hay fever, hiccoughs, insomnia, migraine headache, coronary thrombosis, spur on heel, ankle injury, hot flashes, fallen arches, phlebitis, low vitality, cramping pains in fourth toe, anemia, angina pectoris, backache, bladder disturbances, constipation, coryza, deafness, diarrhea, bronchitis, brachial neuritis, conjunctivitis, enteralgia, epilepsy, epistaxis (nose bleed), falling hair, headache, hysteria, laryngitis, loss of voice, lumbago, morning sickness, mumps, nasal catarrh, nervousness, neurasthenia, neuralgia, optic neuritis, sciatica, sea sickness, sneezing, tumors, pulmonary tuberculosis, whooping cough, writer's cramp, and wry neck.

One way to approach these disturbances via the Zone Therapy Method is through the feet. In the book, *Zone Therapy*, you will find a map of the bottom of each foot, revealing exact areas which correspond to the various body organs. Even without this chart, if you probe deeply all over the bottom of your feet, including the webs between, as well as the sides of the toes, you may discover some mighty sore spots you didn't know you had. Although you may not have been previously aware of foot trouble, by deep kneading you most probably will find some sensitive spots.

The introduction to *Zone Therapy* gives the explanation of just how pressure therapy works on these tender areas:

"The modern theory of Zone Therapy is that crystalline deposits form at the nerve endings. These keep the electrical contact or impulse of the nerves from grounding. You are merely rubbing out these crystalline deposits and thus enabling the nerves to ground in the feet or hands or wherever you may choose to work.

"Modern operators and practitioners use the inward or medial side of the thumb at corner of the nail which is kept trimmed down. The work is usually done on the foot which is held firmly with the opposite hand and the thumb corner is wiggled in a firm, slightly advancing, upward or cross manner at the point of tenderness. This can be done with from 2 to 10 pounds of pressure—the more pressure the quicker the results seem to be. In fact, this will be extremely painful to those with disease symptoms—until the crystalline deposits in the foot are worn down after a series of treatments. . . .

"A still more advanced method is the use of such instruments as an electrical vibrating instrument with its 'needle point' applicator made especially for zone therapy work. In a busy practice the thumb soon gives out—and the electrically-operated instrument can be used for fast and accurate work."

Self-treatment is not simple, nor do people find it easy to be consistent in continuing the treatments. When you first press some of these sore places on your foot, you may find them unbearable. Sometimes the pain is so excruciating, even you, who are gentle with yourself, can scarcely stand it. One explanation is that the soreness represents toxicity at some point in the zone. Five or ten minutes of treatment by deep finger-massage usually helps the soreness to disappear. Perhaps when the soreness is completely gone, some ailment from which you have been suffering will disappear also.

If you have a sudden temporary flare-up of symptoms, don't be frightened. The zone therapists call this a "crisis." They consider it a good sign of a body housecleaning.

So take off your shoes and stockings, grit your teeth, and get started! I have an acquaintance who swears that the secret of keeping her good health is to massage every inch of the bottom of her feet for at least ten minutes every evening. Another method: put dried beans in a pair of socks or shoes. If you can't stand on them at first, sit down, and exert as much pressure as possible as you roll the sole of your feet over the beans.

Dr. F. M. Houston, D.C., uses pressure therapy in another manner: by locating sore spots on the face and head and applying pressure wherever he finds them. His book *Contact Healing* (see Bibliography) includes maps of the face and head showing the centers related to the location of each organ of the body. Thus, according to his findings, a sore spot at any of these points indicates which organs are in trouble. And although his charts are specific, he says you do not *have* to know, though it is helpful, which centers control which organs. He advises you to treat a sore spot wherever you find it.

Dr. Houston's type of pressure is better adapted to the head and face area. He says,

"The method is simple: Once one finds the nerve center . . . it must be held by the end of the finger, preferably the index or middle finger. This stimulates the nerves you hold, clear into the tissues or organs you wish to help or regenerate. Sometimes these nerve centers are so painful, one can scarcely stand any pressure on them, nevertheless this must be done and the oftener and longer one treats them, the sooner will complete healing take place; at which time there will not be even a spark of tenderness on the nerve center. . . . treat gently at first, then as [you] can stand it, more firmly. . . . always remember that *none* of these nerve centers will ever be tender or painful unless *something is in a state of disease or imbalance*. . . . the more toxic a body is, the more nerve centers you will find in trouble. . . . The more these contact nerve centers are stimulated by pressure contact, the sooner results are noted. Personally I always treat an hour on each patient and more if the case warrants it. So find these centers on yourself. Learn what organs in the body they control, prove it on yourself, then help your family and your neighbors . . . I know of *no* illness or condition, aside from death itself, that Contact Healing does not help immeasureably. In some chronic cases where the nerves are very weak it may take several treatments in order to stimulate them alive again, to the point where they will again begin doing the job they were intended to do. This I am sure of—in 25 years of working with sick people, I have never seen a therapy that so consistently gave results and in many cases the healing was so fast it seemed like a miracle."

Contact healing has now been accepted by Midwestern University, which issues a diploma upon completion of the required hours of study and practical application.

A third approach to using pressure therapy is offered by George A. Wilson, D.C., D.Sc., in his book *Emotions in Sickness*. (For source, see Bibliography.) Dr. Wilson provides a chart, showing the location of various possible tension sore spots, not on the feet, nor on the head, but along the zone lines of current which connect the head and feet, and thus lie scattered over the body. He has named these sore spots, Visceral-Muscle-Tension spots. He gives case histories of patients whose physical distress in various ailments has been relieved by pressure. His method: Using the index finger, exert pressure at the Visceral-Muscle-Tension areas, moving the finger (by lifting it up) around until the more sensitive tension sore spot is found. . . . The exact spots may vary in some individuals; therefore use them as places to start looking for the tenderest spot you can find in each of the areas.

These areas are too numerous to describe and can only be located by consulting Dr. Wilson's charts. However, when he does find a sensitive tension sore spot, he goads it with his finger a few minutes, using only the amount of firmness one can tolerate, until the soreness is relieved. If you are doing some probing and find tension sore spots along the sides of your neck, on the shoulder ridges, on your breast bone, under your ribs, on the outline of your hips, or the insides of your thighs (and many, many other places) Dr. Wilson would probably advise you to goad these sore spots daily until the soreness subsides. I am sure he would also encourage you to look for emotional factors as original causes of these tension spots. Once the emotional cause has been removed and finger pressure has been applied, soreness in the spots themselves and body distress should disappear. Dr. Wilson's books are refreshing, and remarkably helpful.

Wrapping up all the methods of pressure therapy, Robert H.

Walker, D.C., in a pamphlet called *Functional Processes of Disease* shows a chart which may explain why and how pressure therapy works. This chart, though extremely technical, seems to show that injured cells are electrically negative, revealing irritation. By applying counterirritation (pressure), positive electrical current is stimulated to reach the cells, bringing about neutralization of the irritation. This in turn, according to Dr. Walker's chart, leads to healing of the injured cells.

In the book, *Zone Therapy*, Dr. George Starr White, when asked if he considered it advisable for people to treat themselves with pressure therapy, answered, "A true physician wants people to be well and does not interfere with self-treatment."

Actually, the pressure therapy concept is not new—it had merely been laid aside and forgotten. Dr. George Soulie de Morant, a brilliant investigator of Chinese medical knowledge stated that this concept dates back as far as the late Neolithic Age. The Chinese discovered the relationship between painful points on the body surface and a disturbed inner organ, even though the painful area was a considerable distance from the organ itself. In A.D. 443 the Emperor of Japan imported physicians from Korea with this Chinese-taught information, and at the beginning of the seventh century a delegation of Japanese doctors went to China to acquire the Chinese method.

ACUPUNCTURE

Science magazine reports that a Canadian physician, Dr. Walter Penfield, recently toured the Chinese mainland and observed modern medicine and surgery as well as traditional methods in current use. One treatment he noted was the ancient method of acupuncture, which he saw used for the treatment of appendicitis. If an appendicitis case is extremely serious, the Chinese employ modern surgery. But in many cases Dr. Penfield observed the substitution of the nonmedicinal, nonoperative acupuncture technique with great success.

The acupuncture method is to insert two slender sterile gold, silver, or steel needles in the lower part of the right leg of the acute appendicitis patient. The needles have nothing in them but are supposed to affect the nerves which control the appendix. And, instead of drugs, the patient is given herbs. The Chinese use this traditional treatment in the hope of avoiding an operation and there are many cases of extraordinary recovery.

Leslie O. Korth, D.O., of England, also reports cases of successful recovery from appendicitis through acupuncture. He says, "Although the very thought of inserting needles into the skin may cause you to shudder, in spite of the thousands of injections that are given almost every hour of the day, you may take it from me as an actual fact that the many patients I have treated experienced either no pain whatsoever, or only such a trifling sensation as to make no odds. They have no hesitation at all in having the treatment repeated as many times as may be necessary, even asking for it because of the excellent result obtained."

A Cambridge-trained London physician, Dr. Felix Mann, author of a new book, *Acupuncture*, worked extensively with European physicians as well as oriental teachers in successfully treating various diseases with acupuncture. Aldous Huxley, in the foreword to Dr. Mann's book, says, "That a needle stuck into one's foot should improve the functioning of one's liver is obviously incredible. . . . It makes no sense. Therefore we say it can't happen. The only trouble with this argument is that as a matter of empirical fact, it does happen."

The *Journal of the American Medical Association* has given acupuncture this blessing: "Acupuncture has for millennia constituted the mainstay of traditional Chinese medicine. In recent years it has by decree become part of medical practice in the People's Republic of China. It has maintained its popularity without compulsion in Japan, and most surprisingly it has taken a firm foothold in such medically enlightened countries as France and Germany. . . .

"No matter how bizarre a therapy is, how lacking in rationale, and how uncertain its value, it is concerned with patients and disease and hence is a phenomenon which must interest the world of medicine."

Acupuncture is hardly a do-it-yourself treatment, but it is based on a principle not unlike pressure therapy.

Pressure therapy is certainly no more bizarre than acupuncture and is probably easier. The best part of pressure therapy is the fact that there are those who have done it themselves.

A small, and helpful first-aid book based on finger pressure therapy applied to acupuncture points is now available. It is quick, concise, easy to follow. For the first time in the English language it presents details of priceless knowledge discovered by the Chinese thousands of years ago. The illustrations indicate the exact location of each point which pertains to such conditions as anxiety, insect bites, hemorrhages, cramp, exhaustion, and many others. The book is *First Aid at Your Finger Tips*, by D. and J. Lawson-Wood (1963), Health Science Press, Rustington, Sussex, England. It is available for $2.00 in this country from Harmony Book Shop. P.O. Box 115, New Castle, Pennsylvania.

11 Autotherapy—the Duncan method

Autotherapy is a simple, almost extinct method of healing, yet it can be available to anyone. It was practiced in the early 1900's by some physicians, evidently with great success. For some reason it has become a lost art. Autotherapy is produced by a unique method of self-immunization.

Charles H. Duncan, M.D., accidentally discovered the principle when he noticed that a dog which licked its own wound recovered quickly without help from antiseptics or drugs. He later reported to the medical world, "The only place a dog ever has severe infection is on his head, where for anatomical reasons, he cannot lick."

At first this speedy recovery was thought to be due to increased circulation to the wound, due to the licking process. Later it became clear that the dog was vaccinating himself with an exudate from the wound, which he swallowed and which set up antibodies within his body and built a natural defense system against the infection.

Intrigued with this discovery, Dr. Duncan next experimented with people. Fresh wounds with infections, as well as long standing chronic cases of infectious diseases which had resisted treatment, sometimes for years, responded favorably in a surprisingly short time. Moreover, the good results appeared to be permanent. After Dr. Duncan reported his therapeutic technique in the medical journals, other physicians tried the method with success.

All manner of diseases have responded to Autotherapy, as documented by physicians in medical journals and in a long out-of-print book, *Autotherapy*, written and published by Dr. Duncan in 1918. After physicians in the United States became convinced of its unique remedial effect, reports began to drift in from other countries including India, the Philippines, and France, where physicians were using Autotherapy with brilliant results.

The principle, though shocking to the average layman at first glance, is so simple, it is a wonder we haven't thought of it before. E. Abercrombie Verner, a civil and structural engineer, who spent 25 years hunting for written documentation of Autotherapy, called my attention to it and was kind enough to put the book in my hands so that I might report on it to you. He was spurred in his efforts by the realization that he had always instinctively "licked" or sucked his own wounds whenever he was where medical help was unavailable. Later, on finding a copy of this hard to find book, he reapplied Dr. Duncan's technique to himself and his family evidently with success. He believes that everyone, for self-defense and self-preservation if medical help is unavailable (or even with the aid of a physician), should know of the technique. I agree with him.

Dr. Duncan states the theory underlying Autotherapy: "Pus

by mouth acts therapeutically at once, and the results tend to be permanent. In some cases, the pus or discharge from the infection is filtered and injected hypodermically."

The explanation is simplicity itself: all localized infections, according to Dr. Duncan, have a discharge which contains *all* microorganisms present in the focus of the infection. This discharge is effective in creating antibodies for the host of the infection if swallowed or injected into the system. There is an old medical axiom, "Disease carries its own cure." Thus Autotherapy is a natural cure brought about by auto-immunization of the individual's own unmodified toxin-complex, which becomes his own, unique remedy, effective for his condition only.

Dr. Duncan reports many case histories of diseases which have responded to this strange yet simple therapy. He writes, "Acute bronchitis was cured within twenty-four hours; pneumonia in the early stages was cured almost instantly; in endometritis, salpingitis, mastoiditis, otitis media, etc., the curative reaction was often apparent within a few hours, and it tended to be permanent."

Hay fever, asthma, rhinitis, influenza, laryngitis, tonsilitis, pulmonary tuberculosis, cholecystitis, and appendicitis have all been known to respond dramatically (see below). Boils, carbuncles, abscesses, pyorrhea, common acne, whooping cough, and even the common cold respond with dramatic success. Long-standing, chronic coughs also disappear, it is said. Sinus trouble is no exception. Mr. Verner stated that he had suffered from a sinus infection for 40 years. He had been unable to breathe through one nostril for this length of time. Autotherapy (by injection) gave him permanent relief within approximately ten days.

I am told that at least one physician in the United States is using the Autotherapy principle (under another name) for the apparently successful treatment of cancer.

Autotherapy toxin drawn from one part of the body often has a mysterious and good effect on another disturbance in a distant area of the body. For example, Dr. Duncan learned that there was a relationship between bronchitis and appendicitis. Cases of appendicitis and other abdominal infections cleared up after injections of a filtrate made of bronchial sputum. Another physician, Edward C. Rosenow, M.D., further proved this finding with animals. When a culture made from tonsils of individuals suffering from appendicitis was injected into animals, these animals developed lesions in the appendix. Conversely, when mucous from an individual's tonsils was injected into his own body, the appendicitis disappeared and an operation was usually avoided.

It is interesting to note that many amputations were also made unnecessary by Autotherapy.

Regardless of the disease, Dr. Duncan states, "The quick cessation of pain and the immediate reduction of swelling are characteristic of this treatment. The more virulent or aggressive the infecting microorganisms, the quicker will be the response and cure. The pain usually leaves within a few hours as if by the action of morphine. Free drainage and autoseptic technic will cause almost any purulent infection to heal quickly. The diagnosis of the microorganisms is often unnecessary as far as a cure is concerned."

Dr. Duncan points out that of 70 different forms of cutaneous bacteria, 56 are some form of cocci. Whatever the form, whether staphylococcus, streptococcus, gonococcus, or mixed forms, the reactions of Autotherapy are strikingly prompt and curative. Dr. Duncan also emphasizes the speed, certainty and comparative freedom from danger (as compared with commercial vaccines) with which these infections may be cured by Autotherapy.

One of the many examples cited came from Dr. Alexander Vertes of Louisville, Kentucky: "A patient, a night watchman, had carbuncles and boils almost all his life. He consulted me December, 1911. After lancing a carbuncle on his arm, I prepared a weak dilution (with distilled water) from his pus, which I gave him internally (by mouth). The parts healed promptly, of course, but that he has had no more lesions seems remarkable. I am using Autotherapy in my practice, when it is applicable, to the exclusion of all other medication, because it gives me results no other medication has given."

Autotherapy has been used, perhaps unconsciously, by soldiers wounded during war. *Scribner's Magazine* (October 1917), contains an article which describes soldiers of the British Army. "After battle, the wounded soldiers sit by the roadside *licking their wounds* aseptically." A celebrated surgeon of the French Army testified that the technique of Autotherapy was well known in and out of their Army. A past assistant surgeon of the United States Navy also reported successful case histories.

Dr. Duncan tells of using the autotherapeutic principle to produce more milk in nursing mothers whose milk was failing. Lactation increased markedly after the mother took some of her own milk.

Autotherapy has been used in endless numbers of cases by veterinarians. Daniel J. Mangan, D.V.S., of New York City, who formerly treated thousands of horses for the City of New York's departments of maintenance, states, "Autotherapy has not only been a boon to the human race, but has extended its usefulness to suffering dumb animals."

Dr. James Law, M.D., D.V.S., former dean and professor emeritus of New York State Veterinary Medical College at Cornell University, has used and praised Autotherapy.

Why is it that this system of self-vaccination is superior to commercially prepared vaccines? Dr. Duncan answers this question. "It is well known that the animal organism has the power of developing antibodies to any foreign albuminous substance introduced into it, which neutralize or destroy the foreign substance."

In the case of commercially prepared or stock vaccines, ". . . the therapeutic effect of all autogenous vaccines is either absent or altered by every step in the process through which it passes in the laboratory during its preparation. Through error in technic, the laboratory vaccine may not include the causative microorganisms. Heat, time, chemical preservatives may alter the commercial vaccine. Change may occur by being grown in foreign culture media; by being grown *outside* the body tissues; or extraneous matter may creep in, rendering the vaccine worthless. . . . Alluring as have been the brilliant cures occasionally obtained with these, it is well known that the plans of nature in curing the sick, do not include immunizing the patient to heterogenous toxins, nor even to modified partial autogenous toxins, nor even to modified partial autogenous toxic substances; but she has foreordained that the patient should be immunized to *his own unmodified toxin-complex* or toxins and toxic tissue substances elaborated with his own body by the action of the infectious agents upon the body tissues.

"The autotherapeutic remedy is the *only* strictly autogenous therapeutic agent we have in fighting disease. Wherever a patient is suffering with an infectious disease, maybe he has his own natural remedy within his body and it often can be obtained. . . . We are forced to the conclusion that microorganisms *should not be grown outside of the patient's body* if the best therapeutic results are to be obtained."

GENERAL RULES FOR AUTOTHERAPY

Here are the instructions for the use of Autotherapy, in Dr. Duncan's own words:

"When the pathogenic exudate or the end product (or a dilution of the same) of any localized, loosely located, and possibly nonlocalized infectious diseases is filtered with a Berkfeld filter and the filtrate injected hypodermically, or placed in healthy tissues remote from the infected area, antibodies specifically corresponding to all of the microorganisms in the locus of infection will tend to be developed.

"In extra-alimentary and extra-pulmonary diseases, if the crude pathogenic exudates or end products are placed in the mouth, specific resistance to all the infection microorganisms in the locus of infection will tend to be developed. The live pathogenic causative microorganisms appear to be especially prompt and curative when given in this manner."

If a physician is administering the treatment, Dr. Duncan advises:

"One teaspoon of pus is thoroughly shaken with two ounces of distilled water. This mixture is then without loss of time, passed through a Berkfeld filter and one cc. of the filtrate injected subcutaneously. The result is immediate and most gratifying both to patient and physician.

"If the best results are to be obtained in giving the autotherapeutic medication, the patient should be watched carefully for any change in his condition. Except in very acute cases, no further dose is given till the patient ceases to improve under the preceding dose; in chronic cases this will often be from the third to the seventh day. . . . The constitutional reaction is usually slight, the temperature seldom rising above 100°F.

"After twenty-four hours, the cutaneous and constitutional reactions will begin to subside; in forty-eight hours, they usually disappear. . . . A thin discharge is the indication that the curative reaction is continuing. No further dose is given, as long as the discharge is thin. If the discharge becomes thick again, another dose is given. Watch your patient carefully, let him be the guide as to when another treatment is needed. No set of rules will fit all cases. . . .

"The doses given are for a strong healthy man. The very young, the very old, and patients with low vitality should receive smaller doses. Never use antiseptics on a wound treated autotherapeutically, for many antiseptics destroy the therapeutic value of the toxins."

In the event that a physician is not available, Dr. Duncan supplies the rule for self-treatment:

"Place from two to six drops of pus on a lump of sugar, or in a little water, mixed with cocoa, if desired, and take in one dose.

"Another method . . . is simply to lick the pus from the infected area. If the infection is very recent, this may be done at comparatively frequent intervals; if it is chronic, this treatment should not be so frequent. When another dose is needed, there is some indication for it in the wound. It feels irritated or the patient's attention is attracted to it. If it is then placed in the mouth and licked, the irritation will soon subside. If it is impossible to reach the wound with the tongue, a part of the stained dressing may be chewed. (Or it may be soaked in a small amount of distilled water and drunk.) In very chronic cases, one or two treatments of this nature is often all that is required. . . .

"In test cases I have practically thrown aseptic technic to the winds and have seldom seen an apparent infection follow this treatment."

Few doctors, certainly those who have received recent training, know about Autotherapy, although it appears that every physician might well try it. One doctor told me he had heard of Autotherapy —that it was the use of the patient's own blood serum. Dr. Duncan explains, "The blood serum from blood with a high leukocyte count may often be employed successfully, although it is not always as reliable as the filtrate of the pathogenic exudate from the source of infection."

One of the earliest issues of *Coronet* magazine (January, 1937) says, "For twenty-five years, Dr. Duncan's method of treatment has felt the stigma of controversy. Today, although it is practiced successfully by many physicians, it is condemned by others, and as a result it is little known by those not familiar with the medical profession. At one time Dr. Duncan was recommended for the Nobel Prize by a group of well-known and reputable medical men. He was decorated by the French Government in 1932 in recognition of his work. Despite this, Dr. Duncan has not received the acknowledgement due him. His method of treatment may be found in any standard medical dictionary under 'The Duncan Method of Treatment.' "

12 Human electronics —radiesthesia

If you were living 50 years ago and someone had predicted tele vision or space travel, you probably would have laughed it off as science fiction. If anyone had told our early ancestors that tele-graph, telephone, radio, automobiles, and air travel would become a common occurrence, they would have snorted, "Impossible!" But these discoveries did happen. They are so commonplace today that we take them for granted—unless they stop working and cause us inconvenience. And then we wonder how we ever lived without them.

Nearly all new, great inventions follow a similar pattern: they are first considered impossible; then when they are introduced the inventor is ignored or ridiculed; finally when the invention is proved successful, everybody wants one!

There is, in existence today, a device for health which painlessly, cheaply, and quickly (as tested in thousands of cases) diagnoses disease; and as painlessly, quickly and cheaply has so often reversed the disease that health has been achieved. But because its use might threaten certain established interests or because orthodox medicine hasn't yet recognized it, it is being kept from the public. Perhaps 1 per cent of the population has heard of it. It is being used quietly by some dedicated members of the healing professions who predict that it will be "the coming thing" in future diagnosis and treatment of disease. Yet the reputable doctors who use the device are terrified for fear of being found out. They know that if they make any claims for the success of the device, or the word gets around that they might be using one, they may be persecuted, possibly imprisoned, and their device seized and demolished. It has happened.

One doctor, who begged me not to give him away, told me, "This radiesthetic device is so marvelous and so effective that I literally treat myself out of patients. They get well and don't have to come back. Because it is simple and painless, many are unaware of *how* they were helped. They just know that I 'did something' and they got well!"

Please do not write and ask me where you can find a doctor who uses such a device. Remember, the whole subject is still hush-hush. I can only give you some possible clues in this chapter to help you find out about it. The public can demand—and get —such help if the demand is great enough. The system is called "radiesthesia." Every physician, every diagnostician, every hospital, should, in my opinion, use radiesthetic instruments, and every patient might own or rent an auxiliary unit for home use under a doctor's supervision. Furthermore, these instruments do not negate the use of nutrition, vitamins, minerals, or homeopathic remedies. It tests them for each individual to see which ones are helpful! Through radiesthesia I have seen, for example, five varieties of calcium tested which were not being assimilated by a patient. A sixth brand tested positively and the patient received immediate benefits. Many people choose vitamins blindly, or by trial and error. The radiesthetic device could help to solve this problem. It has also been useful in detecting food allergies, difficult to locate by other means.

Radiesthesia is defined as sensitivity to harmless radiations. Abbé Mermet, in his book on radiesthesia, says that everyone is sensitive to such radiations. It is only a question of degree. He writes, "One of the greatest scientists of our time, Dr. Alexis Carrel, Nobel Laureate, and perhaps the most famous worker that the Rockefeller Institute of New York has ever had, realized the importance of radiesthesia over thirty years ago, and expressed his opinion in the following words: 'The physician must detect in every patient the characteristics of his individuality, his resistance to the cause of disease, his sensitivity to pain, the state of all his organic functions, his past as well as his future. He must keep an open mind free from personal assumptions that certain unorthodox methods of investigation are useless. Therefore he should remember that radiesthesia is worthy of serious consideration.' "

ALL NATURE EMITS RADIATIONS

Scientists have established the fact that everything in nature radiates energy. Stanford University physicists demonstrated in 1947 that they could pick up a radio signal, by means of a tuning device, from various substances, including atomic material, and that each substance had its own characteristic signal.

Two other scientists, Professor Daniel F. Comstock, of M.I.T., and Leonard T. Troland, of Harvard University, wrote, "According to the modern theory of matter all bodies are complex structures composed of small particles known as electrons. If, therefore, we are familiar with the laws of atoms and electrons we should understand completely all the physical phenomena in nature."

John Mills, research physicist with Western Electric Company, adds, "Atoms of all substances are now known to be composed of small particles of electricity called electrons. . . . All phenomena of matter, such as cohesion, vaporization, capillarity, elasticity, heat conduction, light and heat radiation and photochemical effects, must finally be explained in terms of a matter which is . . . electrical in character."

Robert A. Millikan won the Nobel Prize for his findings in this field. He said, "Recent experiments indicate radioactivity is not confined to the radium series, but seems to be possessed, though in a less degree, by *all* substances."

Some of these electrical radiations from bodies—animal, vegetable, or mineral—are visible to the naked eye, for example, phosphorescent rocks, or the light from glowworms or fireflies.

Electricity generated by the glowworm can be seen. Electricity from the electric eel can be felt. Dr. John H. Heller, in his book *Mice, Men and Molecules*, says, "In a ten-foot eel, about the first ten inches contain all the vital parts of the animal—heart, lungs, intestinal tract, and so on. All the rest is a series of electric batteries . . . used for offense and defense to obtain food. A fully grown eel can send out about 400 to 600 volts and up to one ampere. This could easily kill a man or a horse.

"Christopher Coates, Director of the New York Aquarium, was filling an eel tank with water from a hose with a brass nozzle. His fingers touched the brass, and the current from the eel, flowing back through the column of hose water and into the nozzle, knocked him right across the room. This is an enormous amount of electricity. . . . On this basis the eel is far more efficient than atomic-reactor-produced electricity. . . .

"The waters of the world contain a richness of life which equals, if not exceeds, that of land. We have not even begun to tap the tremendous resources hidden there."

Most radiations, however, cannot be seen or felt. No one can see radioactivity from radioactive materials. Yet a Geiger counter not only picks it up, it measures the amount of radioactivity. In 1948 Dr. Harold S. Burr, of the department of neuro-anatomy of Yale University, demonstrated—and measured—the electrical radiations from maple trees. And at least two vitamins, A and D, have been found to emit some kind of radiation which will affect the emulsion of a photographic plate in the same way that light and X rays do. (*Science*, Vol. 74, No. 1907.)

Scientists are closing in on electrical discoveries in nature in many different ways. For example, an oscilloscope at the life science laboratory of the Goodyear Aerospace Corporation can measure the electrical impulses coming from the eye when it recognizes color. Each color is believed to set off a distinctively shaped wave-form. The instrument, with its many dials, which picks up this electrical information from the eye, does not look greatly different from the outlawed diagnostic machines which detect various conditions in other parts of the body.

In *Nutrition Reviews* (November, 1963) Gilbert B. Forbes, M.D., of the University of Rochester (N.Y.) School of Medicine and Dentistry, calls attention to a "new technique, one which offers promise in the study of certain aspects of nutrition. The instrument in question is a low level scintillation counter designed to measure very small radiations emanating from the human body. . . . There are now 42 such instruments in operation in Europe and 44 in the U.S. and Canada. More are in process of construction."

Although one of the current uses is "for the monitoring of fall-out product accumulation in man . . . a most fascinating nutritional implication of this instrument stems from its ability to measure the body content of potassium."

In 1960 an electronics engineer and a physician discovered that human muscles emit signals of a frequency once used for transatlantic broadcasts. Richard Bittner, an electronics technician for General Electric and Cohu Electronics, and Dr. Walter K. Volkers of the Millivac Instrument Division of Cohu, also accidentally found that *diseased* muscles generated different high-frequency signals than *normal* muscles.

"The discovery," they said, "leads to speculation whether or not [the human body] is capable of actually transmitting these signals and whether another person can pick them up."

A second research team from the University of California Medical School went still further. They not only agreed that malfunctioning organs in the body might be able to send out distress signals, but they implanted small electromagnets in animals which picked up these signals and carried them by a wire to a recording system to show that they did exist and were not a figment of the imagination.

Dr. Alexander Kolin, who presented the experiments to the National Biophysics Conference, pointed out that malfunctioning of any organ might thus be detected long before the clinical symptoms appeared.

As early as 1910 Albert Abrams, M.D., not only had already discovered that the various parts of the body emitted certain electrical signals, which change during health and disease, but he had invented a device which recorded and measured them in their varying states. He then took an exciting step forward. He established which frequencies represented healthy organs, and "played back" a healthy electrical wave-rate to a diseased organ. He could focus this wave length upon the area needing treatment, and he could turn it off when indicated. By saturating a disturbed tissue or cell or organ with the correct electrical wave-length, proper ionization apparently took place, a balance was achieved, and the area treated became normal.

What was the result of this astounding discovery? You already know the answer. He had the choice of giving up research and use of his new discovery and continuing as one of the outstanding medical men of his day—or facing disgrace and ruin. Because he felt that the discovery had untold potentiality for human health, he chose the latter course. As a result, he was driven to an early grave by the denunciation, vindictive treatment, and persecution he received at the hands of the orthodox nonbelievers. Yet, today, scientists from some of our greatest universities have confirmed the findings of Dr. Abrams.

Dr. Ian Donald, professor of obstetrics and gynecology at the University of Glasgow, told an American medical meeting in 1963 that a pattern of "blips" from a sonar machine was being used in Scotland to locate and diagnose internal tumors and cysts. And in Canada, research in this field of human electronics is being subsidized by the government. Corporations embarking upon what the Canadian government considers a sound program for human welfare have been given governmental assistance. One electronics corporation, Sharpe Instruments, has been commissioned by the Canadian National Research Council to perfect a stereophonic "stethoscope." Based on the same principle used to enhance the sound of your music records, this instrument can pinpoint the location of hidden body disorders. A related instrument, also developed by the same firm, is even more amazing. A nurse, seated in front of the machine equipped with many dials, can check the temperature, pulse beat, and respiration of scores of patients and keep an accurate graph chart of their condition without waking, or even visiting, them!

HOW SUCH INVENTIONS ARE RECEIVED IN THE U.S.

What about similar inventions in the United States? Two 1962 news items tell the story: The first: "An electronic-type machine which officials of the F.D.A. [Federal Food and Administration] said 'was supposed to be able to diagnose 55 diseases and conditions ranging from arthritis to cancer' was seized yesterday."

The second: "United States marshals raided chiropractors' offices in Brooklyn and Queens yesterday and seized five electronic machines purported to diagnose scores of serious illnesses."

One chiropractor personally told me that officials raided his office and promised not to bother him if he would smash his electronics instrument before their eyes, at which they handed him a sledge-hammer. He refused and is still fighting them in court. Another man is serving a five-year prison sentence for selling an electronics instrument even though, according to the Franklin Institute *Report* of 1944, this type of apparatus has been used by various well-respected institutions including the British School of Tropical Medicine and the Mayo Clinic. A firm which manufactured and had already distributed to 700 doctors a machine based on Dr. Abrams' "black box" (as his instrument was scathingly called) was forced to discontinue manufacture and go out of business. Other companies have met a similar fate. The excuse that such seizures by officials have been made to "protect the American people" is poppycock. There have been no known adverse effects of treatment by such machines, and medical practitioners in other countries use them successfully.

At least 10,000 United States operators, all properly educated in the various healing professions, have had either to surrender their apparatus or to go underground. They have even gone to jail and are terrified of being found out by federal authorities. Meanwhile there is a rumor that some of the large electrical corporations "are toying with" the development of these devices, because of their great possibilities. One instrument, manufactured by Remington Rand, called Dia-Pulse, and distributed by the Diapulse Corporation, has so far survived. This instrument treats—does not diagnose. I am told it is now used by over 1,000 physicians.

Another instrument, somewhat similar, is apparently being used in some hospitals. It is called Medcalator-Sonar-Ultra Sound. Still another machine is somewhat related to this general field. It employs a technique in which photographs of the infrared radiation that emanates naturally from the human body are used as an aid in the diagnosis of various diseases, including cancer. The instrument is called the Barnes Infrared Thermograph and is described in the *Journal of the American Medical Association*, September 1963.

These instruments that measure human radiations are quite simple to those who understand electricity or electronics. To others they are a mystery. Actually they are no more mysterious than the telephone, radio, television, or the Geiger counter. According to Thomas Colson, writing in *The Electron Theory in Medicine*, "The tuning means is taken from radio engineering practices using inductance and capacity in the same manner as that used to tune radio receiving sets." The delicate radiolike instrument picks up the electrical signals from each organ or tissue. These electrical signals could very well indicate the strength of the vital force in each organ.

How does such a diagnosis feel? There is absolutely no sensation in the patient being tested. A plate, attached by two wires connected to the apparatus, is placed on the patient's midriff or soles of the feet as he sits upright on a chair, fully clothed. The electric energy in the body is picked up and travels through the wires to the apparatus (often no larger than a table radio). The operator can, by turning dials—again, like a radio picking up various stations—detect the strong or weak signals of the various organs and by comparing them with frequency "rates" previously tested of healthy and diseased organs, determine the condition of each area in the patient. Some of the newer instruments constructed by physicists have a meter, similar to that of a Geiger counter. A radiesthesia instrument is actually a modified Geiger-type counter, finely tuned to pick up much fainter electrical energy radiations from the body.

How long does a diagnosis take? A complete diagnosis takes about an hour and a half and costs in some instances about fifteen dollars. Its accuracy has often been found to be far greater than the usual battery of tests. In one case I have witnessed an M.D. receiving a radiesthetic report of a patient and not believing it. So he had the patient retested by orthodox methods (longer, more expensive and in some cases uncomfortable) only to find confirmation of the radiesthetic diagnosis. And, obviously, the radiesthetic method is far preferable to exploratory surgery! In some instances if the patient is not able to come to the doctor, a blood or sputum sample seems to give satisfactory results.

After diagnosis, another instrument, which also resembles a table radio, is plugged into an electric outlet and dials are set according to the patient's condition. A plate connected with wires is again placed somewhere upon the person's body. This time, instead of the electrical energy flowing from the patient's body *into* the instrument, the process is reversed. A correct wave-length is sent back into the patient by the electrically empowered machine. Dr. Colson explains, "Such treatment energy can be produced artificially by a properly built short-wave, pulsed, low-power radio transmitter. Radiant energy of low power, properly tuned and applied, normalizes diseased tissues."

DOES RADIESTHESIA REALLY WORK?

Does this method of treatment work? You will recall the statement made by one doctor who "treats himself out of patients." His experience is not an exception. Case histories by the hundreds, of successful treatment of nearly every type of disease, would fill more than one book. Dr. John Heller of the New England Institute of Medical Research produced photographs showing that radio waves set up an electric field. When the current is switched off, chemical substances or one-celled animals swim around at random. But when the current is turned on, the chemical substances line up in chains and the one-celled animals can swim only in a horizontal direction along the lines of electrical force. In other words, the electrical waves are controlling their behavior.

Dr. Heller says, "As we examined this phenomenon even more closely, I found myself seated one day looking into the microscope at a paramecium that had become trapped in some debris on the microscopic slide. He was wedged in so firmly that he could not respond to the frequency field when it was turned on. However, I noted a tiny particle inside the cell which was flipping back and forth whenever I turned the field on or off. This meant that we had the possibility of affecting tiny structures on the inside of cells irrespective of what we did to the cells as a whole. The implications here were staggering. Could we control vital cell molecules and their processes in this manner? Could we intrude our force field into a cell and selectively affect vital processes or life itself? . . . It also occurred to us that one might conceivably use this same force in order to control malignant and uncontrolled cells such as occur in cancer. . . . Whether it will be useful in cancer or in many other fields, only time and a great deal more work will tell. . . . Perhaps in time this probe [radio frequency] may become a tool of healing for certain nervous diseases, or even mental abnormalities." (See Bibliography for source.)

If similar waves are beamed at cells which are misbehaving or malfunctioning, it may not be surprising if they restore law and order, or balance.

Radiations of many varieties surround us and we have already harnessed some of them and put them to work for us. In health treatment the difference between radiesthesia and sine wave, diathermy, or short-wave diathermy is that radiesthesia is *selective* and tuned to a specific disease or abnormality.

The *British Journal of Physical Medicine*, as long ago as June, 1936, reported the calming effects of high-frequency currents on the nervous system. The report read, "As a therapeutic application method the 'weak intensity treatment' has been developed and gave very good results in over 3,000 cases, which were treated in the last three years. Special portable short wave emitters for the 'weak intensity treatment' have been constructed and can be seen on exhibition."

A Zurich professional report, *An Internationaler Radiolongenkongress* (Vol. II, p. 501), gives the results of over 5,000 cases by doctors using ultrashort waves. Of diseases of the joints, 76 per cent were cured; in gout and gonorrheal diseases of the joints, nearly 100 per cent were cured; 80 per cent of early cases of sciatica were cured and 90 per cent of lumbago and acute rheumatic diseases responded.

According to the *Electronic Medical Digest*, "Reiter found that exposure to ultrashort waves inhibited metabolism in tumor cells. Wave lengths between three or four meters destroyed tumors in his experiments. *He found that very large doses of X ray were required to produce results comparable to those obtained with low intensity.*" (Again the effect of the minimum dose!)

In August, 1963, a Long Island, New York, fisherman, his pulse undetectable, his face blue, was brought back from the edge of death by the fire department which used a little-known device, a batronic resuscitator. The wandlike instrument projects electric impulses through the body from a generator by way of a sponge placed at the solar plexus and a metal plate at the back. "In 15 minutes," according to the New York *Daily Mirror*, "natural color replaced the blue in the fisherman's cheeks and his pulse was discernible. He opened his eyes and said, 'Where am I?'"

RADIONICS

One branch of radiesthesia, as compared with electronics, is known as Radionics. In this technique, an operator picks up the radio signals from the human body by stroking a plate on the instrument and sensing the energy radiations through the finger tips. Not every operator can do this. De La Warr, in his book, *New Worlds Beyond the Atom* (New York: Devin-Adair, 1963), explains that only those qualified can be successfully trained to operate a radionics instrument. "Where living matter is concerned, persons possessing a certain kind of sensitivity, or an extra sense of perception, can become aware of emanations emitted by human beings or animals."

Thus a radionics treating instrument, instead of plugging into electric current, uses the patient's own electrical radiations or energy to "play back" or focus it where needed. Some doctors use a combination of radionics and electronics.

What type of illness has radiesthesia helped? Since the list covers almost the entire range of human ailments, a detailed list would be too long to give. However, the following categories are included:

Glandular disorders.
Diseases of the nervous system.
Infections.
Respiratory diseases.
Gastrointestinal ailments.
Kidney, bladder, genito-urinary complaints.
Certain muscular and bone conditions.
Blood conditions.
Abnormal growths.
Diseases of the circulatory system, including heart.
Headaches.
Allergies.
Skin disturbances.
Insecticide and other poison contaminations.

The number of radiesthetic treatments needed to clear up a serious condition varies in different cases. If the ailment has not existed for long or is not too severe, it has often been cleared up with a few treatments. Stubborn cases or long-standing chronic complaints would obviously need more treatment, depending upon the severity of the case. Additional types of therapy such as vitamins and minerals, some glandular extracts, homeopathic and Schuessler salts can speed recovery. And once health has been restored, the patient must not think he can go gaily on his way breaking all known laws of proper nutrition and normal behavior. Health must be constantly maintained by feeding the body the substances it needs so that its machinery will not break down again.

To find a member of the healing profession who operates a radiesthesia instrument is admittedly difficult. Since the process is known by different names, one doctor may call it electronics, another radionics. Radiesthesia is a general term, and the name may not be recognized by some operators. You are more likely to find such equipment in the offices of chiropractors, naturopaths, and osteopaths, and in a few offices of M.D.'s. It is useless to call on a telephone and ask if a doctor has such apparatus. Fearing it is a "plant" by an official spy, you will probably get an abrupt No! The only method I can suggest is to search for the information from other patients who are receiving this treatment. And when you do find this help, guard the secret or you too may soon be without it!

This system carries many testimonials of improved health, both by patients who have received treatment, and by doctors who have administered it. Sooner or later as more people are able to locate operators who use these instruments, the good reports are bound to travel by word of mouth until they create a groundswell for demand for such therapy.

13 Do-it-yourself radiesthesia —the pendulum

Even though science is slowly coming around to the admission that every living thing generates—and emits—electricity, machines which detect human radiations in relation to health are hard to find. So you might like to have fun experimenting with a simple do-it-yourself device.

I wish to make it absolutely clear that I am making no claims for the following information. I am merely reporting what others have discovered. You may have great success, or you may have none. I can neither promise nor predict. Because it will be a field new to you, and because you naturally do not have the benefit of experience or training, there is no guarantee of accuracy. You will have to proceed by trial and error. The project as a whole may not even appeal to you. But I will place before you the findings of some respectable, unregimented investigators and let you decide for yourself whether or not to make use of the information. My guess is that those of you who do experiment will have lots of fun. Whether you get results is another thing again. But the project, if you are the experimental type, will be undeniably fascinating.

One device used in a branch of radiesthesia is surrounded by a great deal of confusion. This device is the pendulum. Not realizing that its specialized use has attracted serious attention in various parts of the world, the average person assumes that it is a toy. Thus its original use has been lost sight of. Dr. Ernest Thomas Jensen (1873-1950) of England said, "Radiesthesia (including the use of the pendulum) is a rediscovery rather than a product of modern times for there is evidence that it was known and practiced extensively . . . in ancient China, Egypt, Babylon and among the Maya in Central America."

A Catholic priest, Abbé Mermet, wrote an entire book, *Introduction to Principles and Practices of Radiesthesia* as a result of his highly successful tests with the pendulum, which seems to act as a small Geiger counter in detecting radiations of various substances. A generous amount of research, particularly in England, points to the fact that a pendulum may be able to "pick up" electrical radiations from rocks and minerals, metals, liquids, and even foods. This true radiesthetic pendulum is not to be confused with the parlor-game pendulum used to answer personal questions such as, "Should I go shopping today?" or "Should I invest in XYZ stock?" People who have tried the pendulum for those purposes say it is inaccurate and reflects the conscious or unconscious attitude of the operator. These same people contend, on the other hand, that using the pendulum to detect natural radiations is remarkably accurate, providing the operator is sufficiently sensitive to act as a conductor.

The system is related to dowsing for water and metals. Dowsing may be a controversial subject, but those who have not been able to find water or hidden minerals by other means claim its results are incontestable. Not everyone can dowse, however. Nor can everyone successfully use a pendulum. Many of you will consider the pendulum, like dowsing, pure folklore. Some will even write its activity off as a by-product of an overactive imagination. But there are some startling reports of what a pendulum can do.

A cousin of mine, who owned a large ranch in the Rocky Mountains, would often tie a ring on a piece of string and suspend it over a horse or cow about to give birth. By the direction of the swing of the ring, this man could determine in advance the sex of the newborn calf or colt. And he had scores of witnesses to prove that the swinging ring—actually a pendulum—was always right.

Dr. Abel Martin, with a degree of Doctor of Veterinary Science from the University of Paris in 1933, specialized in diagnosis of disease of animals by means of the pendulum. He wrote his thesis on "Radiesthetic Diagnosis in Veterinary Medicine," later published as a book. Dr. Martin was able, in cases of blood poisoning, to test and find the cause as to which store of hay, oats, or clover was the source of the trouble. One test of tuberculosis was made in the School of Agriculture before a jury of Veterinary Surgeons, and those results compared with those obtained by subcutaneous and intradermic injections of tuberculin. There was a difference in only 1 out of 40 cows tested medically and by pendulum.

THE PENDULUM AS A SELF-HELP DEVICE

I take no responsibility for the pendulum as a self-help device, nor can I say whether or not it is effective. I am merely passing on the remarks of others who have tried it. Those who work with pendulums for the purpose of detecting certain radiations in various substances, including food and vitamins, feel that a pendulum can be very simple. It may be made of wood, metal, glass, or even be a wooden or glass bead, a plumb-bob or a fishing-line weight. It may be any shape, although a round, or tear-drop shape is supposed to give better balance. Some pendulum users feel that metal is less acceptable than other materials. Others feel that it doesn't matter.

Those who are expert in pendulum lore tie the pendulum on a cord, fishing line, or nylon thread, 8 inches or so in length. When they find the thread length which seems to give the best pendulum swing, they tie a knot or wooden peg at that point to prevent it slipping through their fingers. They hold the pendulum thread in their right hand, if they are right-handed, or in their left hand if they are left-handed. Pendulum users are very particular not to let anyone else use their pendulum, and they store it in a cardboard or plastic box when not in use.

The operator, according to the rules, may or may not rest his elbow on the table. Strangely enough, if a pendulum is attached to a wooden stick and suspended over an object, it will not work. Transferred to the human hand of a sufficiently sensitive person, it can become very active. Of course there is always the possibility that the operator is unconsciously (or consciously) manipulating it. But, since there is no way of proving this, it is better not to mention the possibility. It always infuriates the operator, who is sincere. I know, because I raised the question to one person whose hand was obviously moving. He said, indignantly, "I am *not* moving the pendulum! The pendulum is moving *my* hand. It is like the tail wagging the dog." And, since I try to maintain an open mind, I did not argue.

Now, according to our informants, if you have a pendulum, are sensitive enough to operate it (it won't even move for some people), you are ready to begin the tests. You should be rested, not recently have imbibed even a drop of alcohol (which supposedly causes loss of sensitivity), and you should approach the tests with reasonable enthusiasm. Place any sample of food, liquid, or vitamin supplements in front of you. One at a time, place a sample in one hand while you hold the pendulum over it with the other. Continue testing at first only 15 minutes at a time. After a week or so this time can gradually be extended, I am told. Warnings are given that the procedure should not be considered a parlor game. The mental attitude should be as serious as with any other type of study, and is said to be of great importance in attaining accurate results.

The sample to be tested may be placed in a dish or, in the case of liquids, in a glass. No metal should be used, or the pendulum may be measuring the radiations of the metal. Neither should there be any other metal close by so that the field of one item will not encroach upon that of another.

According to one report you proceed as follows: "Hold the pendulum three to six inches away from the specimen and at least twelve inches away from your body. Now close your eyes. After about ten seconds, open your eyes and the pendulum should be gyrating. If the specimen is good for your diet, it will gyrate in a clockwise direction; anti-clockwise will indicate the specimen is not good for your diet. . . . If you get pendulum swings to and fro (oscillations) it will indicate that your specimen is of little consequence to your health so far as diet is concerned. . . . Remember the fifteen minute time limit and do not be tempted [at first] to try tests with more than two specimens.

"Many people do not deny that the subconscious could influence the movement of the pendulum, hence the closing of the eyes at the beginning of the test. If you test a substance about which you have no feeling or knowledge, wishful thinking will be less likely to influence the results."

F. A. Archdale, author of *Elementary Radiesthesia—The Use of the Pendulum*, agrees. He says, "Auto-suggestion is Radiesthesia's worst enemy, and you will find that, unless you are very careful, the pendulum will do what you want it to do or what you think it ought to do. You will no doubt meet people who will tell you that Radiesthesia is auto-suggestion, pure and simple and nothing else; a sweeping statement, but nevertheless it has an element of truth in it, inasmuch as the 'idea of the movement creates the movement.' "

In addition to ascertaining which foods, vitamins, minerals, and drinking water are good for them, some people claim the pendulum has helped them locate elusive allergies.

H. W. Trinder in his book, *Dowsing*, quotes the following letter written to him: "A woman in business near here suffered from headaches three times a week, so much so that she thought she would never hold her job. Her lady doctor told her there was no known cure for that kind of headache, which comes out of the blue. She came to your demonstration then tried a pendulum over all her food, with the following result: clockwise (acceptable)

—brown bread, boiled eggs, etc.; counterclockwise (unacceptable) —white bread, fried eggs, sugar, etc. She promptly dieted accordingly. In a day or two she had lost her headaches and has had no return whatever. She told her doctor, who was curious but noncommittal. She offered her the pendulum to try and the lady doctor put it over her palm, whereupon it began to whizz around almost as rapidly as yours does. The doctor was rather scared and said: "What is it doing? I'm not doing this!"

Although the preceding directions apply to most people, there are exceptions. According to Mira Louise, in her book, *In Search of New Horizons*, "Confusion often arises from the fact that irrespective of whether the operator is left-handed or right-handed, the pendulum will gyrate in a clockwise direction for one person and in an anti-clockwise direction for another."

In order to find out which is your positive swing (meaning that a substance tested is acceptable or "safe" for you) you can make this simple test which Mira Louise has developed:

"Sit in a straight-backed chair, avoiding one with arm rests that would impede your actions, and face North, with the knees about eight inches apart. Hold the pendulum about two inches above the right knee and when it settles down to a steady swing, make a note of the *way* it swings, whether clockwise or anti-clockwise. Upon this will rest your whole future. It does not matter which way it swings, as long as you remember in all your testing that it is *Your Positive Swing*.

"Then having established whether it is clockwise or anti-clockwise, move the pendulum to the space between the knees, where it will oscillate backwards and forwards. Then, very gently, move it towards and hold it over the left knee where it should swing in the opposite direction to that when held over the right knee. As the right knee is always positive and the left knee is always negative, and the space in between is always neutral, the same reactions can be expected as if the pendulum were held over the prepared sample.

"Rest for a few seconds between each attempt and do not be discouraged if the pendulum remains stationary at the first trial. Persevere again and again. . . . In an emergency a cotton reel, a button, a bead or even a ring can be suspended by a slender thread, but when setting out to acquire a new technique, it is a wise student who secures the best instruments available."

I am told, though I have never witnessed it, that in some food markets in the southwestern part of the United States it is not uncommon to see people holding a pendulum over fruits and vegetables to test whether they are too green, overripe, or contaminated with sprays—therefore unacceptable.

One of the funniest experiences I have witnessed was that of a well-educated, experimentally minded woman who had just learned about and rigged up a pendulum. We were having lunch at a restaurant one day when the woman took her pendulum out of purse to test the soup she was about to eat.

"It is a good thing my husband can't see me," she said.

At that precise moment, her husband, an executive in a huge corporation, walked in, accompanied by a group of his fellow executives. His wife almost—not quite—dropped the pendulum into her soup.

Consider the pendulum as folklore, if you wish. Perhaps it is a product of the imagination. But to many people it is an informative and helpful gadget. To others it is a source of harmless amusement. For still others it won't work at all. However, if you wish to pursue the subject further, you will find in the Bibliography a list of books written by some throughtful and intelligent investigators, describing its use more fully.

A pendulum is not a substitute for a nutritionally trained physician. It is merely a tool to try when other methods fail.

If someone had predicted 20 years ago that I would have breakfast in San Francisco, lunch 40,000 feet over Denver, and dinner in New York—as I often do—I would have said, "Impossible." If our great-grandparents had received a prediction of fluoroscope, X-ray or electronic stoves which cook food in seconds, they too would have snorted, "Impossible!" I am beginning to wonder if the word *impossible* shouldn't be removed from the dictionary.

As I was writing this chapter, I was invited to dinner at a distinguished university. There were several professors at the table and the subject of dowsing came up. Each man told of an instance in which he had seen dowsing in action. At the end of the discussion, one professor said, "I don't believe it, I don't understand it —*but it works!*" Five Nobel prize winners agree.

An admonition, timely at this point, is, "Help us not to dispose or oppose what we do not understand." (William Penn.)

I will not be surprised, if, in the future, every household should own and consider the pendulum an indispensable diagnostic gadget. As a baby Geiger counter used in proper hands, it might very well, by wagging its head Yes or No, determine which foods and which drinking water are safe; which foods or beverages cause allergies; and which vitamins and minerals are most effective for each individual. It might turn out to be a priceless method of detecting insecticide sprays and poisons as well as dangerous additives and fallout hidden in foods from the unsuspecting consumer. Stranger things have happened!

14   Stranger than fiction—the Edgar Cayce readings

There are unseen forces in this world which we do not understand. Sometimes there is a plausible explanation; sometimes not. Take one example: the effect of music on the growth of plants. The *Houston Chronicle* has presented its testimony, together with photographs, of the effect of music on two nearly identical geranium plants. The owner of these plants placed the two geraniums in pots of the same size and gave them the same amount of water and fertilizer. She also exposed them to similar lighting conditions. One plant, however, was kept cuddled up to an FM radio which played day and night. The other plant was kept in silence. The plant treated to music had more blooms, straighter stalks, and crisper and greener leaves. The plant confined to silence withered and drooped and its blooms appeared wilted. Heat from the FM was not a factor.

An Indian botanist, Dr. T. C. N. Singh, began investigating the effect of music on growing plants as early as 1950. After eight years of study he reported that tapioca and sweet potatoes constantly subjected to recorded music showed an increase of 40 per cent in yield. Rice plants increased by 50 per cent when subjected to classical music, and tobacco plants increased 50 per cent when subjected to violin music. Dr. Singh's explanation is that the vibrations agitate the protoplasm and the nuclei inside the plant cells and cause them to react in such a way that growth is accelerated.

Dairy farmers have already learned that playing soothing music to cows facilitates milk flow. The assumption has always been that the music produces a tranquilizing effect. Perhaps so; however, Dr. Singh's explanation of sound vibrations may eventually prove more valid. A chicken farmer in England discovered that his 2,500 chickens exposed to sensuous mambo music laid eggs at a rapid rate. When the music recordings were changed to whistling ear-splitters the hens refused to lay at all.

John Ott, who is mentioned in the chapter on arthritis, has noted that light waves, admitted through the eyes of a chicken, reach the pituitary gland and in turn step up egg production. Though we do not always understand the mysterious forces of nature, we dare not sit in judgment against them. One doctor told me, "A colleague of mine stated unequivocally in print some years ago that the theory of healing by sound and light waves was not only ridiculous; it was impossible. He has lived to witness the healing results of ultrasonic waves and the bloodless surgery by the laser ray. His face is mighty red."

THE CAYCE READINGS, AN UNEXPLAINED PHENOMENON

Though it is undeniably important, it is questionable that the *only* route to diagnosis and healing is through the doors of the medical school. One great exception was Edgar Cayce who, without benefit of schooling beyond the age of 16 and certainly without medical training, diagnosed thousands of people while he was asleep in a trance state. In his "readings" not only the diagnosis of a disturbance was presented, but its cause and suggested treatment as well.

This treatment was often a home remedy, sometimes an herb, now and then a natural medicine. Osteopathy, with explicit directions for relieving pressure in specific areas, was often recommended. In rare cases surgery was advocated. Many people have testified to the success of the information contained in these readings. Those who did not follow the advice wished afterward that they had, when other methods failed to cure them.

Thomas Sugrue, writing about Edgar Cayce in his book, *There Is a River*, says,

"Over the years certain ideas about health, the causes of disease, and cures, had been repeated over and over again in readings. There was a compound that was given for every person suffering from pyorrhea; there was an inhalant suggested for one of the three types of hay fever; there was a salve for hemorrhoids; there were castor oil packs for appendicitis and intestinal complications; there were grape poultices for intestinal fevers; there was the suggestion to some people that they eat a few almonds a day to thwart a tendency toward cancer; there was the suggestion to others that they massage peanut oil into their skin to head off arthritis; there was a dose which time and again proved efficacious in breaking up a common cold.

"At the hospital these and other remedies could be checked and rechecked until their value was beyond doubt. Then they could be turned over to the medical profession and the public. There were skin lotions, intestinal antiseptics, treatment for stimulating the growth of the hair, diets helpful to certain conditions, and mechanical appliances. . . .

"In commenting on the theory behind this [an appliance], a reading said, 'The human body is made up of electronic vibrations, with each atom and element of the body, each organ and organism, having its electronic unit of vibration necessary for the sustenance of, and the equilibrium in, that particular organism. Each unit, then, being a cell or unit of life in itself has its capacity for reproducing itself by the first law of reproduction-division.

" 'When a force in any organ, or element of the body becomes deficient in its ability to reproduce that equilibrium necessary for the sustenance of the physical existence and its reproduction, that portion becomes deficient in electronic energy. This may come by injury or by disease, received from external forces. It may come from internal forces through lack of elimination produced in the system, or by lack of other agencies to meet its requirement in the body.' "

It was not unusual for the readings to suggest a medicine which was not even listed by a manufacturer. In one instance, a reading helped a chemist perfect a formula, then suggested a use which had not occurred to him, though he had earned his doctorate in chemistry at Oxford University in England.

Even physicians stood in awe of the information which came through a man who did not understand the technical medical terms he uttered. In one instance, Thomas B. House, M.D., summoned Edgar Cayce at the insistence of his sick wife, who was a believer in the Cayce readings. A leading specialist had already given Mrs. House an orthodox diagnosis of abdominal tumor. The Cayce reading, on the other hand, diagnosed the condition as a locked bowel and pregnancy. It recommended warm oil enemas and other remedies. Although he was unconvinced, Dr. House yielded to his wife's request that he try the remedies and recheck the diagnosis. The Cayce diagnosis proved correct; the remedies relieved the locked bowel and in due time a son was born to the couple.

Many years later, after they had watched the results of many other readings, Mrs. House said to her husband, "Maybe science will discover these things someday."

Her husband now agreed with her. He advised the Cayce family, "Keep the records of everything in the readings. Some day they will catch up with us."

Meanwhile other cures were taking place. Hugh Lynn Cayce, Edgar's elder son, suffered from an accident to his eyes when a whole tray of photographic flash powder exploded in his face. The doctors decided that he would be blind in one eye, maybe both, and urged the removal of the eye with the greatest damage in hopes of saving the other one. A reading from the boy's father prescribed a poultice which was made up by a local pharmacist and its use resulted in perfect eyesight with scarcely a trace of a scar.

Edgar Evans Cayce, Edgar's younger son, was given help for serious burns when his clothing caught fire from an open fireplace; and Mrs. Cayce was completely cured of an "incurable" case of tuberculosis as a result of a course of treatment prescribed by the readings. During their lifetimes, both Mr. and Mrs. Cayce developed appendicitis. The reading told one to have an operation; the other one not to. Both recovered to full health. Thousands of others received help through the readings.

It is not surprising that there were those who considered Edgar Cayce a fake and the reading information purely imaginary. In 1928, Dr. William Moseley Brown, head of the psychology department of Washington and Lee University, arrived at the Cayce residence in Virginia Beach, Virginia. He said, "Hugh Lynn is one of my students. I made a statement that I could expose any medium. I have come to expose Hugh Lynn's father."

Edgar Cayce greeted him, smiled, shook his hand, and asked him to sit down. Dr. Brown began asking questions, and examining readings. He stayed to listen to several readings being given by the elder Cayce. Finally he surrendered. "I can't expose you," he said, "and I can't ignore you. I'll have to believe in you." He joined the association and requested a reading for himself and members of his family.

I knew Edgar Cayce personally, and like everyone else, loved and respected him. Actually, he was an uncomplicated man with great integrity. He taught Sunday school, fished off a pier on a pond in his backyard, gave readings and visited with his guests, usually those who had come for readings. He was completely sincere, humble, and religious. The books which have already told his story are: *There Is a River*, by Thomas Sugrue (originally published by Henry Holt and Co., 1942, 1945; now in a Dell paperback edition, 1961); *Edgar Cayce, Man of Miracles*, by Joseph Millard (Wehman Publishers, 1963) and *Venture Inward*, by Hugh Lynn Cayce (published by Harper & Row, 1964).

An association, known as the Association for Research and Enlightenment, a nonprofit research organization, has been organized by and for those who are studying the work of Edgar Cayce.

Since his death, the association continues to grow and accept new members under the able leadership of Hugh Lynn Cayce. The association has followed Dr. House's advice. Every word of the 50-year file of 90,000 pages of readings is being catalogued, indexed, cross-indexed, and the information on diseases assembled and tabulated. Doctors have tested the remedies over the years. One clinic, supervised by two physicians (both M.D.'s), is beginning a new program of thorough research on the treatments advocated in the readings. You can learn more about this fascinating story and findings of the Cayce Foundation (which does not prescribe) by writing to A.R.E. Incorporated, Virginia Beach, Virginia, 23451.

I can personally vouch for Edgar Cayce, his family, and the excellent staff of the association. His passing was a great loss to the world but the wealth of information he left behind is a veritable treasure of health information, relatively untapped. True to the predictions of Dr. House and his wife, science is now just beginning to catch up with it!

PART TWO

HEALTH THROUGH NUTRITION

AUTHOR'S NOTE

Countless studies show that correct nutrition strengthens the entire body, maintains good health and serves as a preventive of degenerative illness. The following chapters present some recent findings.

15 Our "good" American diet?

It is now past the point of conjecture that there is a relationship between health and nutrition. There are many cases of both animals and people to prove that this relationship exists, and they continue to mount. America is *said* to be the healthiest nation in the world and to have the best diet. Statistics show this to be a fallacy. As two prime examples, cancer and heart disease are increasing. Obviously, diet is not entirely responsible, but it makes a great contribution to health or its lack. It is true that America has *more* food, but this does not mean *better* food. Let me give you an illustration.

I can recall earlier times when dining on the train was a luxurious occasion. The tables were set with snowy linen, sparkling silver and glassware, waiters were courteous, and food was cooked to order and delicious. Recently on the Atlantic coast I boarded a train just before lunch. When I made my way to the diner, I reflected that this particular railroad no longer had the wonderful food it used to serve, but I consoled myself that it would at least be hot, and if I chose it carefully, relatively nourishing. But I was due for a shock.

At the threshold of the dining car I glimpsed one waiter only. He was pleasant and courteous, but harassed. He was helping people to make change and choices from a recent addition to the railroad line—a vending machine! No other source of food was in sight. I watched in disbelief as people shoved in a quarter here or a fifty cent piece there and pulled out such items as a dry ham sandwich on white bread—no butter, no lettuce, no mayonnaise.

Wrapped in waxed paper the sandwich undoubtedly had been made days before, and would last many days longer if no one happened to choose it. There were frozen TV dinners which one took out of their cubicle and warmed under a flash heating device. There were canned soups and other canned foods also to heat after opening. A toaster sat on one of the bare tables in case you wanted to toast the already dry bread in your sandwich. Other choices included pies, pastries, canned fruit, dry cereal, canned fruit and vegetable juices, and other foods which would keep practically forever. Of course there was the vending-machine type of hot coffee, tea, and chocolate as well as soft and hard drinks, gum, and candy. Three times while I sat there the coffee machine got stuck and the poor steward had to get down on his knees in order to pry it open to release the machinery.

I must admit that there were two saving graces: a choice of "fresh fruit"—an apple or an orange—and no tipping. Since I was hungry, I finally chose, in desperation, that ham sandwich, sat down at the bare table and toasted each piece of bread separately and tried to choke it down with a cup of hot coffee, which was preferable to a cold bottled synthetic drink. I rejected the fruit because there were no knives for peeling, only plastic ware.

I finished this typical American meal and accosted the steward. I asked him if other people actually liked the changeover to vending machines. He was guarded in his answers. After all he is a family man, he told me, and had to make a living. He said the college students who rode the trains liked the idea because it saved them money; the people in the coach car (where I was riding) were resigned to it, but that the people who had come from a great distance and were riding in the Pullmans were "screaming with anger." I said I didn't blame them. He added with a little nostalgia, "You know, it looks as if the good old days are gone. There used to be a wonderful restaurant in a town where I wait between trains. Now there is nothing but vending machines and a sign on the wall, which reads, 'In case of mechanical failure telephone this number.'"

Even sadder than vending machines on trains, where people are trapped and can't eat anything else, are vending machines in schools. In the area where I live the cafeterias have been closed in the junior and senior high schools and vending machines have been installed. Apparently this is becoming the national rule. An article "Our Starving Teen-agers," published by the *Reader's Digest* as early as 1955, says, "Investigators are now convinced that teen-age malnutrition is nationwide. . . . Teen-agers with plenty of money and allowed to eat anything they like away from home . . . do not get enough protein to build sound tissues, enough calcium for strong bones and good teeth, enough vitamins and minerals for steady nerves, normal blood and efficient vision.

"Result: the boys make a sad showing in physical examinations, as Selective Service records testify; but the nutritional status of the mothers of tomorrow is even more serious. . . . Dr. I. G. Macy-Hoobler, an authority on maternal diets, speaks bluntly: 'A girl whose nutrition is not adequate for her own body cannot expect to develop a good baby.' "

Vending machines in schools contain esssentially the same choices of foods with long shelf life as stocked on train vending machines. Candy and soft drinks are included in schools which allow them.

There are at least two good examples of schools where care is taken, at any cost, with children's bodies as well as their minds. As a result, not only has health improved, but grades too. In North Country School, a private school in Lake Placid, New York, fresh whole wheat bread is baked daily, and hot whole grain cereal is served exclusively. The grains for both are fresh ground on the premises. Vegetables are grown in the school garden and served liberally, and salads are included once a day. The school raises its own poultry, pigs, and beef cattle. Organ meats are served once a week as is salt-water fish. Fresh raw milk is served twice daily and desserts, puddings, and pies only once a week. Dessert on the remaining days consists of fruit, either fresh or dried. Raw wheat germ is placed on the breakfast table so that children can help themselves. Brewer's yeast and ground kelp are added to meat loaves and other recipes. Honey is used instead of sugar, and there is plenty of real butter and cheese, and eggs fresh from the school hens.

What effect does this have on the children? Visitors coming to the school ask what shampoo the school uses to produce such beautiful hair sheen. Ruddy complexions are also common. Fat children lose weight. Thin children gain weight and illnesses have decreased by half, according to infirmary records kept over the years. Epidemics which flare in nearby schools rarely touch the North Country schoolchildren. Sometimes a whole term goes by without a child missing a class or a meal. Cavities are practically unheard of. Walter E. Clark, director of the school, is responsible for this wonderful program. Do the children themselves like it? One ten-year-old wrote home, "The food is wonderful and it is a lot of fun to be here."

Unique? Not necessarily. A similar program is conducted in a public school, Helix High, in La Mesa, California. Here, too, fresh-ground wheat is made into freshly baked bread daily. Wheat germ and the other special nutrients scornfully classed as "food fads" by critics, are, as in North Country School, also on the bill of fare. Fresh fruits, vegetables, and plenty of protein are served. No candies, soft drinks, or gooey desserts are available. The food is delicious, appetizing, and wholesome. Does it pay off not to cut costs? The record at this high school, with its cafeteria run so efficiently by Gina Larsen, proves that it does. Grades have risen so high that the school is actually embarrassed because of the many scholarships granted to the students. And injuries from football and other sports are practically nonexistent. Mrs. Larsen was walking across the campus one day when a student, his arm in a sling, passed her. She looked at him in surprise. He said, "Don't worry, lady. I am not from your school."

People who cut costs in nutrition may later pay those costs many times over. Hospitals are more crowded than ever. According to the *New York Times*, a United Hospital Fund study revealed that patient care costs which were $15.35 a day in 1947, jumped to $40.92 in 1962 and will probably soar to $53.35 per day in 1967.

Incontestable evidence shows that correct nutrition helps to prevent, and often corrects illness. The *American Journal of Clinical Nutrition* (April, 1963) warns, "Excessive consumption of refined flour, refined fat, sugar and alcohol can and does result in serious malnutrition and disease without serious weight loss. During both world wars, the health of England and Denmark improved noticeably. Sherman and others maintained it was because they couldn't get refined foods and ate large amounts of coarse, unrefined foods from natural sources. . . .

"Forgetfulness, confusion, anxiety, depression, delirium, dementia, hallucinations, headache and convulsions have all resulted from dietary deficiency. A certain number of patients suffering from 'senility' have responded dramatically to therapy with essential nutrients. Too often it is assumed that manifest nutritional deficiency is the result of deprivation for only a period of months or perhaps a few years. There is no sound basis for this assumption. . . . Without any doubt, trials of nutritional therapy have been judged to be failures, not because they would not have been successful, but solely on the basis that they were not carried on for long enough periods of time."

Many people ask what vitamin or mineral they should take for this or that disturbance. Although I do not prescribe, I do report, and the answer, based on studies of experts in this field of health-via-nutrition, is that *everything* is necessary. Donald Cooley states, "Vitamins never work singlehandedly, but *in partnership with each other* [italics added], with hormones, enzymes and many other substances."

George L. Siefert, M.D., and H. Curtis Wood, Jr., M.D., state, "It is probably true that minerals may actually be more important than vitamins for good health and resistance to disease, some authorities having stated that many vitamins are functionless in the absence of minerals."

These two physicians, after 20 years of experience with mineral therapy, are convinced that organic minerals are better assimilated than synthetics. They point out, that due to erosion, "every hour of every day, the land is getting poorer and the ocean richer. Therefore, vegetables that grow in the sea are much more constant in their mineral content than are earth-grown plants."

Couple this with the hypothesis that all life began in the sea, where it existed for millions of years before occupying the land, and that the mineral analysis of the human blood parallels that of the analysis of sea water. It is therefore possible that these sea-water minerals are still necessary for the continuation of life and health.

Some evidence of this concept was forthcoming from a study, conducted by Drs. Siefert and Wood, in which they used a form of seaweed, *Macrocystis pyrifera*, harvested from the Pacific Ocean, as a source of trace minerals. Many of the patients who were given these minerals reported the following benefits:

If the symptoms of a cold appeared, the cold did not develop and was gone in a few days' time.

Hemoglobin of 400 pregnant women improved from 65 per cent to 83 per cent as a result of taking three mineral tablets daily.

Improvement of abnormal fatigue was noted.

Color and quality of hair improved.

Fingernails became less brittle.

Less fragile capillaries and less bruising were noticeable.

Relief of certain skin conditions took place.

Increase in virility was noted.

There was marked improvement in arthritic cases.

Eye conditions, such as iritis and cataracts, improved.

Constipation was diminished.

A sense of well-being was experienced.*

Vitamins and minerals, of natural origin, are the equivalent of many pounds of food (and calories); even so these supplements mean just that: supplements. They are not a substitute for good food—and vice versa, unless you want to drag along and feel half alive. Both may be necessary. Those dubious people who still think we can get everything we need from a "good diet" are out of date. We don't get the food our ancestors ate. Refined, packaged—to keep on the shelf, thus purposely depleted—food, and fruits and vegetables picked green to ship great distances; these do not contain the amount of vitamins and minerals found in our ancestors' natural, home-grown food. Furthermore, in these days of ten-

* This information is included in a reprint, available for 25¢ from the National Health Federation, P.O. Box 686, Monrovia, California. The title: "Macrocystis Pyrifera (Sea Weed) as a Source of Trace Elements in Human Nutrition," by George L. Siefert, M.D. and H. Curtis Wood, Jr., M.D.

sions, worldwide wars, fallout, and occupational hurry and worry, our bodies are undergoing so much stress that we need not an *under*allowance but an *over*abundance of nutritional factors to fortify our resistance! It is silly to just scrape through when we need a wide-open door to good health.

As I pointed out in *Stay Young Longer*, synthetic vitamins have a special function: to overcome a disability quickly. They are often used in massive doses by injection, or mouth, as the doctor sees fit. The results are sometimes startling. Large amounts of niacin (a B vitamin), for example, have relieved seriously disturbed mental states and returned the persons to normal within 48 hours. Massive doses of synthetic vitamin C in tablet form for troublesome infections can produce results within a few hours.

But once an acute situation has been eliminated, many nutritionists feel that for day-in, day-out use, natural vitamins and minerals are wiser.

A nutritionally oriented physician prescribed a diet for two of my friends, a married couple, who had been disciples of good nutrition for years and were in above-average health. After testing them, the physician found they were not getting enough special nutrients. He prescribed cod-liver oil. He increased their intake of brewer's yeast to one cup per day for the wife, and three-quarters of a cup for her husband. He prescribed 900 units of vitamin E for the wife to help her through menopause, and 300 units for her husband as heart insurance.* He urged them each to take a generous supply of calcium and a mixture of all the vital minerals plus one-third cup of desiccated liver daily. These amounts were, of course, in addition to a good diet! When I next saw the couple, less than a year later, they both looked five years younger, and had forgotten the meaning of the word "fatigue." I wish you could see the physician himself. He *looks* a robust 40. He actually is 70.

A study conducted in India several years ago, showed that humans can stay alive on low intakes of food if nutrients are fairly well balanced. However, if one vitamin or mineral, or even a food-type is stepped up, other elements need to be increased also.

A voluminous amount of literature is accumulating showing that

---

* The effect of vitamin E on menopause and heart is documented in *Stay Young Longer*.

important interrelationships between vitamins, minerals and amino acids exist in natural foods. When man tries to separate these nutrients, known and unknown, balance is upset and health may suffer.

Incidentally, there is one caution to observe in taking large amounts of brewer's yeast or wheat germ. Both of them, otherwise excellent food supplements, are high in phosphorus in relation to calcium. If taken in continuous large amounts, they might cause difficulty. Phosphorus combines with calcium in the body, and when there is too much it is excreted. Unfortunately it takes calcium with it, creating a calcium deficiency.

Melvin E. Page, D.D.S., considers the correct body calcium-phosphorus balance to be 2.5 parts of calcium to 1 part of phosphorus, or the ratio of 2½ to 1. Brewer's yeast, though being excellent in all other respects, has a calcium-phosphorus ratio of 1:18 and wheat germ 1:13. Dr. Michael Walsh corrects this in two ways: He advises that for every tablespoon of brewer's yeast or wheat germ you should take 8 ounces of skim milk, whole milk or buttermilk, to supply the correct amount of calcium. Or, if you are not a milk drinker, he suggests four tablespoons of skim milk powder to every tablespoon of brewer's yeast or wheat germ. Adelle Davis corrects the imbalance by adding ¼ cup of calcium lactate or ½ cup of calcium gluconate to each pound of brewer's yeast. Mix ahead of time, then you won't have to give it another thought whenever you take your brewer's yeast mixture.

In my humble opinion, those who make fun of nutrition are either behind the times, or are afraid that too many people will find out the amazing health changes correct nutrition can produce —of course, leading to an out-of-pocket loss for the manufacturers or producers of drugs or unnatural foods. This perhaps is why they are trying to silence those who make health claims for nutrition.

According to the *Organic Consumer Report* (October 9, 1962), "Our present federal laws hold that, where foods, food supplements, or plain concentrated vegetable supplements, minerals and natural ingredients are concerned, what can be said on labels is determined by the 'concensus of medical opinion' *not* the

truth of such statements. Hence the manufacturer of natural vitamins and minerals, for instance, may not truthfully label his products, even though he can prove his statements, if the concensus
of medical opinion is in conflict. If he does so, he is guilty of making 'false claim' and subject to fine and imprisonment—for telling the truth!"

To help fight these pressures, the National Health Federation
sponsors a national conference on health monopoly, purposely
planned at the same time, in the same city where the American
Medical Association and the federal Food and Drug Administration sponsor their annual "anti-quackery" meeting. The chief
purpose of the National Health Federation conferences is to try
to determine the extent to which the F.D.A. and the A.M.A.
policies are dominated by giant food, drug, and chemical companies, and to point out where their financial interests have led
them, to the ultimate detriment of American health.

Doctors themselves are not immune to attack. According to
Health Bulletin for April 13, 1963, "Santa Cruz, California, Medical Society has expelled one M.D., a graduate of the University of
Cincinnati Medical School, who recommends that his patients
eat organic foods and use natural food supplements. He also refuses to prescribe drugs. The society action was spurred by his use
of the anthrone test for detection of cancer, one not recognized as
effective by the American Medical Association." (Undaunted, this
physician is still practicing.)

At this writing, many doctors, dedicated to the health of their
patients and who employ natural methods of treatment, are getting tired of being pushed around. George W. Crane, M.D., for
example, a nationally known physician, dissatisfied with present
outside pressure aimed to control M.D.'s and others in the healing
profession, has rebelled. With the help of his two professionally
trained sons, one a psychiatrist, the other a dentist, Dr. Crane is
organizing a new and free medical association. A prospectus is being sent to members of all the healing professions throughout the
country. The hope is that at least 5,000 dissatisfied doctors who
wish to practice as they see fit, will sign up. This is the beginning
of a revolution in medical circles which has been brewing for a

long time. Such action takes courage, is badly needed by sincere physicians and patients alike, and requires cooperation in order to succeed. Let us stand behind them!

SCIENTISTS AS A TARGET

Scientists attempting to warn people of other potential health dangers are an even greater target than doctors. *Organic Consumer Report* (October 9, 1962) reports, "Many such dedicated scientists have been harassed, besmirched, threatened, ridiculed, demoted or fired. Dr. William Hueper, long time member of The International Union Against Cancer, *former* chief (he was mysteriously removed from his job) of Environmental Cancer Research, U.S. Dept. of Health, Education and Welfare, was ordered by a higher government official not to appear before a Senate investigating committee, even as an individual, and give his opinion about environmental cancer and chemicals. When he did so, under summons, he was demoted professionally, and a recent increase of salary was rescinded.

"Dr. Hueper was ordered by officials in the United States not to continue cancer experiments which he had been conducting for years. Interviewed by the press, only one of a group of science writers' reports was carried by the newspapers, although Dr. Hueper openly charged the U.S. Government with conspiracy to defraud the American public by suppressing known facts about cancer and chemicals. . . ."

Such actions make us wonder; are we living under the free-speech, free-press policy of the American Eagle, or under some sort of Gestapo rule? Unfortunately, many people are actually being convinced through "planted" information in magazine and in newspaper articles that correct nutrition and so-called health foods are not necessary for health. We are "assured" that we can get everything we need in our everyday average supermarket diet.

Hippocrates, the father of medicine, said, "Let food be your medicine." There is an ever growing group of physicians and scientists who agree.

NUTRITIONALLY TRAINED DOCTORS NEEDED

William B. Bean, M.D., in his 1963 presidential address to the American Society for Clinical Nutrition, stated, "There is one pre-eminent lesson I should like to hammer home. . . . I wish to emphasize and repeat the statement that the field of clinical nutrition has at least as many and probably more unexplored and readily accessible regions than any other field of clinical inquiry. If only one of every dozen young clinical investigators who eagerly and hopefully enter the well plowed terrain of cardiology [heart disease] were to turn his attention to clinical nutrition, his opportunities would be numerous and his rewards great. In exploring the multitudinous interrelationships of various food deficiencies with signs and symptoms, he could not fail to add useful medical knowledge."

One group of doctors and dentists, known as the American Academy of Applied Nutrition, adds the science of nutrition to the other treatments they use for their patients. Whenever possible they prefer the nutritional approach to drugs.

Sooner or later the medical profession as a whole will accept the nutritional approach, but the time is not yet. Meanwhile, to offset the shocking deterioration in our national health, we should as individuals upgrade our nutrition and resist those behind-the-scenes pressure from big business to buy what they want us to buy and eat what they want us to eat.

CHOOSING FOOD WISELY

Of course our choice of food is often conditioned by habit or taste. Most people choose to eat food—not nutrients. Agnes Toms, author of the natural foods cook book, *Eat, Drink and Be Healthy* (Devin-Adair) explains, "Foods become a status symbol to some people, so they haunt the gourmet shelves of expensive markets and learn to eat the unfamiliar foods which they think will enhance their social position. . . . The mature educated person who wishes to have good health will not confine his food selections to favorite foods or to the blunt insidious pressure of today's advertising which leads to an inadequate diet and poor nutrition; he will learn to like many foods, properly grown, unprocessed and unrefined, which will achieve for him the physical and mental vigor that is his right."

If you are looking for a good diet which prevents as well as relieves poor health, you would do well to consider Dr. Leo V. Roy's diet listed in the chapter "Arthritis." This comprehensive diet combines the better elements of many successful nutritional research studies. It is also delicious.

Remember, the more natural the food, the better. Raw foods, being live foods, contain their own vital or life force which can boost the vital force in humans. This may explain why so many people have found them more effective than the usual lifeless cooked or refined foods.

In this country we are being lured far afield from natural foods. I read of a housewife who discovered that meat, which was a rich red at the supermarket, turned out to be pale pink at home. Suspicious, she returned to the market and discovered an overhead, concealed red spotlight shining on the meat display to "color" it a natural red. Not long after, I personally found a bunch of celery bright green in the market turn pale in natural daylight. I, too, returned to the market and found a hidden green spotlight shining over the vegetable counter giving all vegetables that "natural green" color.

Another example of our "good" American diet: In spite of the extensive research linking tooth decay to soft drinks, *Business Week* notes that the average American drinks about 250 bottles of "soda" a year, of which 100 are cola drinks. The cola manufacturers would like to wean people from drinking coffee, according to this report. One firm's advertising director is reported as saying, "If we can only get 7 per cent of the coffee market we would sell more than if we put our competitor entirely out of business."

According to *Health Bulletin* (September 21, 1963) the soda pop industry is reluctant to list ingredients on the bottle for fear of losing sales. The one ingredient which is apparently constant in all cola drinks is caffeine. Beyond that point the manufacturers are vague. *Health Bulletin* says, "The soda industry asks to be able to put eight different kinds of 'optional' additives in its products. Most of them are synthetic chemicals and non-nutritive. The kinds of additives proposed are: 1. acidifying agents, 2. salts or buffering agents, 3. emulsifiers, 4. carriers (such as ethyl alcohol or glycerine), 5. foaming or anti-foaming agents, 6. nutrients (vitamin C and thiamine hydrochloride), 7. caffeine, and 8. chemical preservatives."

If you're thirsty, drink water.

But this is not always possible. In one large city, architects were ordered—at the last minute—to eliminate all drinking fountains from the plans of a 22-million-dollar stadium so that customers would be forced to buy and quench their thirst with soft drinks instead of water!

Even the zoos know better than this. They have begged visitors not to feed animals unnatural foods for fear of producing illness or death (which has happened). A national park has gone even further; they have warned the animals themselves, as the following sign posted in Yosemite National Park shows:

NOTICE TO BEARS
BEWARE OF SABOTAGE

We want to warn you that certain humans in this park have been passing the biscuits and soda pop to some of your brothers. Keep your self respect—avoid them. Don't be pauperized like your uncles were last year. You remember what happened to those pan-handlers, don't you?

Do you want gout, an unbalanced diet, vitamin deficiencies, or gas on the stomach? Beware of "ersatz" foodstuffs—accept only natural foods and hunt these yourself. These visitors mean well but they will ignore the signs. If they come too close, read this notice to them. They'll catch on after awhile.

IF YOU CAN'T READ,
ASK THE BEAR AT THE NEXT INTERSECTION

16 Nutritional help for stress

Stress can upset a number of conditions in the body including the cholesterol level. To illustrate the effect of psychological stress on food absorption, Dr. Nevin Scrimshaw reported in the *American Journal of Clinical Nutrition* (November, 1962), the case of a woman whose nitrogen balance (a test of protein adequacy) had remained normal on one gram of daily protein which she had been eating for many months. But when she was informed that her son had been wounded in Korea, her nitrogen balance became strongly negative, showing that the same amount of protein was now inadequate. Yet she exhibited no outward signs of the stress she felt inwardly. When she received word that her son was safe, her nitrogen balance became strongly positive for a few days then returned to normal. The episode was repeated in almost identical form several months later.

In Norway, a young man with a normal calcium balance developed a negative balance a few weeks before his preliminary exam. for a Ph.D. degree. Once the examination was safely passed, according to Dr. Scrimshaw, his calcium balance became strongly positive before returning to normal.

Since all of us are exposed to stress of so many kinds, what are we going to do? Elsewhere in this book, we discussed the wisdom of *over*fortifying the diet to offset nutrient withdrawals from our bodies during episodes of stress. Another approach comes from Dr. George A. Wilson, D.C., Chief Emeritus of the Spears Chiropractic Hospital, Research Department. I consider Dr. Wilson nutritionally far ahead of his time. He does not indulge in armchair theories. In his 42 years of practice he tested hundreds of patients before announcing his surprising discoveries.

One of his conclusions is that most people are not sufficiently acid. This sounds startling because we are constantly deluged with commercials advertising pills and potions to counteract "over-acidity."

Dr. Wilson (and Boris Sokoloff, M.D., is in agreement) explains that in former days when people were physically active and ate more natural foods, a general problem of overacidity did exist. But because of the present trend in eating more processed and alkaline foods, and because of mounting psychological stress, Dr. Wilson has found that the pendulum has swung toward overalkalinity. He feels that many physicians are not yet aware of this change.

Dr. Wilson has discovered that: (1) the more alkaline the person, the less healthy; (2) the more acid, the more healthy.

Many people, in Dr. Wilson's opinion, are eating increasing amounts of alkaline foods and wondering why their health is not improving. It may explain the craving for alcohol, coffee, and tobacco, according to Dr. Wilson, since these "props" are temporarily acid but later become alkaline in the body.

Science has established the fact that a healthy body is mildly acid. Dr. Wilson calls this body-acidity balance the "bio-electric force" (perhaps another term for the vital or life force). He points out that when any part of the body is injured, that specific area immediately becomes acid, representing the body defense system or vital force at work trying to speed healing.

Dr. Wilson has learned that the following stresses disturb the acid balance, resulting in alkalinity, and though the stresses may be only temporary, if prolonged they can, unless corrected, become permanent. (This is in keeping with the findings of Dr. Hans Selye, the stress expert, who noted that such stresses can destroy the body reserve of vitamin C, an acid, in the adrenal glands in seconds.) Stresses which disturb acid balance result from:

Shocks.
Keen disappointments.
Intense emotional upsets.

Excess fears and worries.
Overworking.
Under-resting.

Dr. Wilson finds that aging parallels alkalinity. He tested many men and women in their 80's. Those with an acid dominance were healthy. Those with alkaline dominance were not. This ties in with the Gallup Poll which reported that oldsters who had lived long and were still healthy, had an easygoing temperament or had learned to face life's problems with serenity. In Dr. Wilson's opinion, death, unless caused by accident, heart failure, or strangulation, is due to alkalinity leading to decreased nerve (bio-electric) energy which finally becomes too weak to maintain life.

Dr. Wilson finds that many people are:

More acid in the afternoon, more alkaline in the early morning.
More acid in summer, more alkaline in winter.
More acid during exercise, more alkaline during rest.
More alkaline when chilled, tired, chronically sick, or at the onset of illness.

The Wilson booklet, *Nutrition in the Space Age*, lists these rules for correcting overalkalinity:

Eat properly balanced meals (Dr. Wilson presents a new technique, discussed shortly).
Live a balanced way of life, which includes a generous amount of exercise.
Use acidizing aids (also explained shortly).
As a chiropractor, Dr. Wilson considers correction of nerve interference important. If this is impossible, he advocates pressure theraphy. (See chapter 10)

In testing a patient's eating habits and observing consequent health or ill health, Dr. Wilson uncovered some information which not only surprised him but led to changing some of his own eating habits. This information comes from his book, *A New Slant to Diet* (see Bibliography), in which careful graphs of patient's food correlations appear.

In general, he learned that correct nutrition improved the acid balance; that starches and sweets were offenders. The diet which produced good health in his patients included:

Meat once a day. Other proteins were acceptable at other meals.

One piece of whole-grain bread daily.

Vegetables whose leaves are exposed to the sun's rays were found most effective: alfalfa, celery stalks and leaves, dandelion greens, endive, kale, mustard greens, turnip leaves, watercress, parsley, asparagus, red-beet leaves, and carrot leaves.

A heavy meal at night caused tossing and turning as well as weight gain.

Fruit was less helpful when eaten with meals than when eaten between meals. Dr. Wilson's reason: fruits don't energize; they cleanse. Since Dr. Wilson himself had eaten fruit with his meals for years, this came as a surprise.

As for acidizing aids, he noticed that vitamins and minerals especially vitamins B and C, were helpful. He also learned that hydrochloric acid in liquid added to water, or in capsule or tablet form, indirectly aided in restoring body acid as well as helping people to get more from their food. This fact has been known for a long time, particularly in connection with assimilation of protein, calcium, and iron. But Dr. Wilson went a step further. He found out that if HCL were unavailable, vinegar was a reasonably good substitute. He considers apple cider vinegar best, and suggests that those who show symptoms of underacidity take one tablespoon of vinegar in water the first thing each morning and one teaspoon in water after each meal. He also recommends it when you are tired, irritable, when your hands and feet are cold (indicating slowed circulation), when you have aches or are stiff, or when your digestion is upset. He even suggests giving it to other members of the family when they are irritable!

Any acid, even fruit juice, can contribute to erosion of tooth enamel. Vinegar in water is no exception. To protect teeth, sip vinegar and water solution through a straw or rinse your mouth afterward with, or drink some clear water.

Obviously, because of individual differences, not everyone needs vinegar. Many people are sufficiently acid, but, according to Dr. Wilson, such people are in the minority. His theory about vinegar agrees with that of the Vermonters, as explained in the book *Folk Medicine* by D. C. Jarvis, M.D.

But neither Dr. Jarvis nor Dr. Wilson invented vinegar therapy. It has been used for centuries. Here is one proof, taken from *Roots of Strategy*, edited by Brigadier General Thomas R. Phillips, U.S. Army, published by the Military Service Publishing Co., Harrisburg, Penna. (fourth printing, 1955), p. 199:

Marshal Maurice De Saxe in one section, "My Reveries on the Art of War," says, "I should not omit to mention here a custom of the Romans by which they prevented the diseases that attack armies with changes of climate. A part of their amazing success can be attributed to it. More than a third of the German armies perished upon arrival in Italy and Hungary. In the year 1718 we entered the camp at Belgrade with 55,000 men. It is on a height, the air is healthy, the spring water good, and we had plenty of everything. On the day of battle, August 18 there were only 22,000 men under arms; all the rest were dead or unable to fight. I could produce similar instances among other nations. It is the changes of climate that cause it. There were no such examples among the Romans as long as they had vinegar. But just as soon as it was lacking, they were subject to the same misfortunes that our troops are at present. This is a fact to which few persons have given any attention, but which, however, is of great consequence for the conquerors and their success. As for how to use it, the Romans distributed several days' supply among their men by order, and each man poured a few drops in his drinking water. I leave to the doctors the discovery of the causes of such beneficial effects; what I report is unquestionable."

17 The magic mineral, magnesium

Magnesium, a metal which in its mineral form has gone more or less unnoticed, has suddenly been making news. It may turn out to be one of the important discoveries of the century. At least 200 studies show that magnesium may be the missing link in a long chain of baffling diseases.

Because magnesium has always been assumed to be plentiful in the average diet, most authorities have considered a deficiency unlikely. This supposition is false. Mildred S. Seelig, M.D., the author of a monumental study of magnesium requirements in the normal adult, in different parts of the world, states: "Contrary to the consensus, the customary diet in the Occidental countries cannot be relied upon to provide sufficient magnesium to maintain equilibrium."

Dr. Seelig, who reports her study in the *American Journal of Clinical Nutrition* (June, 1964), points out that the orientals are not deficient in magnesium. They are also free of many of our most distressing diseases. She speculates that magnesium may make the difference. Apparently many people are deficient in magnesium and do not know it. According to Dr. Seelig, such a deficiency is hard to diagnose and may easily be overlooked in a physical examination. Only after a prolonged deficiency do abnormalities show up.

EXAMPLES OF MAGNESIUM THERAPY

Kidney Stones. H. E. Sauberlich, M.D., of the Army's Fitzimons General Hospital, Denver, prescribed a 420-mg. tablet of magnesium oxide daily (to provide 250 mg. of magnesium ion) to patients with histories of kidney stones. After a short time Dr. Sauberlich discovered that the patients were free of kidney stones. Two years later they were still free of stones. As long as magnesium was continued there was no recurrence. There were no magnesium side effects. (*Health Bulletin,* June 13, 1964.)

Heart Disease. Hans Selye, M.D., subjected animals to severe or continued stress. Serious heart disease was found in all of these animals *except* those which had been given magnesium and potassium. (*Stress and Your Heart,* Dr. Hans Selye and Fred Kerner [New York: Hawthorn Books, 1961]).

Severe angina and coronary thrombosis have been successfully treated with magnesium sulphate. (*Lancet,* December 9, 1961). *The South African Medical Journal* (October 18, 1958) adds: "We have completed 50 cases of patients treated with magnesium sulphate. . . . We feel that this form of treatment has surpassed other forms, particularly in cases suffering from angina."

A high magnesium diet has prevented the development of hardening of the arteries in rats. (*Lancet,* November 1, 1958). The addition of magnesium salts in any form lowered cholesterol levels in rats. (*Indian Journal Medical Research* [1963], 51; 742-8.)

Prostate. Magnesium chloride has been successfully used in treating prostate troubles, including enlarged prostate and difficulty in urination, especially at night. In one report, 10 of the 12 patients treated with magnesium tablets were cured. A French physician reported that men of his acquaintance (including some physicians) who had been taking magnesium chloride for years had not developed prostate trouble. (*Equilbre Mineral et Santé,* Joseph Favier, M.D., Librairie le François, Paris.)

Polio. Polio has been dramatically arrested by the use of magnesium chloride. According to Dr. A. Neveu of France, a complete reversal of this dread disease has occurred on magnesium therapy within two days to one week, even after early arm and leg paralysis. Long-standing cases have also shown some improvement, though complete normality cannot be expected if atrophy has already taken place. For example, a 20-year-old farmer was paralyzed in both lower legs and one arm. Magnesium chloride was begun 32 days after the attack. After four months of treatment, he was able to walk with crutches. Two years later he discarded his crutches and used only a cane.

On the other hand, when magnesium therapy is given immediately, according to Dr. Neveu, rapid results are realized. He cites 14 cases as proof. One case was that of a 9-year-old boy who contracted polio and was paralyzed in his right lower leg. Magnesium therapy effected a complete cure within one week.

Dr. Neveu claims that magnesium, correctly given, will remove the patient from danger in two days as well as reversing the disease. He believes that every household should keep magnesium chloride in the medicine chest. At the first sign of sore throat and stiff back-of-the-neck, or as late as the first appearance of paralysis, he advises the use of magnesium under the care of a qualified physician. His formula: 20 grams (.7 oz.) of desiccated magnesium chloride added to one liter (about one quart) of water. The dose varies from 80 cc. every three hours to 125 cc. every six hours.

Alcoholism.   An alcoholic was admitted to a hospital. He exhibited wildly combative behavior. Magnesium sulphate produced quieter and more cooperative behavior in this man within a few hours. One month after his discharge from the hospital he was still mentally clear, neurologically intact, and practically free of previous symptoms.

Magnesium seems to disperse the irritability, depression, and disagreeable behavior so often displayed by heavy drinkers. The change is noticeable within a few hours after magnesium is taken.

Mental and Emotional Problems.   A 68-year-old man, following an abdominal operation, suddenly became irrational, noisy, wildly restless, confused, and combative. He experienced hallucinations. His brain and heart pattern were abnormal. Vitamins, dextrose, potassium, and calcium were given, without effect. Then he was given magnesium sulphate, and calcium gluconate was continued. In 18 hours following the first magnesium dose the patient was rational, oriented, and completely free of neuromuscular disorder. By the third day he was up and around, a delightful elderly man, exhibiting no psychiatric or neuromuscular abnormalities. (Both cases from *American Journal of Internal Medicine* [1959], 50, p. 257.)

Nervousness and Hand Tremor. Magnesium can improve hand tremor, according to a study of samples of handwriting. A patient signed his name. The signature was completely illegible. Magnesium therapy was started. Four hours later the man signed his name again and the letters were now distinguishable. For test purposes, therapy was halted. Twenty-eight hours later the signature was exactly the same. Magnesium therapy was resumed and 24 hours later the signature was well formed, the letters clear and legible. Nine days later the handwriting was still legible and normal. (*Journal of American Medical Association*, April 21, 1956.)

Other problems have yielded to magnesium therapy. They include brain disturbances (as revealed by human electroencephalograph and electrocardiogram); irritability, especially to sights and sounds; anxiety; muscle weakness, unsteady gait, staggering, vertigo and twitching; numbness or cramps in hands and feet. Magnesium has also helped epilepsy, kidney disturbance, tetany and eclampsia during pregnancy. It can aid the body with the problem of water retention. A magnesium deficiency produces calcium deposits in kidney, blood vessels, and heart, as established by autopsy on animals.

Magnesium *may* lower the blood pressure. A German study found that magnesium completely prevented high blood pressure in rats, as well as reversing it. Magnesium may also act as a tranquilizer. Adelle Davis points out that when a person feels the need of a tranquilizer, what he may actually need is magnesium.

Dr. P. Schrumpf-Pierron, professor of medicine at the Sorbonne, Paris, studied the health of many thousands of Egyptions. He concluded that magnesium played a role in preventing cancer. Dr. Pierre Delbet, of the French Academy of Medicine, stated that magnesium acts as a "brake for cancer." (*Bulletin of the French Association for Study of Cancer*, July 1931.)

Magnesium, because it seems to improve calcium deposits, may be valuable in arthritis. I am watching several arthritics who are using magnesium. Though premature, the results seem good. A controlled study is needed.

Magnesium deficiency may be caused by a prolonged dietary deficiency, diarrhea, vomiting, excessive sweating, use of diuretics, malabsorption, diabetic acidosis therapy, pancreatitis, emotional disturbance, or a high carbohydrate diet. One of the most common causes is excessive drinking of alcohol.

Magnesium has several peculiar traits. There is a strong relationship between calcium, phosphorus, and magnesium. Apparently magnesium improves calcium utilization. Repeated radiographic examinations have revealed that during magnesium therapy bone lesions do not develop. If there is adequate magnesium, potassium is also well utilized and a slight loss of sodium takes place. Raising the amount of calcium calls for the addition of magnesium. Vitamin D in normal amounts helps the body to absorb magnesium, as well as calcium, but there seems to be no relation between magnesium and acid (as in the case of calcium), nor with vitamin C, B12, or iron.

Kidneys apparently help to regulate magnesium. Men need more magnesium than women. Pregnant and nursing women need more than the average woman. Raising the level of protein in the diet calls for *extra* magnesium! Dr. Seelig has found the average American and British diet magnesium-deficient.

One special caution: Fluorine has a strong attraction for magnesium and can tie up this element in the cells. (*Clinical Physiology*, Spring, 1964.) This raises the question of the wisdom of drinking fluoridated water.

HOW TO TAKE MAGNESIUM

Mildred Seelig, M.D., suggests the following *minimum* intake of magnesium daily: for a 140-lb. woman, 385 mg.; for a 185-lb. man, 500 mg.

However, for those who do social drinking, consume a diet rich in calcium, protein, and vitamin D, a man would require from 580 to 800 mg., a woman somewhat less. This is the amount found in many oriental diets.

Dr. Seelig states, "The diet should be supplemented with magnesium at least until equilibrium is noted and then possibly reduced to meet the body need."

Apparently, magnesium should be made a daily habit for life.

IS THERE DANGER OF TAKING TOO MUCH?

According to Dr. Seelig, there is no danger of taking too much, since in a normal person the excess is excreted. However in cases of kidney failure (renal insufficiency) there is danger of toxicity because the ion is excreted so slowly. Large amounts of magnesium can also be toxic if the calcium intake is low and phosphorus high. This is easily remedied. Toxicity is relieved when calcium is increased. (See rule for adding calcium to brewer's yeast, p. 108.)

WHAT FORM OF MAGNESIUM IS BEST?

There are many forms of magnesium: carbonate, silicate, phosphate, chloride, gluconate, oxide, hydroxide, sulphate and others. Magnesium sulphate is perhaps the easiest to get since it is the same as Epsom salts. Adelle Davis cites the case of the man who was belligerent and psychotic. He became agreeable within a few hours after receiving one-quarter teaspoon of Epsom salts (magnesium sulphate). Magnesium in this form should not be given in large enough doses to act as a purge or cathartic. *Clinical Science* (1961, Vol. 21, pp. 273-284) says, "Oral supplementation seems useful for treating magnesium deficiency providing the quantity administered is insufficient to cause purgation, which causes the magnesium to be recovered in the faeces."

One teaspoon of Epsom salts equals approximately 1,000 mg. One-eighth of a teaspoon would yield close to Dr. Seelig's recommended requirement. The flavor of this amount can be disguised in juice or put into dry capsules and taken with water. Other forms of magnesium are available at health and drug stores. Dolomite is a very popular source, but there are many good choices.

Magnesium occurs in many foods. It is found in dark green, leafy vegetables, due to the presence of chlorophyll. Soy products, particularly soy flour, are one of the richest sources. Nuts, cashews, almonds, brazil nuts, and pumpkin seeds are high in magnesium. Whole grains also contain it. Magnesium is found in sea water. Cooking creates a loss of magnesium. Raw foods provide a richer source.

Since magnesium is involved in so many major diseases, it would seem wise to be sure you are getting enough. If you do step up magnesium, it would be wise to continue to take the other trace minerals, too. Natural sources of minerals, such as kelp or dulse, include them all, both known and unknown. As we have found in the case of vitamins, one may enhance the other. Therefore it stands to reason that in both vitamins and minerals the whole is better than its parts.

18   Macrobiotics

Macrobiotics is an oriental system which is being practiced by a growing number of people all over the world. This system was discovered by a Japanese, Dr. Sagen Isiduka, 70 years ago, and was actually a new biochemical interpretation of a principle dating back 4,000 years. Dr. Isiduka cured hundreds of thousands of people, including many who had been pronounced incurable. He was so famous that letters merely addressed to Dr. Anti-doctor, Tokyo, would reach him. When he died, his funeral procession was reported to be over two miles long. Today another Japanese, Dr. Georges Ohsawa, is his only known successor. He has developed the system a step further to embrace the whole individual, emotionally and spiritually as well as physically. His initial method of promoting health is through the use of certain nutritional principles.

The word "macrobiotics" is concerned with wholeness and with the art of longevity and rejuvenation, or a wholesome creative life. In the Orient, the two forces of nature are called Yin (passive, centripetal, feminine) and Yang (positive, centrifugal, masculine). Macrobiotics is based upon this Yin-Yang principle. Dr. Georges Ohsawa explains that foods fall into one or the other category, and if properly chosen can re-establish balance in an individual who has become too Yin or too Yang, and consequently ill. Dr. Ohsawa adds that a cure often takes place in as little as 10 days.

For those who wish a more scientific explanation for the macrobiotic principle, Dr. Ohsawa explains that the body's nervous system is made up of two antagonistic forces, the orthosympathetic and the parasympathetic. The orthosympathetic helps to dilate or expand all tissues and organs of the body, whereas the parasympathetic controls constriction. Health, according to Dr. Ohsawa, results from a good equilibrium between these two antagonists, whereas illness represents an imbalance. Vegetables (which also contain chlorophyll) are classified as Yin, whereas meat, fish, and fowl are classified as Yang. Scientific analysis, according to Dr. Ohsawa, reveals that Yin foods are high in sodium, whereas Yang foods are high in potassium. A proper balance between these foods is necessary for health. According to the macrobiotic theory, by correcting an imbalance according to the individual's needs, health will return, and often quickly.

Two little books, written by Dr. Ohsawa, can tell the full story much better than I. Dr. Ohsawa promises that by properly observing the macrobiotic dietetic directions you can become sufficiently healthy so that you will not experience the usual fatigue.

He says, "You will have a good appetite, good and deep sleep, a good memory, good humor, and smartness in thinking and doing."

Dr. Ohsawa states, "My medicine-philosophy is really miraculous and wonderful. I cured myself of tuberculosis and many other incurable diseases after having been given up by doctors when I was under twenty years of age. Since then I have seen hundreds of thousands of amazing cures of poor desperate people who applied my medicine-philosophy by themselves and for themselves throughout Asia, Africa, and Europe.

"Over a period of forty years I have cured many patients, but I never chanced to see one eating properly, as one should do. . . . I never saw one patient suffering from lack of food. They eat to indulge their appetites and for pleasure; they eat anything that tempts them and whatever they see. . . . They always eat these foods in excess, and produce one illness or another. I take the position that every disease is produced by excess in diet."

Today Mr. Ohsawa is over 70. I have seen a picture of him and his wife (he lives for the most part in Europe) and they are remarkably young and vital looking. There are Ohsawa centers in England, France, Germany, Italy, Japan, Brazil, and Sweden, and in California and New York City in the United States. The movement has been reviewed in the *New Yorker, Newsweek,* and in the *Herald Tribune.* It has followers from all walks of life. One of his books, *The Philosophy of Oriental Medicine,* was written in French Equatorial Africa at Dr. Albert Schweitzer's hospital. Dr. Ohsawa's method is infinitely simple: he merely corrects deficiencies of the body with natural food. He uses no medicines, no vitamins, no surgery, no "inactivity." In a few cases he uses some time-honored oriental herbs.

Dr. Ohsawa writes, "I am convinced that there is no incurable disease at all in this world if we apply correctly our medical philosophy. Everyone can adopt it in his daily life, everywhere at any time, if he genuinely wants to be free of all physiological and mental difficulties. . . . You have the right to pursue health and happiness. . . . You must be your own doctor. I have never seen a man who did not improve by observing his diet absolutely and strictly."

Those who wish to study the system seriously will need the

help of Dr. Ohsawa's books. The diet is individualized to each person's condition by balancing liquid and salt, and the proportions of cereals to vegetables. (Apparently everyone varies in Yin-Yang balance as his health alters from time to time.) The food proportion for a normal healthy person is usually 5 of Yin to 1 of Yang.

There is one food, however—waterground, brown, natural rice —which, he claims, is perfectly balanced between the two. To achieve rapidly maximum benefits from the macrobiotic diet, Dr. Ohsawa suggests that you eat this brown rice for 10 days, chew each mouthful 30 times, and limit liquids to as little as possible, preferably to one and one-half cups. This liquid may either be the delicious Mu tea (containing 15 beneficial herbs and available at any Ohsawa center) or green undyed tea and must be taken *after* meals.

For those who don't like regular rice or think that it disagrees with them, there is a surprise in store; natural brown rice is delicious! You may eat as much as often as you wish, provided you chew each mouthful at least 30 times for thorough mastication. The rice may be boiled straight or parched first in the pan before adding boiling water and salt. It can be flavored with naturally fermented soy sauce (not the usual commercial variety) or an excellent flavoring called Gomasio, a powdered blend of sesame seed and salt. Gomasio may be purchased from the Centers or you may make it yourself by toasting together 2 teaspoons of sea salt to 8 teaspoons of sesame. Blend in a blender or crush with mortar and pestle until the consistency of salt or coarse flour.

As your health improves, Dr. Ohsawa believes that vegetables, some fish, fowl, salad, and a little fruit may be added gradually. Sugar or refined foods are not allowed, ever.

Macrobiotics is easy and inexpensive to follow. Dr. Ohsawa concludes, "Not only does it heal present diseases, it prevents all kinds of illnesses in the future."

To illustrate, in his book, *The Philosophy of Oriental Medicine*, he tells this story:

"In Nagasaki, there is a Catholic hospital, the St. Francis Hospital, situated on a hill. Nearby in a valley stands the hospital of the Medical School of Nagasaki University. The atomic bomb fell between them, and both hospitals were destroyed at the same time. In the University hospital, everyone was killed—about 3,000 persons, among them professors, nurses, students, and patients. However, at the Catholic hospital, no one was even injured except Brother Alcantola who suffered a slight wound on his knee. Immediately outside the hospital 8,000 people died. The Vatican declared this 'was a miracle of the twentieth century.' But no one looked for the real reason for this miracle. The head of the Catholic Hospital, Dr. Akiduki, and I both knew the reason. For three years before the war, when Dr. Akiduki himself had been cured of tuberculosis by macrobiotics, the hospital people had followed my dietetic instructions very strictly. For this reason, the patients were immune to the Yin damage of atomic radiation."

According to Dr. Ohsawa this "Oriental Philosophy is simply a practical discipline of life that everyone can observe with the greatest pleasure wherever and whenever one wishes. It restores at the same time health and harmony of mind, soul, and body, which are essential for joyful living."

Studies with animals show that a new diet should be adopted gradually. Sudden, complete changeovers may cause temporary digestive upsets.

Even though the macrobiotic diet advocates very slightly cooked vegetables over raw for better assimilation, the voluminous research on the protective value of raw food for cancer and other degenerative diseases already discussed, cannot be ignored. It is true that many orientals have maintained health on their diet for thousands of years, but their genes, and thus their dietary needs, may differ from ours. Animals and birds have maintained health since the beginning of time without cooking food at all!

I do not question that the macrobiotic diet may eliminate a physical disturbance. Once health is achieved in this manner, in light of research, Americans might be wiser to add raw food, protein in some form, as well as natural vitamins and minerals to this Japanese diet to help prevent future illness. Therefore I, personally, try to strike a happy medium between the various schools of thought. All diets should be adapted to the individual race as well as to the individual person.

19 When to begin nutritional therapy

Is it ever too late to try nutrition for health? No. Although prevention is better, it is never too late to begin. Since aging is known to start very early, I urge everyone—whatever his age—to begin *now*, not only to try to prevent further deterioration but to help repair any damage already done. One of the most shining examples of "turning the clock back" I know is that of a world-champion wrestler of the later 1930's, whom I recently had the good fortune to meet. I shall nickname him "Bob."

Bob's health was adequate at the peak of his career, but by his own admission, his diet was poor. When his career ended, and with it, exercise, his health went to pieces. (This indicates that something more than exercise is needed to ensure physical fitness.) Bob finally reached a state where he was crippled with agonizing, arthritic pain day and night, looked 15 years older than his actual age, and his hair had not only turned gray, it was coming out in large patches. After extensive orthodox medical treatment with drugs, Bob was finally told there was no hope, that he had six weeks to live.

Providentially, during that six weeks, he was directed to a consulting nutritionist and six weeks later, instead of being dead, he was playing golf! Obviously, his troubles had not ended that quickly, since they had been long in the making, but he had turned the corner in the right direction and his health was visibly improving. When I saw him he was handsome, lithe, pain-free, rosy-cheeked and his hair had grown in, a beautiful, natural, glossy black. He looked easily 15 years younger than his age, which was 51. The regeneration took between two and three years. I have the before-and-after pictures as proof.

I asked him about his nutritional program. He admitted that the nutritionist had given him the "works"—a complete, over-all abundance of nutrients (including sprouts). He added that in general he followed the program outlined in *Stay Young Longer*, and was kind enough to say that had he read the book beforehand he probably would have been spared his breakdown. When I asked if he knew precisely what had helped recolor his hair, he answered that he thought it was due to blackstrap molasses, which, on top of all the other "wonder foods," he had taken daily. His method was to mix 2 tablespoons each of blackstrap, natural honey and apple cider vinegar, in a jar, shake vigorously and add it to his drinking water, hot or cold, throughout the day. Each day he mixed and drank a new batch.

I later told Bob's story in a lecture and was promptly—and rightly—challenged on the basis that his case might have been an isolated one and that blackstrap might not do the same thing for others. So I began searching for other cases, which I found. To date I have rounded up reports of seven people who achieved similar results with hair recoloring. All were relying on a *complete* nutritional program. In addition, they took 2 tablespoons of blackstrap molasses daily. Some of them considered honey too sweet so they used the molasses with or without apple cider vinegar. A few added blackstrap to a daily protein drink, another mixed it with yogurt. One woman who had been a coffee addict, as a substitute added a teaspoon of blackstrap to a cup of hot water every time she craved coffee, and was surprised to find it palatable.

There is no mystery about the ingredients of blackstrap.* It contains B vitamins and minerals including iron and copper—all components used in natural recoloring of animal fur. Since certain acids help iron to be assimilated, perhaps the vinegar in Bob's mixture helped too. The length of time necessary for hair recoloring in these cases varied. Bob told me he noticed some results within six months. A young man in his twenties lost gray streaks of hair

* An analysis from the American Medical Association appears in *Stay Young Longer*.

within an incredible two weeks (substantiated by witnesses, as are all cases mentioned). For the most part, however, about a year elapsed before most people achieved results. One 40-plus woman, prematurely gray since she was 18, acquired beautiful brunette hair. Another woman turned into a gorgeous redhead and, of course, was accused of dying her hair. The most amusing instance was that told me by a doctor. A patient of his, 83 years old, began eating blackstrap molasses on a piece of bread every night at bedtime and later exhibited a head of flaming red hair, much to the consternation of his relatives.

Blackstrap should be used conditionally. Adelle Davis warns that unless it is diluted (or the mouth rinsed afterward), it can stick to the teeth, and like any other sweet, cause tooth erosion. It is also a powerful laxative* so it must be added gradually until you become accustomed to it. I do not know if blackstrap will re-color hair for everyone. There has not been enough time, or enough people to report. If you have success or failure after a year's fair trial, please let *me* know.

Finally, whatever food you eat, don't eat it unless you are hungry. No matter how good it is or how good it is for you, if you are tired, angry, worried, afraid, or arguing during meal time, proper digestion cannot take place. If you are traveling or eating in a restaurant, be as discriminating as you can. Since you do have choices, you can choose the good and avoid the bad. If, however, you are eating at the home of a friend who has gone to great trouble to prepare a meal (unless you are allergic to something in which case you should avoid it), enjoy your meal. Worrying may be more disturbing than occasional improper food. It is the day-in, day-out, planned correct nutrition that finally pays off.

The American Nutrition Society recommends these steps for better health through better food:

1. Serve as many foods in the original state as possible—fresh fruits and vegetables, certified whole milk, fresh butter, natural cheese, and cold-pressed vegetable oils.

2. Eat a diet high in protein. Include:

a) Meat, including the variety meats—liver, brain, heart—poultry

* See Clark, *Stay Young Longer.*

and sea food. Cook meat as little as possible because protein is injured by prolonged or high heat. Pork, however, must be well done.

b) Dairy products, eggs, unprocessed cheese, and medically certified milk.

c) The legumes, soy and other beans.

3. Use fruits and vegetables (grown without the use of poisonous chemical sprays if possible.) Cook vegetables with a minimum of water, at low heat, and for as short a time as possible. Use the liquid.

4. Use freshly ground whole-grain cereals and flours, for they contain more protein, all of the B complex vitamins, vitamin E, minerals, and unsaturated fatty acids.

5. Use cold-pressed vegetable oils, which are an excellent source of essential unsaturated fatty acids.

AVOID THESE FOODS:

1. Avoid the use of refined sugar. It provides no nutrients except carbohydrates. Excessive consumption is a prominent factor in dental decay and reduces the appetite for nourishing food. Honey may be used with discretion.

2. Avoid the use of white flour. It has had the vital elements of the grain removed, and enrichment replaces only a few of them. Frequently bleaching and preservative agents are added which may be harmful.

3. Avoid the use of foods such as bread, pastries, ice cream, cheese, and cold meats which contain chemical additives. These are often used as preservatives, coloring and flavoring agents, emulsifiers, extenders, sweeteners, stabilizers, etc.

4. Avoid the use of poultry and meats produced with hormones to stimulate growth and add weight.

5. Avoid the use of hydrogenated fats and oils. They contain mainly saturated fatty acids.

6. Avoid heated or processed milk, processed cheese, cheese foods, and chocolate.

See your physician or dentist for diets and menus for special conditions.

This credo appears in a monthly magazine, *Modern Nutrition*, published by the American Academy of Applied Nutrition, dedicated to a program of human betterment through nutritional knowledge. Subscriptions to *Modern Nutrition* are $5.00 per year. Address: 234 E. Colorado Blvd., Suite 503, Pasadena, California.

20   The Star Exercise

I would like to share with you a method of drawing on a source of greater power to intensify your own. It was taught to me many years ago, and those to whom I have passed it on have later told me that it has been an invaluable aid. These people, incidentally, range from hard-headed business executives to average housewives. One day in the same mail came two letters from opposite sides of the United States. One was from a doctor. The other was from a career woman. Both asked me if I knew about this same technique and then included the directions. I mention it to show you that people in all walks of life are finding it practical and helpful. I hope you will practice it sincerely until you, too, derive benefits.

Here are the directions for the Star Exercise: In the quiet privacy of your room, stand tall with feet apart, and hands outstretched to the sides. Your left palm should face up, your right palm down. This places you in a star position. Now say aloud or silently, "Universal Life Energy is flowing through me. I feel it now."

If you remain relaxed you will soon feel a tingle in your finger tips. This is the power flowing into you. It is as simple to tap it as flicking on the light switch to get illumination. If you don't feel it the first day, don't overtry. Wait until the next day and try again. As you are able to relax, you will be able to feel the power more readily. In due time it won't be necessary to stand in the star position at all. You can merely make the affirmation silently, wherever you are and you will feel the power begin to flow.

The originator of the Star Exercise, the late Baron Eugene Fersen, wrote that you can use it for anything and everything. He suggested that you "tune in" before an important conference, a social engagement which you dread, or a business meeting which worries you. He advised tapping the power before visualizing money, housing, or other supplies you need. He suggested using it for guidance in solving emotional problems or health difficulties. Using Universal Power helps when you are frightened; it cheers when you are depressed. Use it to gather strength for any task which faces you. And as you learn to use the power, you will find that it becomes stronger. It is God's power, always available night and day, on which you can lean and find comfort. You can also direct it to solve your problems for you as Aladdin directed the Genie with his lamp. But it must be used only for good, or it will boomerang! I share the Star Exercise solemnly and reverently with you, and I hope you will pass it on to others whom you consider deserving.

By combining many or all of the tools I have placed in your hands, I hope you will get well and stay well—naturally. God bless you!

PART THREE

TREATING DISEASES NATURALLY

Following are suggestions reported from many and various sources for certain common diseases. Because it would take an encyclopedia to list every disease, the degenerative diseases or disturbances have been emphasized. The underlying concept of health, as advanced by those who believe in natural methods, is that a disease is only a symptom of distress somewhere in the body. Natural therapists feel that it is far wiser to build up the body as a whole, and usually, when this is accomplished, the disturbance mysteriously disappears.

21 Alcohol and alcoholism

Alcohol can be a mixed blessing. It can do lots of harm, and a little good. Here are the pros and cons.

The case against alcohol

1. "The chronic alcoholic who would rather drink than eat fails to get enough vitamins. The few vitamins he has acquired are drained out of his system in the process of burning the alcohol in his body." This is the verdict of Dr. Robert N. Baker, University of California at Los Angeles. Dr. Baker reports that the following neurological symptoms, which were found in a study of 50 alcoholics, stemmed from a single cause—vitamin deficiency:

Delirium tremens.
Convulsions.
Neuritis.
Inco-ordination of gait.
Disorders of eye movement.
Impaired memory.

2. Excessive drinking often causes premature graying of hair, due also to vitamin deficiency.
3. Chronic alcoholism causes a depletion of minerals in the body, particularly magnesium. Why is magnesium so important? Because its lack (as determined by studies at the Veterans Administration Hospital, Department of Medicine, Minneapolis, and the University of Southern California), produced these symptoms in alcoholics:

Tremor of hands, feet, and tongue.
Convulsions.
Mental clouding.
Sweating and facial flushing.

4. Doctors at Seton Hall Medical School, New Jersey, are finding more and more young people in their late teens and early twenties who have developed cirrhosis of the liver after 8 to 10 years of heavy drinking.

5. A study in Europe found 27 children aged 1 month to 14 years with liver cirrhosis. Many of them had been given wine or brandy almost daily from the first year of life, together with inadequate nutrition.

6. Dr. Robert A. Felix, director of the Institute of Mental Health, warns that alcohol can cause brain damage.

7. Charlotte and Dyson Carter (see Bibliography), who visited Russia and investigated Soviet health problems and treatments, reported that alcohol may be a cause of precancerous diseases of the mouth and larynx, and continued use of alcohol frequently leads to the development of such cancers. The Soviets did *not* believe that alcohol was a general cause of cancer; they indicated that hard liquor (not beer or wine) may cause cancer in body tissues that it directly touches.

This Soviet view, according to the Carter report, as later confirmed at the Sloan-Kettering Institute in New York City, adds, "Men who drink heavily (6 ounces of hard liquor daily, or more) get cancers of the larynx 700 per cent more often than non-drinkers or light drinkers."

8. The Russians believe that if conception takes place while parents are intoxicated with alcohol, certain forms of mental retardation in children may occur. If this seems far-fetched the Carters quote the study of Dr. Dora P. Nicholson of George Washington University, in which heavy doses of alcohol were given guinea pigs before mating. Nine out of 10 of the offspring were defective. Dr. Nicholson also reports studies which show that defective human offspring often occur in families in which parents are heavy drinkers.

9. What about the assurance that a little bit of daily alcohol is actually good for your heart? Pure myth, according to the *Journal of the American Medical Association* (May 27, 1950) which cites a study by three United States Public Health doctors. They say, "The results clearly indicate that a misconception exists regarding the value of whiskey in the treatment of coronary disease."

They learned that alcohol does *not* dilate the heart arteries as once supposed; it helps to relieve pressure pains of angina, due to its sedative action. The authors warn that if alcohol is used regularly it can create a false feeling of fitness and security which might lead to fatal consequences. Other researchers at the University of Mississippi Medical Center found that alcohol *reduces* blood flow to the heart, actually increasing its work load!

10. What about that comforting assurance that if you smoke, it's all right to drink? Some people contend that smoking tightens up your arteries and drinking relaxes them. Well, apparently this is another myth. It is true, according to the *Journal of the American Medical Association* (November 8, 1952), that smoking definitely constricts the blood vessels and raises the blood pressure. But W. J. McCormick, M.D., of Toronto, found that in the deaths of 151 cases of coronary thrombosis, the victims used *both* tobacco and alcohol. Dr. McCormick says, "Apparently, the addition of alcohol, as advised by some writers to counteract the vaso-constrictor effect of nicotine, did not prolong life in these cases."

11. Does alcohol upset the pancreas? Dr. Donald F. Magee, an expert on the pancreas, one of the body's most important glands, states that a high-protein diet keeps the pancreas healthy. But a low-protein diet, such as that of an alcoholic, tends to shrink it. This may account for the fact that after an alcoholic binge, if the alcoholic eats an unusually good meal, he sometimes dies of acute pancreatitis. It has been noted that pancreatitis victims enter hospitals in large numbers after holiday feasts.

12. Joseph G. Molner, M.D., warns that excessive alcohol can make you fat and cause irritability and impotency.

13. Dr. William Brady reports some effects of even small doses of alcohol:

Typesetters are slower and make more mistakes.
Typists make more errors.
Pianists strike more wrong notes.
Marksmanship with pistol or rifle is inferior.
Needle-threading becomes more difficult.
Sight and hearing are less keen.
Sense of touch, as measured by the delicate Esthesiometer, is impaired.
Automobile drivers are a fraction of a second slower in braking when
    an unexpected obstacle looms in front of them.

ARE SOME TYPES OF ALCOHOLIC DRINKS WORSE THAN OTHERS?

It depends on the individual. The *Journal of the American Medical Association* reports that gin and tonic has been shown to have effects much worse than a hangover. The "tonic" part of the drink is quinine water and many people are unknowingly allergic to quinine and can experience severe reactions from drinking it. The reactions vary with the individual, but the following disturbances have been noted as side-effects: tinnitus (ringing of the ears), deafness, vertigo, visual impairment, headaches, fever, and nausea. One of the most common as well as most serious effects is a type of dermatitis which may lead to death in some patients. The *Journal* cited a case history of a man whose eyes swelled shut after a facial massage with toilet water containing quinine.

The Alcoholism and Drug Addiction Research Foundation, Toronto, compared the results of spirits, wine, and beer (all of which led to death by cirrhosis of the liver). Wine was responsible for 71 per cent, spirits for 46 per cent, and beer for 33 per cent of the deaths.

DOES THE EFFECT OF ALCOHOL VARY?

There are some people who pride themselves on holding their liquor, yet without warning, on occasion get reeling drunk or even pass out cold. Dr. Joost A. M. Merloo explains why:

Drinking in a crowded, unventilated room provides less oxygen to help burn up the alcohol in the blood. There is also less oxygen at high altitudes, so beware of drinking in the mountains or in an unpressurized plane.

Drinking without eating food which slows down alcohol absorption.

The old joke, "It isn't the liquor, it's the soda," isn't so far off. Carbonated drinks speed the passage of alcohol into the blood and stomach.

Some people can't combine drinking with certain drugs (antihistamine, for one).

Others can't drink after a bout with an infectious disease.

And any type of stress, such as fear, or extreme anxiety, or starvation can cause a seasoned drinker to be felled by a small "snort," whereas in past times with larger drinks, under different circumstances, he has remained immune.

CAN YOU PREVENT HANGOVERS?

During World War II, some Naval officers stationed in Washington, D.C., told me that they had discovered a nutritional preventative for hangover. They took a 5 mg. thiamin (vitamin B-1) tablet for every few drinks. Since alcohol, sugar, and other carbohydrates destroy or burn up vitamin B in the body, this formula compensates for such destruction. It works for everyone I know who has tried it. One caution: Large amounts of vitamin B-1, in larger potencies than 5 or 10 mg. can be dangerous.* There is also danger in taking an excess of a single B vitamin alone, without benefit of the rest of the B family. When B-1 is taken for this, or any other, purpose the entire B complex should be added to the diet in corresponding amounts *that* day. For additional help see chapter 40 on magnesium.

The case for alcohol

There is a positive side of alcohol, wine especially. Under certain circumstances wine has not been harmful; in some cases it has proved helpful.

In Rome, a study with diabetic patients showed that there was

* See Clark, *Stay Young Longer.*

no side reaction when a small amount of wine was given to those who were under diet or insulin treatment. Rises in blood sugar did not occur up to three hours after the wine was administered. Results were best when the wine was taken with a mixed meal. (Quarterly Journal, *Studies of Alcohol* [1963], 24, 412-416.)

1. The Wine Institute Research Division of California learned that Roman soldiers who drank wine seemed to suffer fewer casualties from dysentery and other intestinal diseases. This is explained by a University of California graduate student, John E. Gardner, who has isolated an antibacterial substance in red wine which had fermented for only two to six weeks.

2. Luigi Cornaro, an Italian living in the fifteenth century, was given up by physicians to die at age 40. He then decided to take matters into his own hands. He simplified his diet, cutting it down to the barest minimum. Within a few days he noticed improvement and within a year he was completely restored to health. He lived to be 102. He ate 12 ounces of food daily, and he drank 14 ounces of wine. Once when, at a worried friend's insistence, he increased his intake to 14 ounces of food and 16 ounces of wine, within eight days his health began to backslide. He promptly returned to his original routine. In discussing wine, he said, "I found that *old* wine did not suit me, but that *new* wine did."

The Harvard Medical School, has tested certain red wines, including Burgundy and Bordeaux, and found that they contain iron which can be absorbed by the body. French wines tested yielded more iron than American wines. (*Nature* [1963], 199, 922.)

3. Wine is used in some instances as medicine. "Wine is not an alcoholic beverage," says Dr. Salvatore P. Lucia, professor of medicine and chairman of preventive medicine at the University of California Medical School. "It is a most complex biologic fluid possessing definite physiologic values. It has nutritional value due to its content of B vitamins and minerals—potassium, magnesium, sodium, calcium, iron and phosphorus."

Dr. Lucia feels that wine helps the digestion and that the tranquilizing and sedative effects are good for heart, arteries, blood pressure and strengthening the walls of the capillary veins.

4. Charles De Coti Marsh, of England, reports success in treat-

ing fatigue (see "Fatigue" p. 282). He allows a glass of wine with each evening meal. He says, "Wine is a natural drink. A little wine dilates the arterioles, those tiny hairlike veins in the extremities, thereby allowing a free traverse of blood throughout the body. Wine frees the circulation. But spirits I am against in any quantity. They burn so rapidly in the body that vitamins are consumed, producing malnutrition.

"There is another point. Older or crippled folk have little to look forward to in a day, hence the evening glass of wine after dinner provides a much needed sparkle in their lives."

Peter J. Steincrohn, M.D., agrees that a little alcohol can brighten the life of an elderly person. He also considers it far superior to tranquilizers. He cites the case of a 48-year-old executive who refused to drink alcohol on "moral" grounds but was popping more and more tranquilizers into his mouth during the day and taking two sleeping pills at night. Realizing that he was the type who would soon double his intake of tranquilizers, Dr. Steincrohn suggested that he give up tranquilizers and substitute a highball before dinner and a glass of sherry before bedtime.

Dr. Steincrohn adds, "This was years ago. Neither he nor his wife has increased the daily intake of alcohol. He sleeps like a baby. Evening tensions at home have disappeared. He has not had to take tranquilizers."

5. Dr. Steincrohn believes that alcohol is a two-edged sword. He feels that many people over 40 might be better off if they *did* take alcohol. He approves of drinking: if a person is over 40 and not an alcoholic; if he has angina or other coronary disturbance; if he is taking more and more tranquilizers.

He disapproves of alcohol for those who: are teen-agers; emotionally unstable; have high blood pressure, ulcer or gout, liver, or kidney disease; or who expect to drive a car.

Dr. Steincrohn does not believe in taking all the joy out of life, but neither does he believe in being fool-hardy. He recommends a happy middle way.

TO DRINK OR NOT TO DRINK?

To sum up, the question apparently is not should you drink or shouldn't you, but how *much?* As one doctor told me, "Some of the worst cases of drunkenness I have ever seen have been caused by drinking wine." Yet, Cornaro lived to be a healthy 102 on his 14 ounces a day, and De Coti Marsh's patients are cheered by the thought of their evening glass of wine.

Some doctors, as noted, have reported red table wine as acceptable for diabetics and, in addition, if taken in moderation, a possible help for anemia, colitis, spastic constipation, angina, hypertension, neuralgia, and Parkinson's disease. In Italy, which ranks almost solely as a wine-drinking country (France is leaning toward beer and spirits), the alcoholism rate is the lowest in Europe, mostly because wine is considered a food and is taken primarily at meal times as part of the diet. Italian children encounter it as a food and attach no more importance to it than their parents do. In the United States, however, the many average men and women make a ritual of the before-dinner cocktail. Dr. Georgi Lolli, of Rome and New York, an expert on alcoholics, remarked, "If the average American has held himself to a commuter breakfast of a hurried cup of coffee and has not had more than a sandwich or piece of pie for lunch, he may well be in a general state of starvation by the cocktail hour. This means that he is left with little protection against the toxic effects of excessive amounts of alcohol."

Dr. Leon A. Greenberg, associate professor of physiology at Yale, has made an interesting study on rats. *In small quantities*, he finds, it does not seem to make much difference whether the alcoholic beverage is wine or hard liquor. But in larger amounts, there is a difference. Whereas small amounts of alcohol act as a tranquilizer and relieve tension, stepped-up amounts, particularly of plain alcohol, begin to create new tensions.

The type of diet has a great deal to do with it, too. Both the Cornaro and the De Coti Marsh diets allow leeway for a small bit of wine. New wine is apparently richer in vitamins, as well as in a recently discovered antibiotic factor. Many people claim benefits from unpasteurized beer. A French wine connoisseur tells me that while some wines improve with age, others taste better when new.

WHAT TO DO ABOUT ALCOHOLISM

If you are an alcoholic, or even if you are an excessive drinker, you have a serious problem to face. Alcoholics Anonymous is one organization that can help you deal with it. Twice I have heard its originator tell the story of how in his own desperation he discovered the principles, then passed them on to others. Each time I have heard his story, I have been deeply moved. But there is another way out of alcoholism which most people have not heard of.

Here is the clue: Alcoholics, according to the *American Journal of Clinical Nutrition* (July-August, 1961), usually have had long histories of an inadequate diet.

At the department of neurology, Jefferson Medical College, Philadelphia, studies were made with alcoholics (who were also, in most cases, heavy smokers). The men suffered from visual disturbances. Their condition improved when the intake of alcohol was reduced. It improved still further when a high-energy diet plus B vitamins was given, even if drinking and smoking continued. The report concludes, "The *evidence suggests that nutritional deficiency, not the toxic effects of alcohol or tobacco or both,* is the cause of the disorder. . . . It is not clear which nutrients are responsible."

But one person has gone further and learned which nutrients *are* responsible. Dr. Roger J. Williams has conducted extensive alcoholic tests at the University of Texas, and has written a wonderful little book in which he answers questions that have stumped others. For instance, why does one drink call for another? Dr. Williams finds it is due to a deranged physiological craving. Each individual is different. Some persons, due to heredity, have a higher requirement for certain foods and this need causes the person to crave *something* he is not getting. Often he turns to alcohol and becomes doubly vulnerable. His diet then becomes still more diluted. The appetite-control center in his brain becomes more poorly nourished and goes berserk. In turn, it produces a still greater craving for alcohol (one drink calling for another) instead of the normal craving for food, thus creating a vicious circle.

Alcohol is apt to be habit-forming. The more you have, the more you want. The more you drink, the less you eat. Soon the body is out of gear, because it has been getting an inadequate type of fuel.

Dr. Williams states that alcohol addiction *can* be overcome, and he has learned which nutrients can help restore normality. By replacing these missing nutrients— the specific vitamins and other foods—Dr. Williams finds you can reduce the craving for alcohol. The alcoholic, he says, because of a long history of poor nutrition, has nutritional needs far greater than those of his neighbor, who may be able to get away with reckless eating. Because each individual differs, there is no cut-and-dried diet which will suit the exact needs of every person, but Dr. Williams does contend that certain principles are necessary.

The alcoholic needs plenty of high-quality protein. An adult male, he states, should get approximately 2.5 ounces of protein daily.

Dr. Williams warns that the alcoholic should restrict all refined foods possible, in order to build up his weakened nutritional condition. These refined foods include sugar or syrups, white rice, macaroni products, and white flour. Such foods crowd out the more important food elements needed for rehabilitation.

At the research center, University of Texas, Dr. Williams has worked out a specific nutritional supplement containing the nutrients necessary for an alcoholic. In addition to a good diet, this supplement should be taken in sufficient amounts for a considerable time. The supplement is commercially available and Dr. Williams lists the names of the nutrients as well as the addresses where they may be obtained. In my opinion, every alcoholic, nearalcoholic, or member of an alcoholic's family should read Dr. Roger J. Williams' book, *Alcoholism—The Nutritional Approach* (available from University of Texas Press, Austin, price $2.50).*

* Physicians may receive further information from another author: John J. Miller, Ph.D., "Alcoholism, a Metabolic Disease," *Journal of Applied Nutrition*, Vol. 16, No. 4 (1963).

ARE OTHER MEASURES HELPFUL?

Dr. Williams suggests that in addition to good food, proper vita-min and mineral supplementation, and plenty of rest, some out-door exercise is necessary. The healthy condition of the appetite center, which controls the craving for alcohol, is apparently im-proved by exercise.

Magnesium is a must for alcoholics. (See Chapter 17.)

Emotional problems respond to varied wholesome interests and good social adjustment, too. After all, he says, anything which pro-motes good body health also promotes good mental health. Psy-chological problems have been known to disappear when an al-coholic gives up liquor *completely* and stays on good food and supplementation, even for a few days.

Cecilia Rosenfeld, M.D., another expert in nutritional therapy, agrees. She gives an example of a housewife who was a victim of social drinking which led to marital problems. After only five weeks of nutritional therapy, the woman was able to make a good adjustment in her marriage.

Are there any other props or self-helps an alcoholic can use to speed his progress? Although there is more and more agreement that alcoholism is caused by excessive and continued drinking, which leads to poorer and poorer nutrition, there is often a person-ality problem which prompted the drinker to begin using alcohol as a crutch, in the first place. The Chicago Alcoholic Treatment Center, although admitting that the only cure for alcohol is to give up drinking entirely, admits there are people called "dry drunks" who may stop drinking without making any permanent emotional improvement. A feeling of inadequacy, frustration, loneliness, or being unwanted or unloved has triggered many a per-son into seeking refuge in alcohol, since with one drink under his belt, he likes himself better and the world looks rosier. The *Journal of the American Medical Association* (178:1184; 1961) points out that alcoholics are extremely dependent, not only on drinking, but on other people. Many people use alcohol as a mental, emo-tional, or physical anesthetic.

Harold Sherman, in his book, *Anyone Can Stop Drinking* (see

Bibliography) makes it clear that no one can pull a drinker out of his desire to escape life's hurts, except himself. Like the compulsive eater, who eats to escape some problem, the compulsive drinker probably began to drink for escape, too. Dr. Sherman's book helps the drinker to look unashamedly at himself, learn the reason for his compulsion, and triumphantly effect his own cure.

Gerard Littman, who has been working with alcoholics for 13 years, is administrator of Chicago's Warren Clinic, of the Mental Health Department, State of Illinois. He gives the World Health Organization's definition of alcoholism: "A chronic illness that manifests itself as a disorder of behavior."

Mr. Littman adds, "Many alcoholics resent the religious overtones of the Alcoholics Anonymous program. Others find it difficult to reveal problems to a group of strangers. For these, psychotherapy might prove a better way out of their alcoholism. What psychotherapy can give some alcoholics is the opportunity to get at the root of their emotional problems and thereby remove the need to drink. The alcoholic can learn to accept life and gain confidence in his ability to handle difficulties." ("Bright Light on the Alcoholic," *New York Times Magazine*, April 5, 1964.)

Meanwhile, Herbert Brean gives these helps in getting over the hurdle:

Delay a little. Get into the habit of making yourself wait a little longer before each drink.

Take time out. Set aside a time in which you don't take a drink at a certain time of day, or week. Be easy on yourself at first. Make it stiffer gradually.

Skip one. At a party, have one drink, then make the next one a glass of water or carbonated beverage. This cuts the alcohol in half and still gives you the next drink to look forward to.

Drink lighter alcohol. Substitute dry wines and dry beers for part of your hard liquor. The body gets used to a certain amount of alcohol and seems to demand it, but as you cut it down ounce by ounce, it seems easier with the help of lighter drinks, to adjust to less. The enjoyment of wine is considered one of the great pleasures of life.

Mr. Brean concludes: "Each individual must find his own system. But if one who has been drinking too heavily will school himself to take fewer and less frequent drinks, he will be surprised how pleasurable deceleration can be. He will sleep more soundly and wake with more enthusiasm. His interests will expand. He will get more done on his job and at the same time enjoy it more. He will find himself suddenly free of mysterious aches and pains that he had wrongly accepted as inevitable. He will lose excess pounds. And he will find more money in his pocket."

And finally, Dr. William B. Terhune offers a psychiatrist's ten commandments to prevent alcoholism:

1. Never drink when you "need one."
2. Sip slowly and space your drinks. Take a second drink 30 minutes after the first, a third an hour after the second. Never a fourth drink.
3. Dilute your alcohol.
4. Keep an accurate and truthful record of the amount and number of drinks you take. Never take a drink every day.
5. Do not drink on an empty stomach.
6. Never conceal the amount of alcohol you drink. Instead, exaggerate it.
7. Stop drinking on "signal" (signals are lunch, dinner, fatigue, sex stimulation, boredom, frustration, and bedtime).
8. When tired or tense, soak in a hot tub and follow with a cold shower.
9. Make it a rule never to take a drink to escape discomfort—either physical or mental.
10. Never, never take a drink in the morning thinking it will cure a hangover.

22 Allergies

Many people know that they have allergies. Others do not know. Sometimes allergic individuals are mistakenly considered neurotic, hypochrondriac, or downright ill.

There are many types of allergies, many types of individual differences. Foods are only one problem. Jonathan Forman, M.D., an allergy specialist, classifies the others as follows:

Physical: Barometric pressure changes, heat, cold, light, radiations of various sorts.
Chemical: Drugs, poisons, toxins, dust, pollens, etc.
Psychic: Anxiety, fears, and other stresses.

Dr. Theron G. Randolph, another allergist, finds that gas, used for cooking or heating, is one of the most disturbing irritants of all. Some people are unaware of its effect, yet if there is even a minute amount of leakage, he reports, various symptoms can develop. Paint fumes, certain glues, food odors, and tobacco smoke are also suspect. Even cosmetics, perfumes, dentrifices, soaps, and plastics may give off highly disturbing fumes.

Certain foods, in addition to being irritants for some people (strawberries, citrus fruits, raw onions, etc.), can be tainted with innumerable irritating chemicals. Insecticides, fumigant residues, inorganic sulphur, arsenic, lead, chemical preservatives, chemical flavoring or sweetening agents, extenders, bleaches, softeners, certain nitrates, and nitrites are examples. Traces of lacquers, aluminum, tin, and plastic can come from food containers.

Allergies to drugs and medications, of course, are common. Some disturbing substances get into the blood stream without one's realizing it: for instance, bromine from sleeping pills, or phenacetin from most household pain-killers. (See "Why Drugs?" ch. 3.)

Some people are even allergic to colored-paper products: cleansing and toilet tissue, and towels. Others are allergic to perspiration deodorants. Many deodorants contain salts of aluminum. Benjamin Franklin tells how printers who warmed their lead type often contracted paralysis and lost the use of their hands from the lead vapors. Franklin, himself engaged in printing, experienced pains in his wrist before he would believe that metal poisoning could also be picked up from nerve endings in the skin or fingers.

One woman, whose case came to my attention, developed a great underarm swelling after using a well-known brand of deodorant. So, *beware of them*, and search for a brand that does not contain aluminum salts. Safe products are sold at all health food centers. Dr. Joseph G. Molner suggests powdering with baking soda, starch, or talcum, or a mixture of any of these. It will not do as good a job of deodorizing but at least it should not irritate the skin. Or rub on equal parts of olive oil and lemon juice at night after washing arm pits. Mornings, apply lemon juice.

Beware of hair sprays. A year-long study at Jewish Hospital in St. Louis revealed that two women developed enlargement of the lymph nodes in the lungs, which were discovered through X rays. One patient had three nodes removed. These abnormalities were finally traced to hair sprays that contain synthetic chemicals which apparently are stored in certain lung cells. When the women were urged to stop using the hair sprays, the disturbances gradually cleared up. The spray was then tested on guinea pigs, which developed liver and spleen disturbances. In 1941 Dr. Hueper of the National Cancer Institute warned that PVP, one ingredient now often included in hair sprays, can cause malignant growths. *Consumers Research* has also warned against hair sprays in its July, 1958, issue.

To reduce the amount inhaled, the California Medical Association gives this advice:

Spray on only the amount necessary to keep the hair under control.

Direct the spray as far away from the nose and mouth as possible.

Take deep breaths before releasing hair spray and then limit your breathing during the operation.

Move to a different part of the room before taking a deep breath again.

Ascertain, if possible, whether the spray contains plastic material and if so, be doubly cautious.

Perhaps less convenient, but far safer, is the good old wave set, which is a natural product derived from seaweed.

WHAT ARE THE USUAL SYMPTOMS OF ALLERGY?

Catharyn Elwood, in her book, *Feel Like a Million*, says, "The reactions to these foreign substances are various and often complicated. Sometimes they may appear in the form of hives, hay fever, or skin eruptions. Migraine headaches and other hard-to-explain reactions may result."

B. Bendkowski, M.D., has noticed that boils are found in some allergic patients, often in those with underpar health.

Dr. Granville Knight finds that fatigue is one of the most universal reactions. Other symptoms include headache, cough, eye irritation, repeated "so-called" virus infections in the upper respiratory or gastrointestinal regions, asthma, skin disturbances, edema with either rapid weight gain or loss, heart disturbances, excessive perspiration, vague sensations of fear, forgetfulness, mild mental confusion, depression, laziness, inability to make decisions. Overactivity should be immediately suspect in children.

Here are Dr. Knight's suggestions for treatment:

1. Eliminate and avoid any suspect foods, fumes, or chemicals. In some cases an all-electric home may make the difference between health and invalidism.

2. Eliminate possible pollens, mold spores, or house dust.

3. Build up health and resistance through an excellent nutritional program, including a high protein, high mineral, and high vitamin intake. To disregard a patient's observation that certain foods and drugs disagree may court disaster for both physician and patient. Brewer's

yeast is an excellent dietary supplement. For those unfortunates who are allergic to it, give desiccated liver.

4. "When used with discretion, supplementation with vitamins and trace minerals, including adequate zinc and magnesium, is of tremendous help in reducing allergic reactions. To rely on nutrition alone is to deny patients the amounts of relief which may be obtained by a combination of approaches." ("How to Find Your Own Food Allergies," *Journal of Applied Nutrition*, Vol. 16, Nos. 2 and 3.)

Since skin tests are not always accurate, Arthur Coca, M.D., in his book, *The Pulse Test*, helps you to discover your own allergies by a very simple method. He says, "An allergy no longer means merely hay fever or asthma or an outbreak of hives. It can also mean high blood pressure . . . 'that tired feeling,' constipation, stomach ulcer, dizziness, headaches and mental depression, as well as many other disturbances.

"If you can count to 100 and are determined to be well, you can go a long way toward eliminating your allergic troubles. . . . The following are detailed instructions:

"The pulse can be felt at many spots on the body. . . . the most convenient spot is at the wrist an inch and a half above the base of the thumb. Place the left hand (if you are right-handed) in the lap with the palm facing up. Then place two fingers of the right hand on the wrist. . . . Move the fingers around slightly and vary pressure until the pulse is detected. . . . When counting your pulse have a watch or clock with a second hand close in view. Pick up the pulse . . . and wait until the second hand reaches 60. Then count 1 on the next pulse beat . . . until the second hand has made a complete circuit and returned to 60. . . . The number of pulse beats counted in one minute is the pulse rate."

The allergy test "consists essentially of testing isolated foods in order to tell *which* one accelerates the pulse. On the day the test is started, each 'meal' may be limited to a single, simple food. The pulse is counted in the morning before rising and again just before the first meal. Thirty minutes after the meal the pulse is counted, and again at sixty minutes after the meal."

As new foods are introduced, "a record is kept of the foods eaten and of the pulse counts. The injurious foods are recognized by the abnormal speed-up of the pulse. When these foods are dropped from the diet, the allergic symptoms often disappear as if by magic."

Dr. Coca states that the pulse rate of the normal person is not affected at all by digestion or normal activity. It *can* be affected by sunburn or an infection such as a common cold. Otherwise any step-up in pulse rate indicates an allergy. If your highest count is not over 84, you probably are not allergic. Even if your pulse climbs after eating, as much as 16 beats extra, you may still be in the allergy-free group. Smoking as well as food may be tested.

If you suspect allergies, you will want to read this fascinating book, *The Pulse Test*, which is full of case histories and helpful details. Meanwhile, here are the symptoms Dr. Coca has identified and successfully treated as being allergic:

Recurrent headache.	Abnormal tiredness.
Nervousness.	Indigestion (vomiting, gas)
Migraine.	Colitis.
Dizziness.	Neuralgia.
Constipation.	Sinusitus.
Canker Sores.	Hypertension.
Heartburn.	Hives.
Epilepsy.	Heart attacks.
Overweight.	Asthma.
Underweight.	Hemorrhoids.
Irritability.	Psychic depression.
Gastric ulcer.	Diabetes.
Abdominal pain.	Chest pain.
Gall bladder pain.	Gastrointestinal bleeding.
Gastric pain.	Conjunctivitis.
Nervousness.	Nosebleed.

Dr. Granville Knight adds that after allergic foods have been omitted from the diet for several months, they often may be eaten once or twice a week without reproducing symptoms. Diluted hydrochloric acid and digestive enzymes may also be helpful.

Sometimes immunity to a food can be built up by eating tiny amounts of it, gradually increased to a normal serving. The foods you *think* are disturbing may not actually bother you. Foods found most frequently to cause allergy are: protein in some form, wheat, eggs, milk, chocolate, cabbage, tomatoes, oranges, walnuts, strawberries, bananas, potatoes, cauliflower, oats, rice, oysters, salmon, celery, lettuce, squash, apricots, apples, canteloupes, grapefruit, and peaches.

It is possible to be allergic to a vitamin or the factor with which a capsule or tablet is made. However, many physicians find that vitamin therapy plus protein is extremely useful in treating, especially B complex, A, C, bioflavonoids, B-12, E, D, and the mineral calcium. Hay fever has been greatly helped by large doses of vitamin C ranging from 100 to 1,000 mg. daily prior to the hay-fever season, with a maintenance dose of 100 to 300 mg. daily thereafter.

Dr. Vincent Fontana, an allergy specialist, suggests that hay-fever sufferers stay away from liquor, lacquers, floor waxes, insecticide fumes, highly scented soaps and hair tonics, as well as dust. All of these can aggravate sneezing and wheezing.

Adelle Davis, in her book, *Let's Eat Right to Keep Fit,* writes, "It has been found that vitamin C can prevent or cure chemical poisoning. This vitamin has been valuable in correcting the toxic effects of lead, bromide, arsenic, benzene and many other substances. . . . Studies have proved that vitamin C helps to prevent allergies. If enough is given it can detoxify the harmful effects of allergens which have entered the blood, whether they be pollens, dusts, dandruff, or foods. This vitamin seems to be equally effective in treating all varieties of allergies, whether stuffy nose or post-nasal drip, hay fever, asthma, eczema or hives; spectacular relief often results from massive doses of vitamin C. Even the effects of poison oak or poison ivy often disappear when sufficient vitamin C is taken."

Catharyn Elwood adds, "Many physicians have reported that their patients have recovered [from allergy] rapidly when given large amounts of vitamin C; 300 to 3,000 mg. daily are recommended. The most efficient way to take vitamin C supplement is 100 to 300 mg. with each meal and at bedtime and scattered over the day."

It is interesting to understand why allergies thrive in a deficiency of vitamin C. If you could look at your hand in the dark, illuminated with what is known as "black light" you would be able to see the condition of the tissues inside your body. If you are deficient in vitamin C, this membrane will appear as watery. But if your level of C is high, the tissues will be well knit, with a mucilaginous substance called collagen.

Adelle Davis explains, "The collagen serves much the same purpose as cement does in a brick building except that the 'concrete' in a healthy body is in the form of a stiff jelly. . . . Strong connective tissue is not easily penetrated; thus the cells are protected. An undersupply of vitamin C, however, allows this tissue to break down; . . . protective doors are flung open and the pirates are invited in."

According to Dr. Hans Selye, stress can cause allergies, too. This fits into the picture, because stress destroys vitamin C stored in the adrenal gland within a few seconds. So we are back to the vitamin C deficiency again and the need to restore its loss.

Adelle Davis concludes, "Large amounts of this vitamin [C] often act as a diuretic, causing excessive urination, corresponding dehydration, and extreme thirst. These symptoms are largely prevented if calcium is taken with the vitamin. If calcium is not taken, extreme nervousness sometimes results; therefore let us be cautious."

Probably the first step, if you suspect an allergy, is to help yourself, as well as your doctor, by trying to pinpoint the source of the trouble. Where and at what times does it occur? First, examine possible foods according to the pulse-test technique. Next consider a possible emotional cause. Finally, explore chemicals. I have found that the two most helpful books are: for food, *The Pulse Test* by Arthur F. Coca, M.D.; and for possible chemical irritants, *Human Ecology and Susceptibility to the Chemical Environment* by Theron G. Randolph, M.D. (For sources, see Bibliography.)

There are some types of allergies which occur within minutes or seconds after exposure. Out of 100,000 injections of penicillin in this country, 2,000 end fatally. If a particular allergy is known, a patient should carry a card with him stating his serious allergy. This is an *immediate* help to a physician. If an allergy emergency arises, the patient should be kept warm, with his head down, until the doctor arrives. (*Consultant*, January, 1962, p. 16.)

For those who are allergic to bee or wasp stings, scrape off the stinger (in the case of bees) immediately with a sharp object. Don't remove the stinger or sac with your fingernails, because this might force the remaining venom into the skin. People can be de-sensitized to the venom, and those who are made seriously ill can be treated with antihistamine. In case of any unusual symp-toms suggesting severe allergy, call a physician immediately. More people die each year of bee or wasp stings than of snake bites.

Those who are freest of allergy are those who are healthy. Catha-ryn Elwood sums it up, "Remember that allergies usually appear after the body has been through some illness which has depleted it of its critical nutrients. . . . So, strong health must be carefully planned and intelligently worked for. As vigorous health returns, the allergies usually vanish."

23 Anemia

It has been estimated that 5 to 20 million Americans are anemic. Anemic people may feel only half alive, or rundown; may have a poor memory, fuzzy thinking; experience weakness, dizziness, short-ness of breath, or an I-don't-care attitude. They are usually tired, yet rest does not seem to help. Anemia can catapult you into old age. Even a mild case over a prolonged time can change a gay, happy expression into a gray, haggard one. It can ruin your appear-ance with wrinkles, strain lines, pallor, or a yellowish skin color. It can also cause dry, lusterless hair which turns gray prematurely.

Because of the menstrual cycle, women are more inclined to anemia than men. Pregnancy, requiring added iron for the baby, is a drain on the mother's supply of iron. A hemoglobin (blood count) of 100 *is* possible, though rare. According to Dr. E. E. Judy after a study of 7,000 women, most women test about 86, although a woman's standard is 95. If your hemoglobin is 70-85, you have a borderline anemia. If you are below 60, you have true anemia, and at 35 transfusions are given.

Anemia can be caused by: hemorrhage, disease, drugs or poisons which destroy red blood cells, infection, injury to the bone marrow (where red cells are made), DDT and similar poisons, intestinal parasites, lack of hydrochloric acid which is necessary to dissolve and assimilate iron.

Anemia too can be due to lack of zinc as well as lack of iron. (*Clinical Physiology*, Winter, 1963, p. 195.)

Other causes of anemia, according to Nevin S. Scrimshaw, Ph.D. and M.D., professor of nutrition at the Massachusetts Institute of Technology, include: hookworm, excessive phosphates in the diet interfering with iron absorption; abnormal blood loss due to women's disturbances, duodenal ulcer, or blood disorder; loss of iron in sweat. (*American Journal of Clinical Nutrition*, February, 1964.)

Protein, vitamins, and minerals, in addition to iron, are necessary to fight anemia. Anemia is not always due to a poor diet. It can be due to poor absorption of a good diet. Foods high in iron include meat (especially liver), eggs, dried peas and beans, oatmeal, raisins, prunes, and blackstrap molasses. But other factors are necessary.

If you have a vitamin-C or hydrochloric-acid deficiency, you will not absorb the iron you do eat. The same holds true if you lack copper, cobalt, and possibly manganese (all minerals) in your diet.

Beryl D. Corner, M.D., found in some patients that 500 mg. of vitamin C daily for 10 days, then 50 mg. as a maintenance dose, helped the intestinal tract to absorb iron from a good diet, and additional iron was unnecessary. She also used B vitamins for treatment.

A study with rats revealed that those given rice polishings (rich in B vitamins) recovered a normal hemoglobin level in 26 days. The conclusion of the study was that the polishings may promote better utilization of iron.

According to the *American Journal of Clinical Nutrition* (February, 1963) four subjects kept on a vitamin-E-free diet showed a decrease of red blood cells. When 300 units of vitamin E were added daily, improvement took place.

Injections of vitamin E in large doses relieved 12 children of megaloblastic anemia. (*American Journal of Clinical Nutrition* [1963], Vol. 12, pp. 374-379.)

One man, whose blood count had always hovered around 80 to 85, stumbled across a report from a symposium in England stating that blood corpuscles are protected from destruction by an envelope composed largely of lecithin. When he added lecithin to his diet, his hemoglobin rose to around 95 and has stayed there for 15 years.

In order to raise the hemoglobin even ten points, 80 grams or 3 ounces of protein are necessary. Liver is extremely helpful but, again, if you have a vitamin-C or hydrochloric-acid deficiency, you will not assimilate the liver properly. There are also different types of anemia, each attributed to a shortage of the separate B vitamins.

Two B vitamins, folic acid and vitamin B-12, help to prevent some types of anemia. Folic acid is produced by intestinal bacteria, and vitamin B-12 is derived from foods. Liver, wheat germ, brewer's yeast, and kidney provide both vitamins. For those who do not like liver, desiccated liver powder or tablets are available. When deficiencies of both folic acid and B-12 become great enough, the tongue becomes smooth, shiny, clean and bright red around the edges. The entire mouth may become sore. Anemia due to lack of folic acid is not correctable by iron. Furthermore, when there is even a slight deficiency of folic acid, the stomach is unable to produce enough hydrochloric acid, which is necessary for protein, iron, and calcium digestion. If there is a severe shortage of folic acid, the stomach produces no hydrochloric acid at all. Such a condition causes susceptibility to intestinal parasites and food poisoning. In this case hydrochloric acid can be added to the diet. (See "Indigestion," p. 333.)

Folic acid can help to rectify these troubles and even can heal the mouth. However, folic acid in combination with other vitamins in supplements, has been outlawed on the grounds that it may mask, delay, or conceal pernicious anemia. Folic acid alone is available only by prescription. If it is given without B-12 to patients already showing nerve damage from pernicious anemia (difficulty in walking, lack of coordination, loss of equilibrium, etc.), they may become worse. Some types of anemia will not respond to treatment unless folic acid and a substance called "intrinsic factor" is added.

Folic acid has been used successfully in treating some anemia. Seven women, aged 35 to 82, who had been living on poor diets, mostly tea, sugar, and bread, were given folic acid after they failed to respond to vitamin B-12. All patients exhibited a pallor and grayish-brown pigmentation of the skin. Folic acid, 5 mg. two or three times a day, returned the hemoglobin to normal or near normal within two weeks, after which it was kept normal with 5 mg. folic acid twice daily. (*Quarterly Journal of Medicine* [1963], Vol. 32, pp. 243-256.)

Pernicious anemia *must* be diagnosed and treated by your doctor. Injections of B-12, which can usually control it, are necessary.

For the average case of nutritional or secondary anemia, look to your diet. Dr. Daniel Quigley says, "An examination of the food intake of anemic persons will disclose the fact that the sick person has been living on a diet which is largely composed of devitaminized and devitalized carbohydrates, and this has cut down in his diet, not only iron, but vitamins, calcium, iodine and the other trace minerals."

If all other factors have been checked off and anemia still persists, DDT poisoning,* or intestinal parasites may be suspected. One woman I know fought a losing battle against anemia for years. Finally by chance, a physician suggested an examination for intestinal parasites. Sure enough, hookworm was present. Twenty-five worms can swallow a half ounce of blood every 24 hours! For years the woman had been feeding these "critters" food and vitamins she needed herself. When the hookworms (which had been apparently acquired in the South, where they are common) were disposed of, the anemia promptly disappeared. In one study

* See Clark, *Stay Young Longer*.

94 out of 200 people were found to have intestinal parasites, which, when properly removed, caused people who had harbored them, to lose their symptoms of vitamin deficiencies. According to *Nutrition Review* (April, 1962) in a light case of hookworm about 14 mg. of iron is lost per day.

In Finland tapeworm anemia has been reported high and is a great problem in that country. Carriers revealed a marked deficiency of vitamin B-12.

Symptoms of intestinal worms are: itching at the rectum, restless nights with bad dreams, grinding of teeth when asleep, diarrhea, unpleasant breath, darkness under eyes, biting nails, picking nose, children crying out in sleep, constant longing for food which no meal will satisfy.

Following a treatment for parasites, perfect cleanliness is necessary to prevent reinfestation.

Protective measures should include: a daily bath, clean linen daily, washing hands before meals and after trips to bathroom, clean fingernails (parasites can lodge under them).

Often, after a treatment to eliminate parasites, a few eggs may remain in the body and in two weeks or more, a fresh legion is hatched. Treatment is again necessary until the enemy is completely vanquished.

Parasites can be picked up from doorknobs, handrails, public or private toilets; from pets infested with them; from raw meat handled by butchers who are careless in their cleanliness. Children can transmit worms to one another. Hookworm is common in the South and tapeworm can be spread by using raw cess-pit manure on vegetable gardens. Trichinae can, of course, result from eating undercooked pork, which often masquerades as hamburger. Worm eggs deposited near the human anus can be transferred to bed linen, and during bedmaking can join the dust in the bedroom. Worm eggs have actually been found in dust on top of a bedroom cupboard.

HOW ARE PARASITES DETERMINED AND ELIMINATED?

Laboratory tests can reveal their presence in a stool sample. What kind of remedies expel worms? There are drugs which the doctor *can* give you, but I doubt if the doctor himself knows how upsetting to the patient and how serious the eventual side effects may be. I talked with one father who, when his children had been found suffering from parasitical infestation, was given a vermifuge along with the rest of the family. He and one child experienced especially violent reactions to the medicine itself. He told me, "Never again. I would rather have the parasites."

To date, the only commercial product I consider safe is made of a combination of almonds and raw figs, and acts as a nontoxic vermifuge by digesting the parasites. Fresh papaya acts in a similar fashion.

A reader suggests the following home remedy for worms: a garlic water enema. In her case, after the fourth enema the worms disappeared and did not return. "This is so much better," she writes, "than upsetting the whole system by taking drastic drugs."

As with most home remedies exact proportions were not given. Perhaps several cloves of garlic could be crushed or added to the water in an electric blender.

24 Arthritis

Eleven million arthritics in the United States are looking for help. It is not surprising that in their desperation they rush from one reported cure to another. Let me assure you that there is definite hope for relief from pain and even the possibility of cure. But in order to get relief, you should understand how and why you acquired arthritis in the first place. This knowledge should help you to improve your condition so that life will be worth living again. Arthritis, or its cause, is no longer a mystery.

WHAT CAUSES ARTHRITIS?

The natural remedies I shall report have already brought improvement to a large number of people, although they may not be commonly known or yet accepted in medical circles. Obviously, relief from pain is a blessing, but there is a difference between relief and cure. One method merely suppresses the symptoms, while the other both corrects the cause and eventually helps to diminish the pain.

Those physicians and health therapists who are *really* getting results with arthritics, not just patching them up or temporarily masking their pains, consider that arthritis is, for the most part, a nutritional-deficiency disease. Actually, according to Pauline Beregoff-Gillow, M.D., "Arthritis is *not* a disease. It is a symptom that something is wrong in the system."

A close relative of mine whose arthritis was ascribed to aluminum poisoning from aluminum cooking ware discontinued using it and gradually noticed improvement.

Max Warmbrand, N.D.,D.O., in his book, *New Hope for Arthritis Sufferers*, writes, "Most people regard arthritis as a single specific disease affecting only the joints, and fail to recognize the relationship that exists in the organism as a whole, and therefore fail to realize that only as these abnormal conditions are overcome can the body be restored to health." He lists other symptoms often associated with arthritis: constipation; digestive disorders; catarrhal conditions; poor circulation; cold, clammy hands and feet; fatigue; numbness; irritability.

He continues, "As a rule the disease develops slowly, imperceptibly. It may take years before one becomes aware of its serious manifestation. Even when the onset is sudden, with high fever and severe pains, one must bear in mind that the factors that have given rise to it have been operating a long time.

"To begin with, it is well to realize that arthritis is not a purely local disease but a systemic disorder and the outgrowth of many systemic disturbances. These disturbances weaken the functions of the body, impair circulation and create deficiencies. Starvation of the tissues, retention of toxins, chemical imbalance and stagnation, are the factors that affect the joints and give rise to destructive changes. . . . When a body is in healthy condition, it possesses sufficient recuperative powers to protect the tissues against permanent damage. It is only when the body is in depleted condition . . . or its recuperative powers are weakened that it lacks the power to overcome local impairment."

Due to individual indifferences, arthritis takes different forms in different people. Consequently, one may react differently to different treatments. In the main, however, the underlying cause is the same: nutritional deficiency. Specialists in natural treatment and the reversal of arthritic symptoms are in agreement with this general premise.

Nutrition Reviews (July, 1963) states, "Many patients with arthritis are both malnourished and neglected from a nutritional standpoint. . . . as a group, they represent one of the most nutritionally neglected segments of our medical population."

This statement is based on the work of Dr. L. Eising, who has studied the dietary intake of groups of patients with rheumatoid arthritis and degenerative joint disease. Ninety-two per cent of patients tested were found to have a diet which was deficient in one or more vitamins. Dr. Eising found few significant differences between the diets of rheumatoid arthritis patients, those with degenerative bone disease, and those who had other chronic illnesses. But she did find a common denominator in all three groups: faulty dietary habits. (*Journal of Bone Joint Surgery* [1963], 45A, 69.)

Melvin E. Page, D.D.S., himself a former arthritic but now in good health, is director of the Page Foundation,* St. Petersburg, Florida. To my certain knowledge, he has reversed arthritis in hundreds of patients. In general, his treatment is aimed at correcting the body chemistry. He says, "When the body chemistry is out of balance, degenerative diseases manifest themselves in different ways in different parts of the body.

* This foundation and its methods are explained in Clark, *Stay Young Longer.*

"The cause of arthritis may be in an inadequate diet. . . . In my clinic practice it has been found that the diets of arthritics are preponderantly carbohydrate and deficient in trace minerals. Usually a deficiency of B vitamin is found.

"Mechanical conditions can also produce defective chemistry of a part by interference with normal circulation—witness Pemberton's experiment in tying off parts of the blood supply in a dog's leg, which resulted in arthritic deposits. Arthritis in the shoulder may come from a sleeping posture producing interference with the circulation.

"Infection usually affects body chemistry. When infection is the cause, its removal usually clears up the arthritis. Infection, however, is but one factor which may affect body chemistry. The greatest mistake in the treatment of arthritis has been the supposition that there must always be infection at the root of disease. Thousands of mouths have been wrecked by the needless extraction of teeth, to say nothing of the removal of tonsils, gall bladders, appendices, and what-not to no avail. Even if these measures have given temporary relief . . . disillusionment comes later and the search for infection continues."

Dr. Page concludes, "Mental conditions so affect the body chemistry that there is a wide fluctuation of calcium-phosphorus levels. During time of depression many business men develop aches and pains from worry that later disappear with the return of more normal business conditions."

Dr. D. C. Jarvis agrees heartily (as, of course, does Dr. Hans Selye, the stress expert): "It is common knowledge that arthritic patients feel worse when they are under emotional strain which activates their energy-expending mechanism. In some, an emotional upheaval can produce an attack of arthritis, and in all of them the mechanism may be activated by such common emotional problems as chronic resentment, an unhappy marriage, a bitter career disappointment, or some frustration which the person battles subconsciously every day. The first symptoms of arthritis may occur immediately after a siege of family trouble, and will be caused by a mineral [calcium] precipitation in the body which activates the energy-expending mechanism."

WHAT ARE THE VARIOUS TYPES OF ARTHRITIS?

Dr. Jarvis, in his book *Arthritis and Folk Medicine*, writes, "Vermont folk medicine does not recognize a difference among bursitis, gout, rheumatoid arthritis, osteoarthritis, and muscular rheumatism. Vermont folk medicine believes that the treatment of arthritis begins in the stomach."

In Dr. Page's opinion, "There are different type of arthritis. Rheumatoid arthritis is a generalized disease of the entire body that produces inflammation of the joints; osteoarthritis attacks the bone and cartilage in the joints; in gout a chalky substance is deposited, especially in the joint tissues of the hands and feet; with cataracts a [calcium] deposit is put over the eye; while with pyorrhea [due to calcium deficiency] that part of the jaw bone which supports the teeth dissolves, causing inflammation of the gums which eventually necessitates removing the teeth.

"Although faulty body chemistry is the general cause of arthritis, there are a number of causes for this faulty body chemistry. Hence treatment to cure the disease depends on recognition of the factor or factors responsible."

A strong relationship exists between pyorrhea and rheumatoid arthritis. The similarity in the chemistry of these two disturbances has also been found due to excess phosphorus in the diet, pulling calcium out of the body. (*Modern Nutrition*, June, 1964.) For solutions to this problem, see rules for taking brewer's yeast (p. 108). See also, "The Magic Mineral, Magnesium" (ch. 119).

WHAT ABOUT DRUGS?

Dr. Max Warmband warns, "When the early pre-arthritic symptoms become annoying, remedies are usually prescribed to provide relief. These drugs may help to relieve distressing symptoms or lessen discomfort . . . but they do not eliminate causative factors and they have no corrective value. . . . A stimulating drug or physiotherapy may temporarily improve the circulation and provide relief, but unless fundamental corrective measures are employed . . . the diseased condition continues to grow worse. . . . Most persons are under the impression that these remedies possess specific curative powers."

According to Paul Dudley White, M.D., aspirin relieves but does not cure. It also can produce serious side effects. (See "Why Drugs?" p. 11.)

Dr. W. S. Clark, medical care director of the March of Dimes, has charged, "America's drug industry has hidden from the public the dangerous side effects which can be produced by the indiscriminate use of steroid hormones in the treatment of arthritis victims. Steroids, such as cortisone can be extremely effective in relieving the pain and inflammation of rheumatoid arthritis," he points out, "but patients can become wholly dependent on the drugs. Misuse of them can cause a variety of ailments, including softening of the bone, excessive bleeding ulcers and great emotional distress." "I think," Dr. Clark says, "that this is part of the total program of high-pressure selling of drugs." (*Organic Consumer Report*, November 12, 1963.)

Disturbing side effects of other temporary drugs, including cinchophen, codeine, gold salts, and other "miracle" drugs are documented in Dr. Warmband's *Encyclopedia of Natural Health* (New York: Julian Press, 1962).

WHAT ARE THE MISSING NUTRITIONAL FACTORS?

Although arthritis is in general now considered an all-over nutritional deficiency disease by many enlightened practitioners, in some cases certain nutritional shortages may become apparent before others. Consequently, if these missing factors are supplied, pain may eventually subside, and the "disease" may be arrested. Where bone deterioration has already taken place, it is doubtful that it can be repaired (although it has happened in osteoporosis in animals). However, if an arthritic, who has been bedfast, chairfast, and suffering from excruciating pains, can be relieved from pain without taking drugs, and can be assured of being able to move around by himself with comparative comfort, it is something indeed to look forward to. Here are some examples of what the replacement of some of the missing nutritional factors has accomplished for some people. In reading them, you might check up on your own deficiencies.

ARE YOU DEFICIENT IN OILS?

When Dan Dale Alexander first published his book, *Arthritis and Common Sense*, he was hailed on one hand and condemned on the other. In one city I visited, many people who had been unable to walk noticed improvement within a few months after using the Alexander method, which includes cod-liver oil. The good news spread, and he was invited for a return engagement the following year. Supplies of cod-liver oil, meanwhile, could not be kept on the pharmacy shelves.

On the other hand, critics scorned statements such as, "cod-liver oil lubricates the joints," and branded him a quack. In my opinion, Mr. Alexander's motive was sincere. His language was merely that of an untrained medical investigator. In trying to find a cure for his arthritic mother, he had stumbled on "something" which had been overlooked by others.

Then two doctors, perhaps to settle the argument, or perhaps to disprove his theories—I don't know which—conducted a scientifically acceptable study, using the Alexander method. To the surprise of everyone except Mr. Alexander they found in nearly every patient tested that the treatment worked! The furor against Mr. Alexander and cod-liver oil died down.

The study, reported in the July, 1959, issue of the *Journal of the National Medical Association*, was conducted at the Brusch Medical Center, Cambridge, Massachusetts, by Charles A. Brusch, M.D., and Edward T. Johnson, M.D. Here are the facts as they appeared in the study:

98 cases of osteo, rheumatoid, and mixed arthritis types were treated.
92 responded within a period of 2 to 20 weeks.
Subjectively (or as appeared to the patients themselves), there was
    marked reduction in pain, and general improvement was noted in
    the majority of patients.

Objectively (by test)
1. There was diminished tissue swelling.
2. Less fatigue.
3. Better complexion.
4. Skin and scalp improvement.
5. Ear wax increase.
6. Stronger nails.
7. Greater alertness.
8. Improvement of blood chemistry in over 90 per cent of the patients.
9. Sedimentation rate dropped.
10. Cholesterol level dropped, even with the addition of milk, eggs, butter, as well as the cod-liver oil.
11. High white blood count gave way to normal count.
12. Hemoglobin level frequently rose.
13. Blood sugar dropped to lower side of normal.
14. Blood pressure levels were lower after 15 weeks.
15. Body weight remained the same.
16. Acid urine remained or alkaline urine became acid.
17. Urinary mucous threads generally cleared.
18. Constipation was gradually overcome.
19. Extremities became warmer, with less swelling.
20. More energy was evident in four to five months.

The treatment (the Alexander method) consisted of the following measures:

Water was drunk 60 minutes before breakfast or 30 minutes before the evening meal.

The only liquid permitted with meals was milk served at room temperature, or warm soup.

Cod-liver oil (1 tablespoon as Mr. Alexander recommends) was given in 2 tablespoons of fresh-squeezed orange juice or milk on an empty stomach, preferably five hours after eating. This was given daily except in cases of complications such as diabetes or heart trouble, in which case it was given only twice weekly.

Cod-liver oil was given with milk when a patient was sensitive to orange juice.

Complete elimination of soft drinks, candy, cake, ice cream, or any food made with white sugar was observed.

For those who considered lack of coffee a hardship, coffee was permitted at least 15 minutes before breakfast, provided water was given first.

1,800 to 2,400 calories were allowed.

Here are some excerpts from a letter to the editor written by Dr. Brusch*:

"We felt these (*rapid*) improvements were due primarily to the cod-liver oil and unusual arrangements for liquid-drinking intake. While it is true that these favorable objective and laboratory findings would eventually appear with a favorable diet (alone)—'*the relativity of time*' *to obtain these more or less same results—would differ.* We obtained our results in three to six months time. A wholesome diet alone would perhaps take three to thirty-six months to produce 50 to 75 per cent of our results, at best.

"Complete abstinence from white sugar plus a wholesome diet . . . would perhaps automatically give 25 to 50 per cent of the results noted in our paper. This is based on the observation of noticeable skin improvement, hair and scalp improvement, degree of cerumen (ear wax), correction and diminishing of inflammatory ear conditions to name a few of the objective changes. In addition, of course, we noted favorable blood chemistry and urine changes.

"In the need for the matter of unusual arrangement for water intake, we felt it important to our sedimentation rates. . . . The sedimentation rate levels were erratic unless water was thus controlled. . . .

"We feel that it is the *combination* of several factors that we were striving to coordinate:

"a. A wholesome diet free from refined foods

"b. Control of water and fluid intake—so that the rates at which *all food and liquid* 'entered the bloodstream' were more or less constant. The average person's rate of assimilation of their diet varies widely.

"c. We were trying to gain maximum help from the organic iron in cod-liver oil. Medical history notes that this is best done on an empty stomach. Liquid form of cod-liver oil was used intentionally, not perles. Organic iodine *per se* as found associated in the conventional cod-liver oil molecular structure, was more in line with what we wanted to get into the system with the hope of improving the body metabolism. We also found it had a beneficial effect on blood serum cholesterol. We do not believe cod-liver oil perles would have had a fraction of the success.

* Quoted from *Prevention Magazine*, July, 1960.

"In relatively quick time we found results in correcting skin lustre, hair and scalp conditions. We found this working with ordinary cod-liver oil."

Signed:

Charles A. Brusch, M.D.
Medical Director, Brusch Medical Center
Cambridge 39, Massachusetts

In the early 1930's there was some criticism of the benefits of cod liver oil. The explanation has now come to light. According to Francis M. Pottenger, M.D., only when the oil was rancid did it produce problems.

H. E. Kirschner, M.D., also recommends cod-liver oil for arthritis. He says, "I have had many letters from people who have obtained great relief from their sciatic, arthritic or rheumatic ailment by taking cod-liver oil. Failure to get results has often been due to these two factors: lack of sufficient amount or continuance for too short a time."

He suggests starting out with one-third teaspoon a day, gradually increasing to 1 tablespoon. He, too, feels that it is best to take it when the stomach is empty, either the last thing at night or the first thing in the morning before breakfast. He advises keeping the bottle tightly capped in the refrigerator. To make it more palatable, he suggests putting 1 tablespoon of grape juice in a glass, moistening the glass up to the rim, then floating a tablespoon of cod-liver oil on top and drinking the whole mixture quickly. He finds almost without exception that by starting with small doses at night the patient can soon build up a tolerance. For those who have real trouble, a second best (though not considered as effective by some physicians) is the use of cod-liver oil capsules. In this event Dr. Kirschner recommends starting with one capsule which holds 8 minims; the next day, two. Later increase the size of the capsules. A mint-flavored cod-liver oil is available for those who dislike it straight. Others prefer it mixed with orange juice.

ARE YOU DEFICIENT IN B VITAMINS?

A deficiency of pantothenic acid—a B vitamin—has been found in arthritics. The greater the deficiency, the more pronounced the signs of rheumatoid arthritis. (*Lancet*, 1963 ii, 862-3.)

ARE YOU DEFICIENT IN CALCIUM?

The fact that calcium is deposited in the joints frightens most people away from using it. And yet, eating calcium apparently does not *cause* arthritis. Rather, a lack of it can be the cause! Dr. L. W. Cromwell of San Diego found that 500 older people, victims of osteoarthritis, suffered from a prolonged calcium deficiency and exhibited more bulges at finger joints and other arthritic signs than people who had eaten plenty of calcium. Adelle Davis says, "The lack of calcium necessary to help vitamin C in forming normal cartilage around the joints appears to be the major cause of the disease."

Medical Letter on Drugs and Therapeutics (September, 1963) comments, "It is simpler and probably less hazardous and more effective to rely on intensive calcium therapy than on hormone therapy."

As further proof of this statement, a study with rats at the Albert Einstein Medical Center, Philadelphia, found that when rats were subjected to little or no calcium, osteoporosis was established in 38 days, as confirmed by X rays. When a supplement of calcium was given for 400 days, bone was restored to normal. The study suggested that similar treatment might be applied to humans.

At the Department of Zoology, Oregon State College, Dr. Rosalind Wulzen and Alice Bahrs induced arthritis in guinea pigs by giving them pasteurized milk. They developed muscle stiffness followed by "great emaciation and weakness." Autopsies showed that the muscles were streaked with white lines of calcification. Lumps of tricalcium phosphate were found deposited under the skin, in joints, and in other organs as well. Other animals fed whole raw milk were healthy and on autopsy revealed no abnormality of any kind.

All possible substances for reversing arthritis were then tried. The guinea pigs had reached the point that when laid on their sides they were unable to get up by themselves. Finally, only two remedies reversed the symptoms: raw sugar-cane juice (similar to blackstrap molasses) and raw cream.

In this connection here is a true story of an arthritic whom I have interviewed, and whose story I have checked thoroughly. The story also appears in the Peekskill *Evening Star*, Friday, April 29, 1960, from which I quote here.

"James S. Puellen, a state industrial safety worker, became afflicted with arthritis and his symptoms became increasingly worse until he became bed-fast and unable to move without help. He had been a victim of arthritis for four or five years before becoming bed-fast and and immobile. He said, 'It began to cripple my hands, legs and back. I went from doctor to doctor, from hospital to hospital, from clinic to clinic. I took drugs of all kinds, with no results except that my condition became successively worse.

" 'Finally, I found it impossible to get on my shoes. I hobbled around in a pair of rubbers. My fingers began to close. I was only able to get around with the aid of canes and crutches.

" 'Then came the time when even this was impossible and I became bedridden.'

"When he had been bed-fast five or six months, a friend visited him and asked him if he had ever tried goat's milk. Mr. Puellen laughed at the idea, but the friend assured him that the milk would at least improve Mr. Puellen's general health and might help combat the arthritis. He did not promise a cure.

"Mr. Puellen began to drink at first a pint of fresh, unpasteurized goat's milk daily and as his pain began to lessen, two quarts a day. In two weeks he was feeling better. One day his wife raised her husband's arms for him, at his request, since he was unable to move them himself, and crossed them over his chest. At that moment he discovered he could move his index fingers. From then on his improvement was rapid. Three months later, he was back to work.

"He is now about 98 per cent pain-free (after a long day or continued exertion, he notices a little pain now and then). He is a picture of health and he can lift a 100-lb. bale of hay with no trouble or discomfort. Since regaining his health, he has gathered information about goats from the county agent and Cornell University. He now raises goats to supply milk for himself and others."

One of his arthritic friends noticed definite improvement after drinking the milk, but decided the milk was too expensive (on the East Coast it sells for about 75 cents per quart; on the West Coast for about 45 cents). He started buying canned goat's milk and his improvement ceased. Not until Mr. Puellen learned of the Wulzen study of the effects of *raw cream* on arthritis and realized that goat's milk which is naturally homogenized is similar, did he understand the reason. Canned goat's milk is heat treated, not raw.

I interviewed another of Mr. Puellen's friends who had been stricken with arthritis for five years. He is a garage owner and he told me that at night he could scarcely sleep because he felt as if his arms were being pulled from their sockets. Three months after beginning goat's milk—one quart daily—his pain ceased. His condition remained under control until a temporary shortage of goat's milk forced him to give it up. Then his pain returned. Two weeks after the supply was continued and he resumed drinking his quart a day, his pain once more disappeared.

People who turn up their noses at the idea of drinking goat's milk are in for a surprise. Goats (the females) are clean and fastidious and, contrary to belief, are not smelly. If their feed or hay falls to the ground, they will not touch it. Milk which comes from carefully tested, and carefully tended, animals is disease-free. One large international food laboratory tested samples of Mr. Puellen's goat's milk, and to its amazement found no bacterial count at all the first day after milking. Even after the milk had stood at room temperature for several days, it was still 90 per cent lower in bacteria count than pasteurized cow's milk.

According to the *British Medical Journal* (July 13, 1958), "Goats rarely suffer from tuberculosis, but their milk may contain Brucella melintensis, which causes a rather more severe form of undulant fever than does the Brucella abortus found in cow milk."

I checked this with my county veterinarian. He agreed that it would be a wise precaution for goats to have the blood test for Brucellosis, and as an added precaution, the tuberculosis test as well.

Both tests are simple. Any veterinary doctor can take a sample of goat blood and send it to the laboratory for analysis. If Brucellosis *should* occur (which is very rare) then you will have to find another goat. Pasteurizing the milk, of course, destroys the infection, but this defeats the purpose, as I have pointed out. The usual treatment prescribed for undulant fever in humans is several weeks of massive doses of an antibiotic, tetracycline, which can be dangerous. (F. M. Pottenger, Jr., M.D., has reported good results in treating human cases of undulant fever naturally with trace-mineral therapy. He uses a combination of minerals which includes iodine, manganese, copper, and zinc.) So by taking reasonable and simple precautions, you can drink goat's milk without concern.

For those who cannot get *certified* raw cream (considered safe by health authorities) or raw goat's milk, calcium tablets are recommended by many physicians.* As a matter of fact, the pain of arthritis or any other pain can be gently minimized by calcium tablets, according to Adelle Davis. She says it is so effective a painkiller that she can't understand why more physicians do not recommend it instead of dangerous drugs. She recommends taking calcium tablets to minimize pain—for everything from dentistry to childbirth!

ARE YOU DEFICIENT IN DIGESTIVE ACID?

This lack may prove the clue to many, many cases of arthritis.

Dr. Jarvis says, "People with arthritis are usually classified as calcium deficient. Although they do tend to accumulate calcium deposits, Vermont folk medicine says they are not making hydrochloric acid in the stomach, or else the amount made is too small. Normal calcium metabolism is so highly dependent upon this acid that when there is a lack of it a disturbed calcium metabolism is inevitable."

Biochemists know that calcium cannot be assimilated without acid. This means that older people, even tense people, who secrete a gradually diminishing amount of hydrochloric acid may find the cause of their trouble here. Perhaps vitamin C can provide some of

* See Clark, *Stay Young Longer.*

this much needed acid. Dr. Jarvis recommends adding hydrochloric acid to your diet (see "Indigestion—Gallstones—Kidney Stones," p. 333) or two teaspoons of apple cider vinegar to a glass of water sipped before or during a daily meal. If you will try a little experiment you will discover for yourself the dissolving effect of acid on calcium. Line up several water glasses on a window sill. In one, put regular (pasteurized) milk. In another put plain water. In still another, add two teaspoons of vinegar to water. Drop a bone-meal (calcium) tablet in each. You will notice that in the vinegar water, the bone-meal will begin to dissolve almost at once. In plain water the dissolution is slow. In milk, even after standing an hour or more, the bone-meal tablet will be as hard as at the minute you dropped it in.

Since the calcium, without acid, cannot be properly dissolved in the body, it may pile up in unwanted places including the joints, and lead to arthritis.

ARE YOU DEFICIENT IN VITAMIN C?

Since the average arthritic is deficient in vitamin C, this vitamin is extremely necessary. But it should be taken in tablet form rather than in large amounts of citrus fruit juices, which, for some reason, seem to aggravate arthritis. Royal Lee, D.D.S., says, "Very often the arthritic patient on citrus juices is killing himself by inches. Immediate improvement in the symptomatic reactions follows in these cases if the citrus foods (juices) are dropped from the diet."

One woman, a piano teacher and a friend of mine, developed severe joint pains and stiffness in her fingers, a condition which seriously interfered with her livelihood. She discovered that the condition grew worse during the summer while she was drinking large amounts of grapefruit juice in an attempt to beat the heat. But when she discontinued the juice and substituted vitamin C (ascorbic acid) tablets in massive amounts, according to Adelle Davis' formula for arthritis (1,000 mg. plus a calcium tablet every two hours for three days, followed by a maintenance dose of 1,000 mg. plus a calcium tablet daily), her pain stopped within two days and her stiffness disappeared within a month. (See "Infections," ch. 39.)

Some specialists use bioflavonoids (a name for the entire vitamin C family) instead of ascorbic acid, a single member of the same family. They feel that by combining the two, or using bioflavonoids alone, similar results can be obtained with a lower dosage.

Dr. James R. West of Morrell Memorial Hospital, Lakeland, Florida, treated 21 patients with rheumatoid arthritis with 300 mg. of bioflavonoids daily from two to six months. Improvement in pain, digestion, blood pressure, and action in joints was noticed in a matter of weeks. Bursitis also responds to bioflavonoids.

Dr. Morton S. Biskind and Dr. W. Coda Martin used 200 mg. of bioflavonoids three times daily (making 600 total) for a case of bursitis in a 38-year-old man. Swelling and pain diminished within 24 hours and except for a slight local tenderness, the lesion had subsided almost completely in 72 hours. (*American Journal of Digestive Diseases*, Vol. 21, No. 7 [July, 1954], p. 177.)

Catharyn Elwood reports the case of a young mother suffering with agonizing pain from bursitis. Then she took 100 mg. of bioflavonoids and 100 mg. of vitamin C combined every hour of the waking day for three or four days. Using the bioflavonoid-vitamin C formula, the mother felt better the first day, much better on the second, nearly well on the third, and on the fourth day had no soreness in the joint at all.

To relieve bursitis, put ice cubes in an ice bag or plastic refrigerator bag, wrap in a towel and use for 20-minute intervals, resting 10 minutes between applications. This is not a cure. It merely alleviates the pain while the vitamin treatment is taking hold.

ARE YOU DEFICIENT IN MINERALS?

Calcium is not the only necessary mineral. Curtis Wood, Jr., M.D., has reported relief from pain in arthritic patients by the use of kelp tablets rich in many minerals.

Charles B. Ahlson, B.S., an agronomist for the U.S. Department of Agriculture Conservation Service for twenty-three years, has written a book, *Health From Sea and Soil,* in which he reports the health giving value of sea water on plants, animals and people. He cites the testimony of various physicians to the effect that drinking small amounts of sea water can help to prevent many deficiency diseases. He reports that both arthritis and bursitis respond to sea-water therapy. George W. Crane, M.D. says, "In fact it is entirely possible that the water-soluble trace elements may prove the greatest medical innovation in preventing such ailments that have appeared in the twentieth century." He reports the work of several M.D.'s who are prescribing sea water for various ailments.

Dr. Crane tells of the effect of sea water on arthritis in his own family—that of Mrs. Crane's 96-year-old father. This very elderly man had been bedfast or chairfast with an arthritic hip for nearly 10 years. In four months, Dr. Crane reports, Grandpa got out of his invalid chair and began hobbling around. He perked up both physically and mentally. Dr. Crane observed, "It seemed as if some miracle had happened. Maybe ocean water is the real 'fountain of youth,' for it contains all the water soluble chemicals on this earth."

I have learned of a woman, a veterinarian, who was obliged to give up her practice because of arthritis. After less than a year of sea-water therapy, her arthritis disappeared and she resumed her work.

Sea water *must* be taken from sewage-free ocean areas, must be clear, clean and blue, preferably filtered and not boiled. This processing, to insure safety, explains why sea water sold by some companies (see Bibliography for Sources) is so expensive. It is well worth it. The average supply also lasts a long time.

Actually, sea water is not as salty to drink as you might think, due to the presence of other minerals besides common salt. Furthermore, in taking it, you don't fill a glass and drink it. Most people start with a few drops a day and work up to a maximum of three teaspoons before or during each meal. Robert F. Marx, who crossed the Atlantic in 77 days in an attempt to duplicate Columbus' journey, existed on sea water and wine for two months. So if you should get more than three teaspoonfuls three times daily, don't worry about it.

Dr. Crane calls attention to an analysis of sea water by Sverup, Johnson and Fleming, which disclosed 44 elements, all vital nutrients. One of these, magnesium, may be a major breakthrough for arthritis.

IS MOST OF YOUR FOOD COOKED?

Dr. O. Stiner, an investigator for the Swiss Board of Health in Berne, Switzerland, took a large number of guinea pigs off their normally raw diet and fed them food cooked in a pressure cooker. The animals developed softened teeth, gum disturbances, goiter, and anemia. When two teaspoons of pasteurized milk were added daily, arthritis appeared. These findings were supported by Dr. Francis Pottenger in his study of cooked *vs.* raw food with several generation of cats. (For details, see *Stay Young Longer.*)

WHAT ABOUT THE WEATHER?

For those who claim that the weather has something to do with arthritics, there is support. Tests show that the arthritic notices sudden barometric changes, temperature extremes, and humidity. Pain increases on a falling barometer; decreases or disappears when pressure rises. Arthritics seem to be most comfortable at a steady temperature of 78°.

Heat applied to painful local areas is definitely helpful. Hot-water soaks, hot-water bottles, electric pads, and heat lamps can provide relief.

SOME GENERAL HELPS

An American medical journal describes relief obtained in osteo-arthritic cases by giving doses of vitamin B-12 for three successive weeks. Doses ranged from 30 to 900 micrograms per week.

Cherries have been credited with success. In *Texas Reports on*

Biology and Medicine, Ludwig W. Blau, M.D., cited a study of 12 cases of gouty arthritis on a nonrestricted diet. Improvement occurred in all 12 cases as a result of eating about one-half pound of fresh or canned cherries daily. *Food Field Reporter* (November 10, 1958), reported the successful effect of cherry juice on arthritics. One physician, J. D. Walters, M.D., cautions that cherries should be eaten raw and *not* doused with poison spray. A food analysis finds four types of acids, an unsaturated fatty acid and pectin in cherries. To date, however, I can find no other explanation for the success of cherries.

Michael Rabben, D.D.S., has something to say which may be of help. "Refined carbohydrates (including sugar) intensify pain." (*Modern Nutrition,* September, 1959.)

Dr. Royal Lee D.D.S., points out that alkalinity increases pain; acidity decreases it.

Bernhard Spur, Ph.D., reporting information from a German publication says, "It is a well-known fact that raw potato juice has a curative effect on arthritis."

Numerous people report that alfalfa tea or alfalfa tablets have proved helpful.

Dr. Jarvis says, "Honey helps to alleviate pain in arthritis. It also helps to bring about a disappearance of muscle cramps in the body. Two teaspoons of honey are taken at each meal, either from the spoon or combined with vinegar and water."

Dr. Beregoff-Gillow warns that eating too fast, washing food down with liquids, eating on the run, can cause many deficiency conditions. Primary digestion starts in the mouth. Chewing activates the secretion of saliva which has a ferment ptyalin that digests starches. Liquids may be taken at the end of a meal but never with a meal. Taken with a meal they can dilute what little stomach acid exists.

Exercise of some kind is helpful, even if you are at first only able to tense your muscles, area by area, while lying in bed. It stimulates circulation and brings oxygen to the stagnant tissues. If you can walk, so much the better. According to Dr. Hans Selye, a walk of at least 10 minutes a day will help you to manufacture your own natural cortisone.

A combination of royal (bee) jelly and pantothenic acid, a B vitamin, has relieved rheumatoid arthritics of pain, according to the British medical journal, *Lancet*. The treatment is given by injection.

Remember, there is no single cure for arthritis. *All* nutrients— not just one—should be employed. Leo V. Roy, M.D., of Orlando, Florida, lists the following diet fundamentals every arthritic should follow.

Eat as many fresh raw vegetables, fruits, and as much protein as possible.

Masticate thoroughly so that saliva is mixed with food and better utilized.

Eat slowly. Avoid large quantities.

Proteins: Every meal should contain a protein. One-fourth of the daily food intake should be protein. Best sources: Fish, eggs, nuts, cheese, raw certified milk.

Meats: Use internal organs, rich in vitamins and minerals. Avoid all canned and processed foods. Fowl, lamb, steak are good.

Dairy Products: All kinds of cheese, natural and fermented; yogurt, and natural buttermilk.

Raw Vegetables: All. Especially celery, cucumbers, and carrots. Make salads using oils for dressing.

Cooked Vegetables: Baked potatoes and brown rice are nutritious. Use raw bean sprouts and other sprouts. *Do not overcook any vegetable.* Steam, bake, broil, or use as little water as possible.

Fruits: Especially apples, grapes, bananas, or local varieties.

Juices: Fresh-squeezed or bottled grape juice—no sugar added. No tomatoes. No citrus fruits except as flavoring. Maximum of one teaspoon lemon juice for salad dressing.

Cereals: Try the fresh-ground combination—wheat, rye, sesame seed, flax and millet. Do not boil. Soak 15 to 20 minutes in hot water over a double boiler, or soak overnight and warm. Raw sunflower seeds, raisins, or shredded coconut may be added before eating.

Bread: Use sparingly. Only stone-ground fresh whole wheat or rye.

Soups: Bouillon or consommé.

Acid Drink: Where there is insufficient acid or where there are calcium deposits, use 1 tablespoon apple cider vinegar to a glass of water (with or without honey—1 teaspoon) at least twice daily.

Molasses and Cane Sugar Syrup: Old-fashioned blackstrap (not sulphured) and pure cane syrup available from health food stores. Only one sweet daily, and that in small quantity.

Oils: Especially sesame, safflower and sunflower oil. All seeds and raw nuts.

Avoid all of the following:

Tea.	Commercial Cereals.	All hydrogenated (hardened)
Coffee.	Processed foods.	fat.
Alcohol.	Canned meats.	Roasted nuts.
Canned foods.	White flour.	Stale nuts.
Stale foods.	White sugar.	Stale wheat germ.
		Stale wheat germ oil.

Overcooked and reheated foods.
Jams, jellies, syrups, ice cream, soft drinks, tobacco.
All chemicals added to your food. This means sweeteners, emulsifiers, thickeners, fluoridated water.

Read your labels carefully.

The preceding diet is believed to prevent as well as relieve arthritis.

WHAT ABOUT YOUR EMOTIONS?

Rebecca Beard, M.D., says, "Arthritics are the kind of people who go after something and never give up . . . gently it is true, with no outbursts of temper and without nagging, but persistently and consistently pushing toward a goal of perfection. . . .

"I know a woman who has not stopped for ten years trying to make her husband use proper English. . . . Why this should disturb the woman, I don't know. But it has and she had had arthritis in all the small joints of her body. . . .

"This is what I should like to say to every arthritic. Relinquish self. Relinquish too much pride in accomplishment for yourself and those whom you love." (See Bibliography.)

Remember Pemberton's dog whose leg was tied off—leading to arthritic deposits? In a similar manner, tension can impede circulation to joints.

Optimism, according to Dr. Roy, speeds progress in improvement. A 13-year study at the Cornell University arthritis clinic found that such emotional disturbances as broken homes, financial problems, and long-hidden resentments could cause the disease.

Another study revealed that emotional upsets decrease the retention of calcium. The amount of decrease was in exact ratio to the amount of tension experienced. (*American Journal of Clinical Nutrition*, November, 1962.)

This revelation helps many parts of the arthritic puzzle to fall into place. As already established, stress or strong emotion can both stop the manufacture of hydrocholoric acid in the stomach, and destroy vitamin C reserve in the adrenals, within seconds. Result: no body acid to dissolve calcium. It piles up; proteins are not digested; toxins accumulate and infections can take hold. Illness and aging are invited.

Try to learn to be easygoing and to drain off your grievances in some wholesome way. Use work, play, reading, or hobbies to sidetrack your worry. Prayer can help, too.

And whenever you suffer from any emotional disturbance whatsoever, *your body needs instant help*. Supply acid in some form. (See p. 333.)

THE EFFECT OF DAYLIGHT ON HEALTH AND ARTHRITIS

Lights are turned on early in some chicken houses to increase laying. It was formerly assumed that this light kept the chickens awake, thus causing them to lay more eggs. But later research found that increased egg production was a direct result of the light reaching the pituitary gland (a master gland), through the chicken's eyes.

John Ott, a photographer who did time-lapse photography for Walt Disney, tells in his book, *My Ivory Cellar*, how he began to apply this principle to himself. He found that his arthritis improved when he spent long daylight hours outdoors *without his glasses*. His vision also improved, he says, and sore throats and colds became less frequent. His friends who tried it reported success with other disorders ranging from bleeding gums to bursitis. One man, a photographer who had spent many hours in the dark room, was a diabetic. For four years he had been troubled with hemorrhaging eye blood vessels. He decided, on Mr. Ott's suggestion, to try spending as much time outdoors as possible. At the time he was almost totally blind and could barely distinguish between day and night. After being outdoors as much as possible for six months, his eye blood vessels ceased to burst and he could see the vague outline of the sidewalk on which he walked. Mr. Ott is convinced that spending much time behind windows, spectacles, and windshields, causes trouble. He also thinks artificial light is deleterious to health.

He says, "If the theory of the importance of the full spectrum of sunlight energy proves to be true, it will necessitate some changes in our present way of living. However, it will not mean that everyone will have to go back to living in caves or grass huts. It will mean using certain types of plastic or glass which will permit the transmission of ultraviolet and shorter wave lengths of light energy. . . . It will also mean that artificial lights will have to be developed that more closely give off the same distribution of energy as natural sunlight. . . ."

Mr. Ott has built himself a house with windows made of plastic instead of glass; he spends as much time outdoors as possible, without wearing glasses; and the canes which he formerly used for help with arthritis have now been discarded.

REMEDIES WHICH HAVE GIVEN RELIEF

Leo V. Roy, M.D., finds that deep breathing can help arthritis. Whenever stiffness comes on, he says, breathe fast and deep for five minutes.

Massage, correctly applied, is another aid. It can help unused muscles to improve in tone and circulation. Its greatest usefulness is in cases where joint function and muscular activity have been impaired. Finally, Dr. Roy considers hydrotherapy (water treatment) an excellent relief. It has a beneficial, stimulating effect on the blood circulation, relieves muscles, reduces pain.

Mildred McKie, M.D., suggests the following uses of hydrotherapy.

Soaking is used to relax the body, and for muscle fatigue or strain. Hands or feet can be soaked for 10 minutes three times daily or oftener to relieve pain. Keep stirring the water with the hand to supply a fresh current to the skin.

Wet Compresses are made by dipping a cloth in water, squeezing, and applying to the part. They are usually used for small areas such as the eyes and should be changed every two to three minutes.

Sitz Bath is taken the first thing in the morning or the last thing at night. It consists of sitting in three inches of water for three minutes. A *hip bath* is taken before the noon meal, sitting in eight inches of water for eight minutes. In both of these baths the feet and body are kept warm and dry. Says Dr. McKie, "These baths are helpful in all kinds of acute conditions such as infections of the intestinal tract as well as chronic conditions like constipation, etc. . . . They are good for low-grade temperature following fevers of unknown cause." (See Bibliography.)

Wet Pack: To reduce a high fever, draw out inflammation, infection, or poisons from the body, she advises wet packs. "Short, frequent packs are stimulating, longer packs are sedative. In subnormal body temperature . . . packs are indicated to relieve inner congestion and pain [and] to induce sleep or promote elimination. . . ."

Wet Packs:

Cleanse the skin of waste products thrown off in perspiration.
Secure better elimination and circulation.
Promote heat radiations through the skin and regulate the temperature.

"Every time the pack is removed, the part covered by it must be washed with fresh water, dried with a coarse towel and rubbed briskly with the hand to stimulate circulation and prolong the effect. If the body is not washed, the waste products are reabsorbed by the skin and go back into the body."

Wet packs may be used on the throat, abdomen, chest, arm, leg, or wherever necessary, but the all-over body pack is the most effective.

Here is the method: Put a plastic sheet on your bed to keep it
Boil water in a large enameled bucket to remove chlorine and
mpurities in the water. While it is cooling slightly,

fold several thicknesses of blankets lengthwise so that you can roll them over you quickly when you lie down. If you have someone to help you, so much the better. Peel off all your clothes. Take two single white sheets, dip them in the bucket of hot water and wring them out. Wrap one around your back, and put the other wet sheet across the front of your body.

Now lie down quickly while the sheets are warm and tuck them around every crevice, under arms, groin and bottom of your feet, up to your neck until you look like a mummy. Free one arm long enough to reach for the blankets at your side and spread them over you, tucking them in as best you can. At first the wet sheets will feel cold but within a very few minutes, they will begin to warm up and lull you into a delightful, drowsy state of relaxation. Set an alarm clock for one hour to one hour and fifteen minutes. This must be no longer, since some therapists feel that the poisons which have been drawn out of the body will be reabsorbed.

When the time is up, rub yourself all over briskly with a bath towel, while you are running a tub or shower of warm water. While under the water—for a few minutes only—rub your skin again to remove any waste products, which have been brought to the surface. Drop your wet sheets into the bucket and leave them until morning. Then get into bed for a good night's sleep!

The next morning boil your sheets (in the same bucket), hang them in the sun to sterilize, and then carefully examine the water left in the bucket. It may be all shades of color, depending upon the amount of poisons secreted by your body. It may contain flecks of mucous and other impurities. A friend of mine who is a heavy smoker was incredulous to discover that the color of the water after using the body pack was a dark chocolate brown which gradually became lighter on subsequent use of the pack.

ULTRASONIC WAVE TREATMENT

Ultrasonic or "silent" sound waves (see also "Human Electronics—Radiesthesia," ch. 12) apparently break up microscopic adhesions which cause pain. Dr. William Bierman, former chief of the department of physical medicine at Mt. Sinai Hospital, New York tested this treatment on a 52-year-old woman who had been crippled by severe neuritis for three years. After all other methods of treatment had failed, only three treatments of ultrasonic sound, during which the patient felt merely a mild vibration, removed all pain.

Still more impressive: Dr. John H. Aldes of Cedars of Lebanon Hospital in Los Angeles, conducted a seven-year study with 7,000 people. They were treated with ultrasonics for various disorders including degenerative spine, hip joint disease, bursitis, and arthritis. Here are the results as reported in *Medical Clinics of North America*, Vol. 42, p. 1205:

96 per cent of tennis elbow experienced complete relief.
91 per cent of gouty arthritis showed "marked relief of symptoms."
78.6 per cent of spinal arthritis patients were relieved of symptoms.

DESERT INDIAN REMEDY

Still another treatment for relief from arthritic pain is a desert tea which has been used by the Indians of the Southwest. This particular tea is made from the leaves of the Creosote Bush (*Larrea divaricata*) and is called by the Spanish name "Gobernadora" meaning governor (of the body). It has apparently helped many people, including a man, who makes regular pilgrimages to the desert, picks the leaves and ships them for tea-making. He prefers to supply this herb through health food stores who can order it. However, if this is not feasible, you may write for prices.* This supplier *is not legally allowed to answer letters or ship the herb if the purchaser mentions by letter that the herb is intended for the treatment of any disease, including arthritis.* The supplier makes absolutely no claims for the tea. So inquire about prices only.

Meanwhile I have heard from, or talked with many people who have received beneficial effects from the tea. One of these is a nationally known ordained minister, also a former chemist who was undergoing orthodox medical treatment for his painful arthritis without receiving permanent cure. Hearing about this Indian desert

* For the source of the tea, see Bibliography.

tea, he tried it. He writes, "I have not been back to the doctor since; members of my congregation have been helped too."

The tea is strong-smelling, strong-tasting. Those who take it begin with as little as one-half teaspoon and work upward to a soup-spoonful. Doctors, nurses, and laymen have themselves experienced relief from pain this way. I have watched an arthritic friend respond to it; after years of agonizing pain, he is pain-free. He says, "Except for a neck that is still stiff, I feel wonderful. When I first began taking the tea, I couldn't walk." Some people are relieved of pain within a few weeks, although they notice some improvement sooner. Others improve in two or three months, they tell me.

BEE VENOM

According to Joseph Broadman, M.D., bee venom often relieves certain types of arthritis and rheumatism. This therapy has long been accepted and reported in medical journals in many countries in Europe. In Dr. Broadman's opinion, the causes of arthritis are multiple, but impaired circulation and inadequate oxygen supplied to the tissues are among the major problems. He says, "It is for this reason that the oldest cures for arthritis and rheumatism— exercise, massage and heat—were often successful. They increased the circulation and therefore oxygen to the tissus."

Dr. Broadman's explanation of the bee-venom therapy (which is given medically by injection, not by the bees themselves) is that it mobilizes the body's protective forces and stimulates reconstruction by the adrenal and pituitary glands. He thinks that the bee venom's curative powers are best explained by its stimulating effect on blood and blood vessels—in short, its ability to increase circulation.

He says, "In many of the newer cases, where no joint changes have yet occurred, improvement and recovery are so rapid that it is difficult for the average person, even the physician, to believe it."

The first treatment with bee venom includes a test for allergy to the venom, which takes a few seconds. If there are no allergic reactions within 15 minutes, the patient can proceed with treatment without danger of complication. Dr. Broadman concludes, "The technique is simple. Any physician can readily grasp it either by reading my book or by observation at my clinic. In his book, *Bee Venom*, Dr. Broadman lists 40 case histories of people who were cured and have remained free of symptoms since treatment.

COPPER BRACELETS

Copper bracelets for arthritis have long been considered a huge joke by critics who assure the public that if they experience any relief from wearing them, it is a coincidence.

If, as they claim, it is a coincidence, then there are many coincidences! I, too, was somewhat skeptical until two physicians assured me that copper did indeed help beginning arthritic pain. Such a verdict from two individuals in good medical standing started me on a search for people who might have benefited. The search has been a fascinating one. Here is some information which came to light: Primitive man, including Egyptians, Scandinavians, South American and North American Indians, wore copper bracelets for the relief of aches and pains. In Peru the Incas wear copper today and natives claim they have no rheumatic troubles.

A. J. Tuck, an artist and designer, and his daughter Mary have made copper jewelry for many years. When letters arrived from hundreds of customers, convinced that copper bracelets helped their arthritis, the Tucks were naturally intrigued. At first they treated the idea lightly. But after making the jewelry for nearly ten years, Mr. Tuck decided to try it for his own arthritic condition. When he first started wearing copper bracelets, he was stiff from head to foot. Relief came gradually. In about six to eight weeks, he was climbing steps and picking things off the floor to demonstrate how limber he had become. The Tucks have never made any claims that copper bracelets can cure. It is their customers who have reported that pain stopped, swelling abated. Apparently, most results began to occur in from four to eight weeks, although some people reported quicker results. People who were unable to get up out of a chair or a bed or to walk up and down stairs testify they were able to do so after a period of wearing the bracelets. Some report they regained the use of their hands. The Tucks merely say: Make this a do-it-yourself project. At least no one has ever reported any harm from wearing a copper bracelet.

Doctors have ordered bracelets and some have recommended them to their patients. Since the Tucks no longer are in the jewelry business, they feel free to pass on some of the theories they have picked up over the years from their former customers:

The more copper one wears, the better, especially at first.
Many people wear two bracelets, day and night. (Some even wear them around their ankles.)
If you seem to have results and are not sure what is responsible, do not wear the bracelets for 30 days and see what happens.
Lacquering does not seem to interfere with the action of the copper.
To clean (if not lacquered), remove grease with soap. Then plunge into a solution of 2 parts of vinegar to 1 part of salt added to water. Keep in a wide-mouth jar. Drop the copper bracelets into the solution for a few seconds once a week.

I too have letters in my files from people who claim they were helped by wearing copper.

ANOTHER NATURAL REMEDY:

Dr. George Ohsawa writes in his book, *Zen Macrobiotics*, "Arthritis is very easy to cure. Observe the macrobiotic diet very strictly (see "Macrobiotics," p. 125).

HOMEOPATHIC REMEDIES:

The homeopathic physician does not prescribe for a disease but for the patient. He prescribes the indicated remedy in the smallest possible dose, which often effects a prompt and permanent cure. (See "Homeopathy," ch. 38.) Schuessler Cell Salts have also brought excellent improvement.

So if you are an arthritic, do not despair. Get to work on these suggested remedies and practice good nutrition. There *is* hope.

25   Asthma

Asthma can be due to an allergy. Discovering the offending allergy, and treating it accordingly, is discussed in the chapter on allergies.

Asthma is, in some cases, due to psychological problems. Peter G. Edgell, M.D., of the Department of Psychiatry of the Montreal General Hospital, says, "Asthmatics have a deep-seated emotional insecurity and an intense need for parental love and affection." Children who have not yet learned to disguise emotions are apt to reveal these traits. They cling to their mothers, are self-centered, usually have a high I.Q., but often fail to perform well in school due to fear of failure.

Dr. Leon Unger and Dr. Albert Howard Unger, of Northwestern University Medical School, warn that oversympathy on the part of the family may make symptoms worse.

Although some drugs give temporary relief, they can also cause trouble. The *Journal of the American Medical Association* (October 11, 1952) states that aspirin (acetylsalicylic acid) may cause severe asthma in some people.

When climate and weather are suspected as a cause, many experts urge asthmatics to investigate allergies before pulling up roots and making unnecessary geographical changes. It may be an allergy—not the weather. It is true, however, that some people, apparently, are sensitive to changes in barometric pressure, temperature, humidity, altitude, and wind.

Diet can definitely play a part in the asthmatic's improvement. In *Body, Mind and Sugar*, Dr. E. M. Abrahamson, reports that asthmatics have a consistently low blood sugar. This condition is *not* corrected by eating sugar or sweet foods. They give the blood sugar only a temporary lift to be followed by a lower drop again, thus creating a vicious cycle. The preferred treatment is to supply protein foods, which raise the blood sugar and keep it high for an extended period of time. Nuts, cheese, meat, fish, fowl, and dairy products are preferable to sweets or coffee. For a complete diet list, I recommend that you see *Body, Mind and Sugar.**

Edward Podolsky, M.D., Brooklyn, New York advises the use of calcium for asthma. He says, "Carefully controlled experiments by clinicians in an eastern clinic reveal that the use of calcium gluta-mate causes apparently definite improvement in asthmatic patients with whom other types of treatment have failed." (*Let's Live*, June, 1964.)

One of the most dramatic reliefs from asthma I have ever seen was that of a teen-age boy. He had been an asthmatic victim since he was three and his frantic mother had taken him from specialist to specialist. The boy had been given every type of drug available with no lasting results. I gave a copy of Adelle Davis', *Let's Eat Right to Keep Fit*, to his mother, hoping that nutritional treatment might help to build up the boy's general resistance. In the book she found this statement about asthma: "Large amounts of vita-min (C) are usually needed at first to saturate the tissues; the quantities can later be reduced. Persons suffering from arthritis, asthma and other chronic diseases have often taken drugs for months, even years; these drugs must apparently be detoxified be-fore vitamin C is available to the tissues."

Acting on this information, the mother gave her son several thousand milligrams of vitamin C daily plus a calcium tablet for every 1,000 mg. Within a surprisingly short time, the boy's attacks ceased. He now uses a smaller daily maintenance dose, in addi-tion to a completely well-rounded nutritional regime. His asthma is under complete control.

The mother was overwhelmed at such a simple, quick, and ef-fective measure. She took the copy of Adelle Davis' book to her physician, a personal friend, and asked, "Why didn't you tell me vitamin C was such a wonderful help for asthma?"

He looked a little sheepish and answered, "I didn't know about

* The diet also appears in Clark, *Stay Young Longer.*

it." The doctor is not to blame. Unfortunately, nutrition is not yet taught, as such, in medical schools.

Breathing exercises can be of help during an attack. Dr. Ernesto Escudero, a chest surgeon of Buenos Aires, found that breathing exercises helped 400 asthmatic cases, including his own son. He urges his patients to inhale in short gasps, rather than deep slow breaths. He encourages parents to use the "wheelbarrow" technique, helping the patient walk on his hands while someone else holds up his feet.

An easier way of getting the head lower than the feet is suggested by the Asthma Research Council of Great Britain which advises, "When you get up in the morning, kneel on a chair and let the upper part of the body bend over, head nearly touching the floor. While in this inverted position, you are to cough continuously for three to five minutes. While doing this, mucus is usually coughed up, which is followed by a great deal of relief."

SOME NATURAL REMEDIES

Fenugreek seed—1 teaspoonful used either in 1 cup of boiling water as a tea or ground dry, fresh daily, and added to foods—is an old remedy for dissolving mucous.

Eric F. W. Powell, in his booklet, *Health Secrets of All Ages*, says, "A partial fast (under doctor's supervision) followed by a starchless and sugarless diet, will usually clear up most cases of asthma. [See "Overweight and Fasting," ch. 42.] I have cured many dozens of bad cases by this method alone. Deep breathing is necessary. The following herbal infusion can be taken at frequent intervals. It is harmless and any quantity may be taken. Use during the night if necessary. For best effects take hot:

Liquorice	½ oz.	Ginger root (powder)	1 tsp.
Horehound	½ oz.	Lobelia seed (powder)	1 tsp.
White Pine needles	½ oz.		

Place the mixture in two pints of cold water and cover. Bring very slowly to a boil. As soon as the boiling point is reached, remove from fire. Keep covered and allow to stand 15 minutes; then strain off liquid. Sweeten with pure honey. Take a tablespoon at frequent intervals, as needed or desired."

Eleanor Amend, D.C., adds, "Asthmatics generally have a calcium deficiency. Tend to this."

She suggests first aid to relieve attacks:

Towel wrung out of ice water placed on chest for three minutes, then a vigorous massage with hands dipped in cold water, on throat and chest.

Place on the chest a six-fold cloth dipped in hot water and vinegar; replace every 15 or 20 minutes.

One teaspoon brown apple cider vinegar in one pint of water; heat and inhale fumes with towel over the head.

Comfrey leaf (an herb) has been found helpful. As an example, H. E. Kirschner, M.D., quotes from a letter he received. "A farmer friend casually nibbled a comfrey leaf in the front garden of Mrs. D. H. Johnson of Cambridge, New Zealand. As a result she is now being overwhelmed by requests for the leaf. . . . [The man] had suffered from asthma for thirty years. His first night of unbroken sleep followed. Trying to trace the reason for this unusual experience, he thought back over his action of the previous day. He decided it must be the comfrey leaf he had eaten and he sent for more. Now he eats some every day and has not suffered from asthma since."

Comfrey has brought relief to asthmatics in other countries, including the United States. Dried comfrey leaves may be purchased at health food centers. For sources of fresh plants (which are easy to grow and remain green all winter even in cold climates) see Bibliography.

26 Backache

The first thing to remember in treatment of backache is that separate parts of the body are not isolated; they work together as a whole. They have the same blood stream which links them together, the same nerves, and the same quality of tissue, muscles, and bones. Although your back may bother you most, you may also have other such related disturbances such as fatigue, nervousness, irritability, constipation, and possibly arthritis. Often when general health is improved, several of these complaints also disappear. So, to help your back the first thing to do is to build up your general health.

WHAT CAUSES BACKACHE?

It may be caused by:

Acute or chronic disease (kidney or prostate infections, flu, arthritis, etc.).
Women's complaints.
Injury, stress, strain (long sitting, improper lifting).
Mechanical problems (one shorter leg, poor posture, high heels).
Emotional problems (painful muscle cramping resulting from tension).
Poor nutrition.
Insufficient exercise and relaxation.

These are sedentary days. Typists sit for hours; commuters have been known to acquire "railroad spine" from sitting in uncomfortable train seats. Even children who wiggle and squirm at school may do so because of too much sitting. Too long periods of watching movies or television can take a toll, too. Riding for hours in a car without getting out now and then to stretch can create a tense back.

To reduce strain, check on the angle of your automobile seats and the amount of leg and knee room.

Check also on your chairs at home. One chair does not suit everyone. Tall people need a deeper chair; short people a more shallow one. Provide both.

A housewife may be leaning over a too-low stove, sink, or ironing board; a typist over a too-low desk. A woman may carry all her paraphernalia—vacuum, clothes basket, groceries, even babies, on one side only. She may lean sideways as she carries, instead of keeping her spine straight.

Men may not lift properly. They should not lift suddenly. They should lift with their arms, transferring the strain to their legs, not their backs. If two people are lifting, they should agree to pick up their burden at exactly the same moment. Otherwise one person's back becomes overtaxed. If you move furniture, lean against it and shove; don't push with your arms. If you pick up anything, bend your knees. In other words, keep your spine as straight as you can as often as you can. At all times, watch your posture; keep your head high, chin in, shoulders down, abdomen in. You will protect your spine and look more attractive at the same time. When you sit to work, sit with spine straight, preferably on a hard chair.

WHAT IS A SLIPPED DISC?

A disc is something like a thick-skinned grape. It has a tough outer coating and a soft pulpy interior. It serves as a cushion between vertebrae. Sometimes these grapelike cushions rupture and the pulp protrudes a little. The process is inaccurately known as a "slipped" disc. If the cushion disappears entirely, the result is known as a degenerated disc. In slipped-disc trouble, the nerve is affected in such a way that the pain radiates down the thigh and leg. If the disc "slips" in the neck area, it causes numbness, and pain radiations to the arms.

Contrary to the usual belief by those who swear that a sneeze, a twist, or a bend was responsible, disc trouble does *not* come suddenly. It has been building up for a long time. The final twinge is only the last straw.

W. J. McCormick, M.D., considers a slipped disc a result of a vitamin C deficiency. (See "Infections," ch. 39.)

Our ancestors fared better than we do. They had fewer labor-saving devices. They did less riding, less sitting, and got more exercise. In their day, slipped discs were unheard of. Many specialists now believe that 80 per cent of all backaches are caused by muscles which are too weak or too stiff to do the work they should be able to take in normal stride.

WHAT TO DO ABOUT BACKACHES

Weak abdominal muscles often result in chronic backaches. Physicians at the State University of Iowa, College of Medicine, prescribed an exercise for 58 of their chronic backache patients. Forty-two were relieved of pain. The exercise is simple: Lie flat on your back. Clasp hands behind your neck. Tuck your toes under a bed or sofa. Sit up 10 to 12 times each day.

Another method of strengthening abdominal muscles resulted in a significant improvement in a study of 889 patients with low-back pain. This study was conducted at Madigan General Hospital, Tacoma, Washington. The exercise was a modification of the sit-ups recommended by the Iowa physicians. Instead of keeping legs straight, hips and knees were kept at a 45° angle during the sit-ups. When patients were discharged, they were urged to perform the exercise 15 to 20 times daily, at least five days per week.

Dr. Hans Kraus, of New York University, after examining 5,000 cases of back pain also believes that backache is mostly due to lack of exercise. Whether for prevention or for treatment, he recommends these safety measures for people in sedentary occupations:

A few minutes of exercises daily.
Changing chairs from time to time.
Five-minute breaks for walking around, or simple exercises if possible.

Dr. Michael Newton, of the University of Mississippi School of Medicine, has with the help of Mabel Lum Fitshugh, a physical therapist, devised this simple exercise to relieve backache during pregnancy: Stand 18 inches from the kitchen sink. Bend forward at hip joints. Keeping arms straight, place your hands on the edge of the sink. Inhale, and at the same time, allow your back to curve inward or to become as "sway back" as possible. Then exhale, round out your back, tuck buttocks under and keep knees slightly bent. Repeat three times. Now stand straight, shoulders relaxed, knees flexed slightly, buttocks tucked under. Carry weight evenly on both feet—a position in which the pelvis is level. This posture should become a habit, provide relief from physical fatigue, and improve appearance.

Another clue to backache: Take off your shoes and strip to the waist. Have someone look at your back critically. Does one shoulder lean in one direction, curving the spine with it? Fold several thicknesses of newspaper and slip under the heel of the foot on that side until shoulders are level. Then ask your shoemaker to attach a raise to the heel of the shoe the thickness of the newspapers. Your backache may be over.

Sleeping on a firm bed helps many a backache. Or, putting a bedboard under the mattress may help. In addition, you should relax your back at least once a day—preferably before going to sleep. For best results, according to Harry Clements, D.O., of England, it is necessary to be flat on your back, *not* on a sofa or a soft bed, but on a hard floor. (see Bibliography). This allows the pressure of the whole body gradually to straighten out the spine. Those who try it may find they will sleep much better, since an unrelaxed back can often stay tense all night.

And remember, the physician of the late President John F. Kennedy prescribed a rocking chair.

To relieve neck tension after long hours at your desk or behind the wheel of your car, Dr. Ann Wigmore, D.D., suggests:

Rolling your head around on your shoulders, first one way, then another.

Pulling in your chin as far and as hard as you can, at the same time stretching the back of your neck.

Leaning your head on one side, then another, pulling the cords of your
neck until they hurt.

These exercises relieve strain, according to Dr. Wigmore, stimulate circulation, and whisk away cobwebs from the brain. They may
also help to achieve a prettier chin line.

High heels are a major cause of backaches. Try lower heels, except for festive occasions and see if your back doesn't agree. Back
experts suggest that if a woman takes regular exercises to
strengthen her back (which automatically strengthens her front),
relaxes flat on the floor at intervals, gets plenty of rest, wears working heels, and increases her intake of corrective nutrients, her backache will probably disappear.

Change your position as often as you can. A large manufacturing
plant discovered that in 15 months it had paid $20,969.91 in work-
man's compensation and lost 1,203 man days because of backaches.
The company started a plan of two-minute stretching exercises on
the job. Result: During the next 15 months, payments were reduced to $2,448.88 and man days lost to 119. (*American Practi-
tioner*, September, 1958.)

Your backache may be caused by misalignment of the bones in
your feet. To correct this problem (and many enthusiastic people
have) read and follow the explicit directions in Dr. George A.
Schroeder's book. (See "Feet," p. 288.)

WHAT ABOUT NUTRITION?

Calcium and protein are a *must*. Dr. Richmond W. Smith, Jr., at
Henry Ford Hospital, Detroit, Michigan, studied 72 women with
back pain associated with osteoporosis and compared them with
40 who did not have the problem. The healthy women consumed,
on the average, 862 mg. of calcium and 76.6 grams of protein
daily, whereas the less healthy averaged only 584 mg. of calcium
and 61 grams of protein.

Joseph C. Risser, M.D., professor of orthopedics at the College
of Medical Evangelists in Los Angeles, says, "Materials for bone
matrix as well as the necessary mineral salts are essential. Proteins

and vitamin C are necessary for development of bone matrix. Vitamin D, calcium, phosphorus, and the essential trace minerals are necessary to make bones of good quality. Foods that have been processed for storage and shipping to avoid spoiling have little of these nutrients and should be eliminated from the diet." (*Journal of Applied Nutrition*, Vol. 13, No. 4.)

Vitamin C has proved helpful in relieving low-back pain, and averting spinal-disc operations, according to James Greenwood, Jr., M.D., of Baylor University College of Medicine. Dr. Greenwood claims that 500 to 1,000 mg. of oral vitamin C daily, has successfully relieved pain and averted the need for operations. He has treated more than 500 disc-injury patients, including himself, with vitamin C therapy. (*Health Bulletin*, October 3, 1964.)

Backache can be caused by sustained tension arising from emotional problems. Thomas H. Holmes, M.D., and Harold G. Wolff, M.D., point out that a backache can develop in an individual who faces a threatening life situation involving conflict, anxiety, and other strong emotions. This tension may locate in the neck or back. Some people may also exhibit a tense back ailment in their attempts to maintain security or to get along well with other people. (*Life Stress and Bodily Disease*, Vol. 29 of the 1949 *Proceedings*.)

Drs. T. L. Dorpat and T. H. Holmes write: "In an attempt to restore comfort and productivity to patients with backache of muscle tension origin, one must take a broad perspective which considers the patient's many problems as an interrelated whole. One must not think of the illness in terms of either psychiatric or orthopedic disease, but must consider that both factors are combined and entwined to produce the clinical picture. Management of the patient with emotional disturbances should include an attempt to deal with the personality features that bring about the pattern of muscular hyperfunction. The patient should be allowed to ventilate his suppressed and hostile and guilty feelings and helped to understand something of his emotions, reactions and attitudes." (*Postgraduate Medicine*, Vol. 25, No. 6, June, 1959.)

Give your body, and your back, all the help you can. Don't pamper it; strengthen it through proper nutrition, exercise, and relaxation. Then when you need it most, it won't complain.

27 High blood pressure —hypertension

"In reading blood pressure," writes Herman Pomeranz, M.D., "the doctor mentions two numbers. The first, known as systolic, refers to the contraction of the heart by which the blood is driven onward and the circulation kept up. The second, known as the diastolic pressure, and frequently the more important, indicates the amount of pressure exerted by the blood on the walls of the arteries."

Of great interest to many practitioners is the difference between the two pressures, known as the differential. If you subtract the lower number from the upper number, this difference may give a clue to the state of the arteries. Dr. Russell Sneddon says it is generally understood that the differential should vary between 40 and 50 points; however, he feels this is too high. He prefers a differential of 20 to 30 points. He adds, "A low differential pressure means a less vigorous circulatory flow, and also decreased tension in the arteries with a reduction in the wear and tear of the circulatory system."

But in a survey reported in the *Medical Journal of Australia* (May 24, 1958), of 15,000 healthy individuals age 65 or older it was found that the average blood pressure for all persons studied, from ages 65 to 105, was 145/82 for men and 156/84 for women. This study seems to disprove the old advice that your systolic blood pressure (upper figure) should be 100 plus your age. Actually, blood pressure should remain basically the same throughout life.

Dr. Pomeranz feels that a single blood pressure reading is inconclusive. Nearly everyone's pressure goes up many times each day for many reasons. "Until 1950," he says, "a person whose systolic pressure [upper figure] was consistently above 140-160, and whose diastolic [lower figure] was repeatedly higher than 90, was considered to have high blood pressure or hypertension. . . . A patient after the age of fifty may have a systolic pressure of 160-190 and a diastolic pressure of 100 to 110 and still be in good health."

The law of individual differences operates in blood pressure readings. Medical interpretations of readings can vary, too.

WHEN IS PRESSURE TOO HIGH?

Dr. Pomeranz considers blood pressure too high if it ranges from 150/100 to 200/120 variable pressure with few noticeable physical changes; or 170/110 to 250 with certain body disorders beginning to show up; or a diastolic pressure (lower figure) higher than 140, if it is accompanied by certain physical changes. As to what these physical changes are, it is better for your doctor to diagnose them. It is too easy to imagine symptoms. Remember Job who warned that what you fear may come upon you. So, let the doctor take over this function.

WHAT CAUSES HIGH BLOOD PRESSURE?

Those practitioners who use the natural approach to health do not consider high blood pressure a disease in itself. They consider it a *symptom* of some disturbance within the body.

A specific cause may be kidney malfunction, body toxins, constipation, glandular inbalance (adrenals especially), excessive smoking, alcohol, emotional tension, or nutritional deficiencies relating to any or all of these disorders. The condition of the arteries may be at fault, too. Dr. Sneddon writes, "If for any reason, the arterial walls have become hardened, the resistance to the passage of blood will naturally be very much increased, and a higher pressure required to force the blood to a distant part of the body . . . this tends to raise the blood pressure."

Melvin E. Page, D.D.S., agrees that arteries may be a factor in hypertension, but he also believes that the tension of the arterioles can be due to maladjustment of the nervous system. The main general cause of high blood pressure is, in Dr. Page's opinion, a faulty body chemistry.

Dr. Arthur F. Coca has discovered still another—and previously unsuspected—cause: food allergy. He writes, "The idea that high blood pressure can be a consequence of food allergy did not come out of the blue. It arrived as a result of routine examination of the blood pressure . . . in two patients."

These cases aroused his suspicion and the chase was on. Other cases were tested and that early chance finding led to a major discovery: that food allergy could indeed raise blood pressure in some people.

Dr. Benjamin Sandler cites evidence that low blood sugar can play a part in hypertension; and in a study by five scientists at Creighton University School of Medicine, Omaha, findings revealed that on-again, off-again dieting was another cause.

Dr. Lester Morrison states that tobacco can cause blood pressure to soar. (See p. 316.)

WHAT ABOUT SALT?

This brings up a fascinating debate. There is too much research to show that salt *can* intensify high blood pressure in *some* cases to ignore it as a possibility.

It is also true that some people, suffering from high blood pressure, given as little as one-tenth teaspoon of salt daily experience a drop in blood pressure. Raise the salt in those people and up goes the pressure. Lawrence Galton, a medical reporter, has found that the elimination of salt has helped only about one-fourth of the hypertensives.

In Japan, people who use rice only, in spite of a lower salt intake, are more prone to high blood pressure than those who eat barley. A study with rats provides an explanation. Barley contains more pantothenic acid (a B vitamin) than rice does. Rats given pantothenic acid had a lower pressure than those who were denied it. (*Tohoku Journal of Experimental Medicine* [1963], Vol. 78, pp. 347-351.)

Studies of rats fed high-salt rations for long periods show considerable variation. Selective breeding has produced a strain of rats in which hypertension (and high blood pressure) develops as a result of a high salt ration; another strain shows no change in blood pressure when fed the same ration; a third strain reveals hypertension on no extra salt at all. (*Nutrition Reviews*, May, 1964.)

Raymond Bernard, Ph.D., denounces salt. He feels that salt can rob the body of calcium, disturb the kidneys, and act as a poison. He explains, "If there is too much salt for the kidneys to eliminate, the excess is deposited in various parts of the body, especially in the lower part of the legs. In order to protect itself from these deposits, the body automatically seeks to dilute it by accumulating water in these areas. As the tissue becomes water-logged, the body tends to swell up. Feet and ankles bloat painfully."

But Walter C. Alvarez, M.D., points to the difficulty of the saltless diet as a remedy for many cases of high blood pressure. He adds, "My patients, when placed upon it, would rather die of their high blood pressure than live on the tasteless food that is given them."

George W. Crane, Ph.D. and M.D., surprisingly recommends the use of sea water to provide natural organic salt. One starts with a dosage of several drops a day and works upward to not higher than 1 to 3 teaspoons daily.* Sea water is said to contain 44 natural nutrients. It has long been known to have a chemical constituency almost identical to healthy human blood. One family of my acquaintance puts carefully filtered, condensed sea water in a cruet on the table along with the oil and vinegar and adds it judiciously to food.

Kathleen Hunter of England says, "To make common salt nontoxic it is necessary to add a small percentage of potassium chloride to it." Dr. Henry Gilbert, who studied the subject deeply, said that

* See discussion of sea water in "Arthritis" chapter, p. 180.

when the balance between sodium and potassium is upset by eating common salt . . . it cannot be restored except by potassium salts. . . . Dr. Gilbert also made some careful calculations as to the amounts of potassium salts that must be combined with sodium chloride to make it non-toxic.

Many people use sea salt, which contains a number of minerals in addition to the sodium chloride of ordinary table salt.

WHAT IS THE BEST TREATMENT FOR HIGH BLOOD PRESSURE?

For a disturbed body chemistry, Dr. Page uses corrective nutrition. He eliminates all refined sugar, white flour, refined foods, alcohol, and coffee. He allows weak tea or de-caffinated coffee. In extremely resistant cases, he supplies the body with infinitesimal amounts of certain hormones. I have heard him remark that when a body chemistry is in perfect balance, the blood pressure *can't* rise above normal. And he has cases on file to prove it.*

Losing excess weight can help to reduce pressure in some cases.

Certain special nutritional elements have been found helpful. Edward Podolsky, M.D., cites a study in which 55 patients were given eight grains of calcium lactate in water one-half hour before meals. High pressures were reduced to normal. (*Illinois Medical Journal*, August, 1939.) Calcium is the calming mineral. Vitamin B complex also helps to calm nerves. The two together, or separately, can be gradually increased to provide a sedative effect. Lecithin can also act as a natural tranquilizer.

The Drs. W. E. and E. V. Shute of Canada warn that vitamin E, although a help for circulatory disturbances, must be used with caution in certain cases of high blood pressure.

Bicknell and Prescott, in the English classic, *Vitamins in Medicine*, report success with the use of rutin in restoring capillary fragility to normal. Labels should be checked to see that rutin is added to bioflavonoid complex.

Blood pressure has been lowered by the use of a protein supplement. Dr. W. M. Ringsdorf, Jr., and Dr. E. Cheraskin, of the Uni-

* Dr. Page's method is discussed more completely in Clark, *Stay Young Longer*.

versity of Alabama, significantly lowered the blood pressure among a group of dental students in only four days by giving them 40 grams of a protein supplement every day. (*Journal-Lancet*, Minnesota State Medical Society publication, February, 1964.)

There is evidence that magnesium may lower blood pressure. (See "The Magic Mineral, Magnesium," ch. 17.)

Many people have reported normal blood pressure as a result of eating garlic perles. I had planned to mention this purely as a folk remedy. I found, however, scientific confirmation of its value in a European publication, *Praxis* (July 1, 1948). Dr. Piotrowski of the University of Geneva conducted a study of 100 subjects and found that blood pressure began to drop after about a week of garlic treatment. Dr. Piotrowski used high amounts of oil of garlic (it is available in perles which produce no after-taste or odor), gradually decreasing it over a period of three weeks, then following with a small maintenance dose until the blood pressure remained at its correct level. There are two medical theories for the success of garlic: (1) that it contains a germicidal agent; (2) that it dilates the blood vessels, an action which is considered responsible for its success in lowering high blood pressure.

To avoid breath odor, you can mince fresh garlic fine and swallow it *without* chewing. Put it in a teaspoon and place on back of tongue. Swallow it with a glass of water. These instructions assure us that no one will detect it—the chewing is responsible for the after-odor.

WHAT ELSE CAN YOU DO?

Emotions play a great part in keeping blood pressure high. An emergency of any type—fear, worry, rage—usually activates the adrenal glands. This is a natural body defense, but the victim of high blood pressure is often inclined to be a constant worrier, thus maintaining a continual state of emergency. His adrenals remain in a chronically overactive state and it is difficult for him ever to relax completely. If he does, he often goes from continuous excitability, a state not unlike a constant whipping of an already tired horse, to the other extreme—extreme lethargy and fatigue. If a person is driving himself relentlessly, he should *not* take tranquilizers; when the hypertensive is in a slump he should *not* take pep pills. Such treatment merely masks the condition, and does not correct it. (See "Why Drugs?" ch. 3.)

There are things you can do to help yourself—or your husband, if he has high blood pressure. If you, as a wife, feel inclined to put any type of pressure on your high-pressured husband, ask yourself first, "Is it necessary?" Nagging, piling chores or problems on an already overtired man the minute he comes home, is not the way to encourage relaxation. Overfussing is just as bad; be as serene as you can.

A husband should not use his wife as a whipping girl either. He must face himself, realize his own weaknesses. He must learn how to say No and how to get away by himself if family tensions temporarily bother him. He must find relaxing, wholesome activities. Sports (if they are not allowed to become too competitive) and escape reading both help. One man I know, when ready to blow his top as a result of frustrating encounters with people, takes refuge in a woodworking shop set up in his basement. At the end of the day he works off his frustrations there. By bedtime, he is calm and relaxed again. His blood pressure remains at a normal level. At the Yale School of Medicine, Dr. H. M. Marvin provides handiwork and reading material and avoids talk about symptoms or problems. Usually, no conversation at all is allowed. Patients who have registered a high pressure for five years have returned to normal on this program.

A Texas doctor, L. A. Whitehall, M.D., has discovered that people with high blood pressure often forget to breathe properly—a factor which raises the carbon dioxide in the blood stream. He found that if patients breathe slowly and deeply before blood pressure tests, the pressure readings are often reduced.

A treatment in England some years ago was based solely on breathing exercise. Those who did regular deep-breathing exercises without any other change in their treatment registered a definite drop in pressure for six weeks, at which time they maintained that level. Letting all the air out of the lungs, refilling, then letting it escape slowly as if one were whistling, is an excellent breathing technique.

One of the most helpful books I have found is, *There Is an Art to Breathing*, by Virginia Zoros Barth (Llewellyn Publications Ltd. [1960], 8921 National Blvd., Los Angeles 34, California).

Exercise can be a help. Clement G. Martin, M.D., says, "Even men in middle age who have not exercised regularly in many years can achieve a marked reduction in blood pressure through a carefully graduated increase in their daily walks. An hour's daily walk not only exercises your blood vessels, but the long continued contracting of the muscles increases the flow of blood in the body and its return to the heart. The heart responds with a greater contracting force calling forth better circulation within the heart itself and the opening of more blood vessels. The increased number of channels for blood to flow through results in less resistance to flow and as a result, reduction in blood pressure."

A Japanese physician, Dr. Takashi Sugiyama, has reported that whole or partial bathing is a popular form of therapy for high blood pressure in Japan and other oriental countries.

And here is more good news for those who worry about high blood pressure. Perhaps your diagnosis has been wrong! Physicians at Henry Ford Hospital on checking 355 patients who had had blood pressure readings greater than 150/90, retested them. To relieve nervousness during testing, each patient was asked first to rest on a comfortable bed or cot. A technician took pressure readings every five minutes for a half hour. Fully half of the subjects showed no hypertension at all! This means, according to the physicians who conducted the study, that there may be 10 million of the presumed 20 million hypertensives in the United States who are needlessly treated for high blood pressure. (*Postgraduate Medicine*, Vol. 24, p. 26.)

The most successful and most lasting treatment of high blood pressure is aimed at the body as a whole, not at relieving the blood pressure alone. By clearing up the general condition of the body, many disturbances may fall by the wayside, high blood pressure among them.

It is a tenet of the natural approach that the patient himself is responsible for gaining and maintaining health; that nature alone heals. Particularly is it necessary in treating high blood pressure to strengthen the vital force so that it can help. This can be done in a multifold manner: through correct nutrition, exercise, deep breathing, relief from emotional tension—even prayer.

FOLK REMEDIES

Eric F. W. Powell (*Secrets of All Ages*) suggests this remedy for high blood pressure due to arterial causes: "It is doubtful whether there exists a better remedy than the common stinging nettle. While nettles act better when they are used fresh, they may also be used when dry. Nettles are a harmless remedy for removing the 'fur' from the arteries and making them elastic. They are rich in chlorophyl, which is much praised as a rejuvenating remedy. When using fresh leaves, pour a half pint of hot water over a tablespoonful cut up fine; let stand for twenty minutes, strain and drink before meals. Make fresh each time. When using the dried leaves, infuse a dessert spoonful in a pint of water and simmer gently for fifteen minutes. Strain. A cupful before meals."

If high pressure is due to "clogged arteries" here is another remedy: According to R. Swinburne Clymer, M.D., it promotes bile flow and digestion and thus eliminates build-up of cholesterol. In *Nature's Healing Agents*, he gives these formulas to be taken in water after meals:

Tincture of Barberry (*Berberis vulgaris*)	5 to 10 drops
Tincture of Oregon Grape (*Berberis aquifolium*)	10 to 20 drops
Tincture of Goldenseal (*Hydrastis canadensis*)	8 to 10 drops
Tincture of Mandrake (*Podophyllum peltatum*)	sufficient for proper elimination

—or—

Tincture of Fringe Tree (*Chiolanthus virginica*)	7 to 10 drops
Tincture of Yellow Gentian Root (*Gentiana lutea*)	5 to 20 drops
Tincture of Oregon Grape (*Berberis aquifolium*)	10 to 20 drops
Tincture of Goldenseal (*Hydrastis canadensis*)	8 to 10 drops

Tincture of Mandrake (*Podophyllum peltatum*)

sufficient for proper elimination and/or bile salts in conjunction with these formulas

28 Cancer

Freedom of speech and the press is growing weaker every day, particularly on the subject of cancer. Nearly every month newspapers hint that a cure is just around the corner. But none is forthcoming. Perhaps the following opinions of courageous people—some of them reluctantly anonymous—who are still not afraid to speak up, will help to explain why. Try to maintain an open mind until you have read them all. The final acceptance—or rejection—of this information is undeniably yours. If all cancer remedies had been given unbiased hearings, this section might possibly be mercifully blank.

SOME OPINIONS ON THE CANCER PROBLEM BY VARIOUS REPORTERS

Remember, I am merely reporting the views of others.

1. R. A. Holman, M.D., honorary consultant bacteriologist,

United Cardiff Hospitals, and senior lecturer, School of Medicine, University of Wales, has summed up the cancer problem in a startling and significant manner. He is one of the leading authorities in the world on the bacteriological approach to cancer.

"Cancer is, of course, a condition which has been recognized in man for thousands of years. . . . In recent decades we have become aware that there is an ever increasing number of physical and chemical agents which can cause cancer in laboratory animals and in man, e.g., X-rays, ultra-violet light, radium, certain dyestuffs, soot, tar, etc. . . . In my opinion, *the only common denominator is the cell upon which these agents act* [emphasis mine]. . . .

"As a result of the rapid technological advances, large numbers of physical and chemical agents have been placed or released into man's external and internal environment with little thought about the possible long term effect of these on his own cells. . . . On top of these the body may manufacture certain cancer producing chemicals as a result of other stimuli. . . . Alexander Berglas regards the notion that we could control these environmental agents as utopian, and, therefore, demands an all-out attack on finding a cure for cancer a truly defeatist attitude. . . .

"Our two main therapeutic weapons at the present day are amputation of the growth by surgical means, and a variety of forms of radiation. Numerous workers have pointed out that such measures are merely temporary and restricted stop-gaps, and this is borne out by the poor survival rates after the use of such measures. The real attack on the treatment of malignant growths must come from intelligent interference with the catalase-peroxide mechanism [catalase is a body enzyme]. . . .

"Almost thirty years ago, Maisin succeeded in controlling certain animal tumors with dihydoxymethyl peroxide. Motawei, in Cairo, reported significant results in animals and humans with hydrogen peroxide alone or combined with X-ray. Certain American workers, who have been working along the same lines with H_2O_2, have caused rapid destruction of tumors in periods as short as seven days. . . .

"To develop a far more effective cure it is essential that the catalase-peroxide mechanism be exploited in order to determine the most efficient way of over-oxidizing the catalase-deficient cells. A perfect method of doing this is going to be very difficult to produce because, in certain sites, e.g. the liver, where the catalase concentration of normal cells is high, it will be extremely unlikely that the cancer cells growing there can always be affected when so well buffered by the surrounding catalase.

"Louis Pasteur emphasized that it is far more important to prevent a disease than treat it. . . . The direct treatment of such diseases by chemotherapeutic and antibiotic agents has not been, and never will be, responsible for their elimination. . . . We have a terrible disease which is one of our worst killers; and to stop this we must prevent the tumor starting. It is the only sure way. . . .

"The plan for prevention of cancer should be threefold:

"1. To increase our intake of catalase.

"Catalase, as well as many other enzymes, is destroyed by heat. Civilized man now lives primarily out of the can, the bottle and the package. . . . The agents used to destroy the bacteria invariably destroy the catalase in the food. . . . No other species of animal has such a diet. It would be to everyone's advantage if the consumption of fresh fruit and vegetables were to be markedly increased, thus ensuring a far greater intake of catalase and peroxidase. There are numerous references in the literature to the fact that garlic-eating people have an increased resistance to cancer. This is not surprising when one realizes that garlic is very rich in the catalytic systems containing catalase and peroxidase.

"2. To increase the manufacture of catalase by our own cells.

"It was shown many years ago that if a normally active creature is forcibly imprisoned in a cage so as to limit its normal activity, then after some weeks the catalase content of the body decreases. Conversely, normally inactive creatures can be made to develop more catalase if forcibly exercised. It is very probable, therefore, that the chronic habit of limiting the muscular activity of man, by encouraging him to imprison himself in cars, trains and other forms of mechanical locomotion . . . is doing much to diminish his normal catalase level. . . . In general, a higher concentration of catalase implies an increased consumption of oxygen which provides a catalytic system of prime importance in the detoxification of our bodies.

"3. To curtail the intake of agents which destroy or inhibit the action of our cell catalase.

"This is probably the most important mode of attack. . . . The main pathways are ingestion. . . . Chemical agents have been added to food and drink in order to kill bacteria, resulting in a longer shelf life; to color the products, resulting in increased sales; to act as sweeteners, flavoring agents, etc.; to accelerate the growth of chickens, bullocks, fish, etc. . . .

"It has been estimated that there are now more than 1,000 additives to our food and drink. Many of these interfere with the catalase-peroxide balance, e.g., sulphur dioxide, sodium nitrate, sodium fluoride, certain hormones, insecticides, fungicides and dyes. . . . The deliberate addition of that poisonous substance Sodium Fluoride to public water supplies, with the intent of delaying the onset of dental caries, is a most unscientific and unethical measure. Sodium Fluoride is a potent catalase poison and is cumulative. Its use is not backed up by sound medical facts, and in any case, it does not deal with the prime cause of dental decay . . . [which is] a chemically adulterated food supply. . . .

"It is [also] obvious that the control of air pollution demands our most urgent attention. . . . A good oxygen intake is essential for good health. . . . Oxygen is essential for the removal and destruction of many toxic agents present in or on our cells. . . .

"Many drugs now used can interfere with cell respiration. . . .

"X-rays and other forms of irradiation are known to inhibit catalase.

"Chemical filth (pollution) is the major public health hazard of time. . . .

"Cancer prevention, the only effective scientific method of controlling the disease, can show results if we pull together and reform some of our bad habits so prevalent in our civilized way of living."

These excerpts are quoted from Dr. Holman's monograph with his permission. They were also published by *Prevention* (May, 1963) and labeled by that magazine as one of its most significant articles.

2. "Malcolm Lawrence," pseudonym for a well-known reporter:

"Economically, cancer is one of the most important diseases to both doctor and patient. To the former the flow of money is 'in'; to the latter the flow is 'out.' It is no less than astounding that a surgical procedure which hardly has one long-term survival to boast of is still followed if the patient can afford it. Some students of the subject believe that a poor cancer patient has a better chance for survival than a rich one because the poor man might escape the full surgical treatment.

"To dispel any doubt, consider the interview given some time ago by a non-conformist surgeon, Dr. Paul R. Hawley . . . president of the American College of Surgeons. He told a reporter that one '. . . would be shocked at the amount of unnecessary surgery that is performed.' (*U.S. News & World Report*, February 20, 1953.)

According to this article, the reporter asked: "Why do you suppose a doctor makes an unnecessary operation?"

"Money," Dr. Hawley replied.

"Just plain dishonest money-making? . . . Do you think there are doctors who would do this just for the sake of money?" the interviewer pressed.

Said Dr. Hawley, "I don't think it, I know it, and I can prove it."

Dr. Hawley may or may not have been talking about cancer surgery; however, no more lucrative field for the surgeon's knife exists in the entire kingdom of medicine.

Why is it that independent researchers in the field of cancer who believe they have something worthwhile can never get any place with the American Cancer Society? The Society spends millions of dollars to tell the public that it is looking in every nook and cranny for the answer to cancer. But as soon as a scientist comes along who is not a cog in the finely meshing wheels of organized medical research, he is put under the thumb of the "recognized" researchers. He either has to sign away personal rights to his discovery, or (more likely) he is stalled and ignored.

3. Excerpts from Hearings before a Subcommittee of the United States Senate, conducted by Senator Claude Pepper, July 1-3, 1946:

Dr. M.: ". . . A survey made by Dr. Stanley Reimann of cancer cases in Pennsylvania over a long period of time showed that those who received no treatment lived longer than those who received surgery, radium or X-ray. The exceptions were those patients who had received electrosurgery—in other words, the surgery with an electrical knife—and lived approximately as long as those who received no treatment whatsoever. The survey also showed that following the use of radium and X-ray much more harm than good was done to the average cancer patient. This is a conclusion which is not generally accepted and is highly controversial among leading cancer workers. It would appear that none of the routine measures employed today to combat cancer is as effective as their proponents would have us believe."

4. W. A. Dewey, M.D., former professor of medicine at the University of Michigan Homeopathic Medical College, said, ". . . In a practice of nearly 45 years I have yet to see a single case of cancer, save a few semi-malignant epitheliomata, cured by surgery, X-ray or radium."

5. Professor Hardin B. Jones, Department of Biophysics, University of California Medical School, declared that there was evidence to indicate that untreated cases of cancer survive longer than those that are treated. (From "Demographic Consideration of the Cancer Problem," *Transactions of the New York Academy of Science*, Series II, Vol. 1, No. 4 [1956], pp. 298-333.)

6. F. Allen Rutherford, M.D., who received his training from Johns Hopkins and University of Pennsylvania Medical Schools, and has served as coroner of Lebanon County, Pennsylvania, as well as on the teaching staff of the University of Pennsylvania, Department of Urology, says, "Surgeons can only hope that their operations will be effective in removing cancer; radiologists can only hope that they have been able to burn out the cancerous areas; doctors who inject various chemicals can only hope that the cancer will be eradicated before the patient dies. None of them can look at a patient and say with any surety that the treatment they plan to use will be effective." (From an interview with *Prevention* magazine.)

7. *The FitzGerald Report:*
A Report to a Senate Committee on the Need for Investigation of Cancer Research Organizations, carried in the Congressional Record of August 28, 1953, Pages 5690-93.

From: Benedict F. FitzGerald, Jr., special counsel to the Committee on Interstate and Foreign Commerce.
To: Hon. John W. Bricker and members of the Interstate and Foreign Commerce Committee of the United States Senate.

Subject: Progress report on study requested by the late Senator Charles W. Tobey.

"Pursuant to the above, the undersigned commenced a collection and study of material covering the operations of foundations, hospitals, clinics and government sponsored organizations specializing in cancer problems, . . .

"I have approached this problem with an open mind. Recognizing the importance of men skilled in the science of medicine, who are best informed, if not qualified, on the question of cancer, its causes and treatment, I directed my attention to the propaganda by the American Medical Association and the American Cancer Society to the effect: namely, that radium, X-ray therapy and surgery are the only recognized treatments for cancer.

"Is there any dispute among recognized medical scientists in America and elsewhere in the world on the use of radium and X-ray therapy in the treatment of cancer? The answer is definitely, Yes; there is a division of opinion on the use of radium and X-ray. Both agencies are destructive, not constructive. In the alleged destruction of the abnormal, outlaw or cancer cells both X-ray therapy and radium destroy normal tissue and normal cells. Recognized medical authorities in America and elsewhere state positively that X-ray therapy can cause cancer in and of itself. Documented cases are available.

"If radium, X-ray or surgery or either of them is the complete answer, then the greatest hoax of the age is being perpetrated upon the people by the continued appeal for funds for further research. If neither X-ray, radium or surgery is the complete answer to this dreaded disease, and I submit that it is not, then what is the plain duty of society? Should we stand still? Should we sit idly by and count the number of physicians, surgeons and cancerologists who are not only divided but who, because of fear or favor, are forced to line up with the so-called accepted view of the American Medical Association, or should this Committee make a full scale investigation of the organized effort to hinder, suppress and restrict the free flow of drugs which allegedly have proven successful in cases where clinical records, case history, pathological reports and X-ray photographic proof, together with the alleged cured patients, are available?

"Accordingly, we should determine whether existing agencies, both public and private, are engaged [in] and have pursued a policy of harassment, ridicule, slander and libelous attacks on others sincerely engaged in stamping out this curse of mankind. Have medical associations, through their offices, agents, servants and employees engaged in this practice? My investigation to date should convince this Committee that a conspiracy does exist to stop the free flow and use of drugs in interstate commerce which allegedly has solid therapeutic value. Public and private funds have been thrown around like confetti at a country fair to close up and destroy clinics, hospitals and scientific research laboratories which do not conform to the viewpoint of medical associations.

"How long will the American people take this?

"In this connection this Committee should investigate the advertising agency which controls all advertising in the Journal of the American Medical Association as well as the various State Journals. Why is the stamp of approval, by the so-called nutrition experts and their Council on Foods, placed on certain foodstuffs, denied to others, and others condemned without a reasonable investigation? Is there any relationship between approval by these experts and the operation of the advertising agency in the offices of the American Medical Association?"

Respectfully submitted,

Benedict F. FitzGerald
Special Counsel

WHAT CAUSES CANCER?

1. J. R. Davidson, M.D.: "I decided to make the assumption that cancer was a deficiency disease and to follow this line of research wherever it might lead me. . . . In 10 years of experiments with white mice it was possible to observe cancer in rapid development during several generations, a thing which could not be done in the case of human patients. . . . One strain I fed on a diet of high vitamin content and the fourth generation was a fine, healthy animal with no trace of cancer whatever. . . . [Another strain] I fed on a very poor diet, and at the end of the fourth generation . . . I succeeded in developing a strain of mice with 100 per cent cancer. Then taking the offspring of this strain, I fed them a high vitamin diet and eventually developed a strain which would resist cancer. . . . This established to my satisfaction . . . that cancer is directly dependent on diet. . . ." (*Cancer, A Nutritional*

Deficiency, Reprint No. 18, Lee Foundation for Nutritional Research, Milwaukee 3, Wisconsin.)

2. Two teen-agers, in joint research at Yeshiva University, also uncovered information that cancer is linked with nutritional deficiency. The research was conducted under the supervision of Dr. Robert D. Barnard, a consultant to the Cancer research division of the Department of Health, New York City, and was read to the Fifth International Congress on Nutrition. The conclusion of their investigations was summed up: ". . . that cancer is merely a local manifestation of a body-wide deficiency and can sometimes be treated by feeding patients substances that accelerate cell growth." (*New York Times*, September 3, 1960.)

3. Other factors found by investigators to contribute to cancer are:

A. Viral infections.
B. Trauma (accidental or surgical injury).
C. Hormone imbalance.
D. Radiation.
E. Malnutrition.
F. Constant irritation of latent bacterial (and spirochetal) infections and chemical irritations.

"Alexander Berglas, member of the Cancer Research Foundation of the Pasteur Institute, indicates that *anything* which serves as a constant irritation is capable of causing cancer. He states as examples, 'Irritation and deficiency factors will cause the regulatory mechanisms to fail' . . . factors such as 'industrial noxae' [poisons], denatured nutrition, artificial fertilizers, production of adulterated foods, accumulation of insecticides in foodstuffs." (Report: *The Public Wants to Know* Independent Citizens Research Foundations, 71 West 23 St., New York City.)

4. Smoking, air pollution, and stress have also been found to be contributing factors.

5. D. T. Quigley, M.D., late of Omaha, Neb., and a cancer specialist, says, "One of the few things we do know at the present time about cancer is that it is a disease which follows another disease. It is never primary, but always secondary. It never grows on healthy tissues, but always on previously diseased tissues. The part

of a body on which a cancer grows has a special soil on which the invader finds a favorable environment. If the soil is not prepared in advance, the cancer simply cannot and will not take root and grow. . . . Whether the immediate cause of cancer may be ultimately found to be a virus, a fungus, a bacillus, or a chemical compound makes little difference in the question of prevention. The important fact is that the diseased area on which the cancer finds its suitable soil must not be allowed to exist. *By the prevention of locally diseased areas in the body, we may prevent cancer.*" (*The National Malnutrition*, Milwaukee 3, Wisconsin: Lee Foundation for Nutritional Research, 1943.)

In 1949, Dr. Quigley showed many slides at a meeting of the American Academy of Applied Nutrition, of patients before and after surgical removal of cancer. He said that in over 30 years of experience, *not one of his patients who had followed his dietary recommendations had had recurrences of cancer!*

6. Irritation. There is no such thing as a common 'carcinogenic' factor—the mechanism of action of 'carcinogenic substances' being always and solely a matter of constant irritation. . . . Irritation and deficiency factors will cause the regulatory mechanisms to fail. . . ." (Alexander Berglas, *Cancer: Nature, Cause and Cure* Paris: Pasteur Institute, 1957.)

SOME SPECIFIC IRRITANTS (CARCINOGENS)
Sugar

Albert Brandt, reporter: "There is a great deal of evidence connecting the excessive consumption of sugar, refined or not, with cancer. Nobel Prize-winner Dr. Otto Meyerhoff of the University of Pennsylvania Medical School called attention to 'the appetite of tumors for sugar' and suggested that the growth of cancerous tissue might possibly be stopped if biochemists could find a way of curing this appetite." (*Refined Sugar Can Wreck Your Health*, Reprint, Lee Foundation for Nutritional Research, Milwaukee 3, Wisconsin.)

X Rays

"Some states have outlawed the use of fluoroscopy in the fitting of shoes. The United States Public Health Service has recommended that the widespread use of the photo-chest X-ray survey be discontinued. The hazards of X-ray exposure were emphasized by measurements reported from the Department of Radiobiology at the Massachusetts General Hospital." (*The New England Journal of Medicine,* January 29, 1959, p. 197.)

The American Public Health Association recommends that before submitting to any X-ray examination you should ask the doctor these questions:

Is the examination necessary?
Who is to make the examination?
Has he received formal training in radiology?
Is the assisting technician certified or qualified by formal training?
(*Changing Times,* February, 1959.)

"X-rays should definitely be avoided during the early months of pregnancy, four experts warned. This means that they should be avoided whenever possible in at least the first three months, and there should be no such thing as 'routine' X-rays. . . . It has recently been discovered that one of the largest doses to the reproductive organs is received in the dental chair where 15 to 20 exposures are shot in a sitting position and the rays are directed downward toward the pelvis." (*Science News Letter,* August 22, 1959, p. 118.)

"Dr. Milton T. Edgerton of the Johns Hopkins Hospital, Baltimore, presented data at the National Cancer Conference in Minneapolis showing that in more than eight of every ten cases of thyroid cancer in children under 17 years of age, the patient had received substantial X-ray exposure of the head, neck or chest region years earlier for some non-cancerous condition such as acne, sinusitis or enlarged thymus gland. These exposures Dr. Edgerton said, are very many times more severe than those received in chest X-ray and in dental diagnosis. The interval between the X-ray treatment and the development of thyroid cancer, he said, ranged from about three to twelve years, with the average around eight. The data suggest, he added, that the thyroid gland of infants and children is markedly more suscepitble to cancer-producing effects of radiation than is the thyroid gland of adults." (Science section, *New York Times,* September 18, 1960.)

Excessive Sunlight

"Excessive exposure to sunlight and ultraviolet rays can change certain chemicals on the skin to cancer-producing substances, warns Dr. T. R. Allen. More than 90 per cent of all skin cancers occur on exposed areas. Most susceptible are the fair-skinned who should be particularly careful to avoid overexposure." (*Nature's Path.*)

Emotions

Psychological tests given to 127 cancer patients, who did not yet know that they had cancer, revealed that emotions had apparently played a role in their illness. The official journal of the American Cancer Society reported, "The results were consistent with the observations of others who have described the cancer patient as unable to express his angry feelings and as covering them up with a facade of pleasantness." Yet the patients themselves did not seem to realize they possessed this trait. Involved in the psychological study were 34 patients with lung cancer, and 19 with cancer of the prostate, as compared with 74 subjects who were healthy or had other diseases.

Lest this sound too far-fetched, Dr. Bernard Roizman, Johns Hopkins University School of Medicine, provides the explanation. Many people may harbor a "sleeping" tendency to cancer. Under normal conditions symptoms do not appear. But when the body is subjected to an emotional upset, a physical disturbance of some type, or a generally run-down condition, the sleeping cancer tendency may flare. Thus, emotional as well as physical upsets may trigger cancer in some people.

NATURAL IMMUNITY AND SPONTANEOUS REGRESSION

Dr. Weston Price in his worldwide search for healthy people found no cancer except where people were eating civilized and refined foods, while Dr. Albert Schweitzer reported no cancer among the Africans he observed, until civilized foods were introduced. The late Vilhjalmur Stefansson reported no evidence of cancer among Eskimos until the introduction of civilized foods, and Sir Robert McCarrison, M.D., found the Hunzas, who live on natural foods, to be free of cancer.

Dr. Cornelius P. Rhoads, late director of the Sloan-Kettering Institute, New York, reported that some persons threw off cancer as easily as they did a common cold, whereas others were easy victims. The first definite proof that the human body possesses a special defense system or immunity against cancer was found when cancer cells were injected into healthy volunteer prisoners, at Ohio State Penitentiary. The prisoners experienced only soreness similar to a smallpox vaccination. But when cancer cells were injected into volunteers already suffering from cancer at Memorial Hospital, New York City, instead of minor soreness, cancer flourished. Dr. Rhoads's belief was that the natural defenses of the body can be made more effective if they are given a chance.

Dr. Warren Cole and associates at the University of Illinois report that they found 55 cases out of 400, dating back to 1890, which had fulfilled the requirements for true spontaneous regression, i.e., that the body, for some unknown reason, cured itself.

Dr. Tilden C. Everson of the University of Illinois College of Medicine, cites 130 documented cases of cancer classified as "probably examples of spontaneous regression." *The New York Times*, October 22, 1963, reporting Dr. Everson's findings, says, "In some of the cases documented, it seemed that something happened inside the patient's body within a matter of weeks, sometimes almost overnight, that made conditions unfavorable to cancer."

A study, reported in the *Journal of the American Medical Association* (November, 1961) conducted by Drs. Peter A. Herbut, Theodore T. Tsaltas, and William H. Kraemer, found an active agent in tumor-inhibitory principle (TIP) in the liver. The

Journal stated, "It appears that the normal human liver produces an inhibitory principle which it imparts not only to the bloodstream, but also to the bile."

An extract was made from guinea pig muscle, spleen, kidney, heart, brain, and liver. The researchers found TIP only in liver.

One substance apparently to help the body develop immunity to cancer is found in shark liver. Dr. John H. Heller, of the New England Institute for Medical Research, which is sponsoring a shark hunt, explains, as reported in *Medical World News* (June 19, 1964), how the shark liver substance works.

The hard-to-come-by shark lipid is a potent stimulator of a number of the body's defense activities. Its most important property is its effect on animals with either viral or nonviral tumors.

"The lipid reduces or delays the incidence of tumors, retards tumor growth, increases the life-span of tumorous animals, shows metastasis, and brings about tumor regression."

More tests are needed, but the outlook appears hopeful.

CAN CANCER BE PREVENTED?

Dr. Harry Rubin, of the University of California Virology Laboratory, feels that in the war against cancer, it is more practical to build up the body resistance and defenses against cancer than to fight it. (*Modern Nutrition* [June, 1961], p. 8.)

The late Dr. D. T. Quigley, mentioned above, and whose patients had no recurrence of cancer, provided they followed his dietary advice, agreed that the best way to prevent cancer is to build up the body defenses through excellent nutrition. In this way the tissues, cells, and organs are kept in such a healthy state that, in his opinion, cancer cannot take hold. His dietary advice is to avoid absolutely all refined, synthetic, and processed foods. He bans white flour, enriched fortified foods, white sugar and foods with chemical additives. He recommends natural foods, whole foods, raw vegetables and fruits, generous amounts of protein, raw certified, instead of pasteurized milk, whole grains, plus all the known natural vitamins and minerals. Dr. Quigley wrote:

"A return to normal food alone will never bring health up to normal standard. To make up for past dietary sins, concentrated vitamins should be taken for six months to two years, in order that the individual may reach a point where, with his reserve restored, he can carry on with a balanced diet. . . . It is essential that the concentrate contain all of the vitamins, both known and unknown. . . . For this reason no synthetic preparation can completely replace the vitamins in which the average person may be deficient. Such foods as yeast, liver and wheat germ are excellent sources. . . ." (*The National Malnutrition.*)

Dr. J. R. Davidson (now retired), former associate professor of clinical medicine at the University of Manitoba says, "I believe cancer, a deficiency disease, can be prevented and controlled by a suitable and balanced diet, high in vitamin content.

"I do not pretend to be able to benefit patients in whom the disease has reached advanced or terminal stages, because that does not give any treatment a fair chance. In the patients whom I am treating, however, some of whom have suffered from clearly diagnosed cancers of a severe degree, I can claim some improvement in many cases.

"The diet I prescribe, varied to some extent in each individual case, includes one pint of vegetable juice per day, such as carrot, lettuce and celery juices, prepared freshly, plenty of raw vegetables, particularly peas, beans, carrots, spinach, lettuce, whole wheat bread, supplemented by wheat germ, meat cooked rare, raw milk, and concentrated vitamins of various kinds." (Reprint 189, Lee Foundation for Nutritional Research, Milwaukee 3, Wisconsin.)

Consumers Bulletin (September, 1957, pp. 18-22) gives excellent advice for cancer protection:

"It is known that diet is an important factor in preventing the development of bodily conditions that tend to favor the beginnings of a cancerous condition, and with care and willingness to go to a little extra trouble, we can modify our eating habits in ways that will reduce the likelihood of cancer striking us and our families.

Avoid:

Dyed oranges.
Dyed potatoes, both sweet and white.

Dyed or colored nuts.

Margarine colored with anything except carotene, a natural color.

Caponized poultry.

Turkey and chicken necks.

All dyed foods, including colored desserts and bakery goods.

Burned and fatty foods, especially overtoasted bread, buns, overbroiled steaks, hamburgers, chickens. Remove any charred or tarry substances, burned edges and fats.

Since obesity tends to cancer, cut down on calories and alcohol, fat, sugar, starches. Eat instead, high quality proteins: meat, fish, eggs, natural cheese.

Avoid processed, refined foods, excessive intake of foods, too hot beverages and an over-consumption of pepper and spices."

Read Labels.

WHAT SUBSTANCES PROVIDE PROTECTION?

At the Sloan-Kettering Institute for Cancer Research, four groups of rats were fed rice and butter yellow (a known cancer producer). One group was given nothing to protect them against the butter yellow. All animals developed cancerous livers within 150 days. Brewer's yeast was given to a second group. "The results showed that the addition of 15 per cent yeast to unpolished rice had a distinct protective effect against the pathologic changes leading to the development of liver cancer. *All* the rats receiving yeast, examined between 100 and 200 days after beginning the experiment had smooth and practically normal livers grossly and microscopically."

In a second experiment, desiccated liver was substituted for yeast. Liver in the amount of 10 per cent of the diet was necessary to prevent cancer, but prevent it, it did. When the amount was cut to only 2 per cent, protection did not occur. Dr. Kanematsu Seguira, who supervised the experiment, said, "These dietary influences (liver and brewer's yeast) may prove to play a large part in the causation, prevention and treatment of human cancer." (*Journal of Nutrition,* July 10, 1951.)

Dr. Forbes Ross, a British surgeon specializing in cancer, reported that during his entire practice none of his patients ever developed cancer. He attributed this freedom from the disease to a liberal use of potassium salts which he incorporated in his prescriptions. Potassium occurs in green leaves, blackstrap molasses and other natural foods. Potassium salts are available through homeopathic physicians. (See "Homeopathy," ch. 7.) (F. W. Forbes Ross: *Cancer, the Problem of Its Genesis and Treatment* [London: Methuen and Co., 1912].)

Catharyn Elwood reports, "In 1938 Drs. Max A. Goldzieher, E. Rosenthal and Z. Mizuna inhibited cancer growth in mice and delayed its appearance by the addition of calcium lactate to the diet. After injections of this calcium food, mouse cancers calcified and growth ceased, showing that calcium has a definite inhibiting power on the growth of certain cancers." (*Feel Like a Million*).

WHAT IF CANCER ALREADY EXISTS?

1. The Right to Try a "Quack" Cure
The *San Francisco Chronicle*, Tuesday, June 11, 1963 reported as follows:

"Three irritated women demanded the right yesterday to choose unorthodox methods of combatting cancer without governmental interference.

"The three were among an audience of 12 who attended a State Department of Public Health hearing on 'cancer cures' it says is worthless and a cancer test it says has no scientific validity.

"The Berkeley hearing was one of two scheduled to consider regulations that would ban the use of the Koch, Mucorhicin and Lincoln Agent 'remedies' and the Bohlen Test for cancer.

"The three women insisted they had the right to select what treatment they wanted even though that treatment might be labeled 'quackery.'

" 'I lost two brothers in eight months from cancer,' one woman said. 'I could get it myself. And I want to know why not let people take what treatment they want? I want to know why after a doctor says he can't cure you, you haven't the right to do what you want.'

"State officials attempted vainly to persuade the irate woman that cancer, to be cured, must be diagnosed and treated swiftly. But after protesting against 'governmental interference,' she flounced out of the meeting.

" 'We must fight this thing,' she said angrily."

2. The Page Foundation, Inc., of St. Petersburg, Florida, dedicated to research in the causes and prevention of degenerative diseases says, "We do not claim a cure or treatment for cancer; we cannot diagnose its presence through our blood tests; but those who are reviewing our cases can show definite correlation between endocrine patterns and the presence of family history of cancer. Furthermore, where correction of inefficiency of body chemistry has been achieved in patients with active cancer, the indirect effects upon the disease are startling and gratifying." (*Health Versus Disease* [St. Petersburg, Florida; Page Foundation, Inc., 1960.])

3. Donald C. Collins, M.D., writing in the *American Journal of Proctology* (12:1; February, 1961), reports complete recovery in some patients. *Modern Nutrition* (January, 1962) states, "Five of his patients who had extensive malignancies of either the gastrointestinal tract, or the blood (leukemia) or sarcomas, all proven by adequate biopsies, were found to have no evidence of these diseases when they died many years later of entirely different causes.

"Dr. Collins stated that on five different occasions in his thirty-six years of practice, he has observed this marvelous phenomenon. In all five cases, through painstaking autopsies performed by highly competent pathologists, no discernable pathologic evidence could be found that such patients had ever had the various malignant diseases previously noted.

"It was found that these five patients had one factor in common—all ate home-raised, organically grown foods that were free from various chemical preservatives and pesticides."

4. According to the *Medical World News*, yogurt apparently has an anticancerous effect. "The harmless rod-shaped organism which makes yogurt out of milk, Lactobacillus bulgaricus, turns out to have a potent anti-tumor activity, according to researchers at the Bulgarian Academy of Sciences in Solla. Injections of LB

extracts, they say, can cure several types of experimental cancers and appear to be effective against human skin tumors.

"Hundreds of mice have been 'completely cured' of usually lethal advanced sarcomas and ascites tumors," reported Dr. Ivan Bogdanov of the Scientific Research Institute for Anticancer Antibodies of the Academy of Science. "Moreover, animals thus cured are immune to further transplants of the same tumor. . . ."

5. The *Journal of the American Medical Association* (August 14, 1954), tells of German doctors who observed a vitamin A and C deficiency in 10 patients with cancer located in various areas of the body. When massive doses of C (1,000 mg.) and A (300,000 international units) were given daily, the natural defenses of the cells were strengthened and cancerous ulcers of the cervix and rectum were healed within three weeks. The patients' general condition was also improved. In more advanced cases tumors became smaller but did not completely disappear.

In Germany, in 1960, 218 patients with inoperable or metastatic tumors were treated with vitamins A and C. "For from 14 to 21 days 300,000 I.U. vitamin A was injected intramuscularly and 1 g. vitamin C intravenously. Then smaller amounts were given parenterally and large amounts by mouth for 3 to 6 months. The effect was generally good and growth of the tumor became stationary or regressed. The treatment should be regarded as auxiliary, not as in itself curative. No side effects of excess of vitamins were seen." (*Nutrition Abstracts and Reviews* [April, 1961], No. 2804.)

6. W. J. McCormick, M.D., Toronto, Canada: "The most definitely established physiological function of any food substance is that of the role of vitamin C in the maintenance of ability and elasticity of connective tissues generally and the growth of new scar tissue in wound healing, and this would include the bones, cartilages, muscles, vascular tissues, subcutaneous tissues and submucous tissues. . . . Deficiency of this vitamin results in instability and fragility of all such tissues by reason of the breakdown or liquefaction of 'the intercellular cement substance (collagen) with easy rupture and ineffective healing of any and all such tissues. . . .

"All forms of physical and chemical irritation predisposing to malignancy, including trauma, thermal and electric burns, ultraviolet ray, X-ray, radium, atomic fission, chronic infections and inflammatory lesions, or exposure to cancerogenic agents, are known to increase the body requirements for vitamin C, the lack of which increases vulnerability of body tissues to all such agents. Accordingly, vitamin C therapy is effective in minimizing tissue damage in all such conditions, thus serving to reduce potential malignancy.

"Schneider cites Eckhorn as finding the vitamin C deficiency of cancer cases very pronounced, while his non-cancerous controls averaged [a much lower deficiency]. On the basis of these findings, he [Schneider] applied intensive vitamin C therapy, 1,000 to 2,000 mgs. daily, supplemented by vitamin A, in some hundred early and advanced cancer cases. He reports marked general improvement as shown in reduction of size of tumors, increase of body weight, lowered blood sedimentation rate, delayed cachexia, reduction in hemorrhage and ulceration. He obtained no complete cures. . . . He considers [the vitamin C therapy] harmless. (From *Cancer: The Preconditioning Factor in Pathogenesis, A New Etiologic Approach, Archives of Pediatrics*, 71:313-322; October, 1954.)

LEUKEMIA

A discovery of leukemia virus particles in human tissues and blood, and the fact that leukemia in mice can be caused by a virus, points to one possible cause of this disease, according to Dr. John B. Moloney, of the National Cancer Institute, Bethesda, Maryland. He emphasizes that there is "no direct evidence" that the presence of leukemia virus particles in humans means that they will cause the fatal disease. *Science News Letter* (March 14, 1964) says, "Even if the virus theory is proved as the principal cause of leukemia, it is known that radiation in high dosages such as followed the bombing of Hiroshima also can cause the disease, as can some chemicals."

X rays of one or both parents may cause leukemia in children. Dr. Morton L. Levin, Roswell Park Memorial Institute, Buffalo, New York, reported a three-year study in which X ray of either parent, or both, often dated back several years before the affected children were born. Dr. Levin based his findings on detailed medical and dental records which included routine dental X rays and chest X rays for detection of tuberculosis. He also warned against the well-known dangers of X rays of pregnant women and irradiation of male or female reproductive organs. He pointed out that X ray cannot be the only cause of leukemia, however, since the disease was known before X rays were discovered.

Heavy exposure to an insecticide spray may also be a cause of leukemia. Acute myelogenous leukemia appeared in a mother and son after heavy exposure to an insecticide spray blown through an open window during elm spraying.

The first symptoms were immediate choking and coughing. Leukemia was diagnosed in the son eight months later, and in the mother four and one-half years later. (*Proceedings of the Mayo Clinic,* 38: 523-531; 1963.)

Leukemia was once thought of as a childhood disease, but it is now found in all ages and takes the lives of more adults than children. It may be acute or chronic. Acute leukemia progresses rapidly; chronic leukemia more slowly. *Science News Letter* (March 14, 1964) reports that acute leukemia is more common in children under 15.

Drs. Karl M. Kolmeier and Edwin Bayrd, of the Mayo Clinic, report, "Many chemicals and drugs have been shown to induce leukemia in animals, but only benzene has been established as an etiologic agent in man. However, other toxic agents, especially the aromatic hydrocarbons in solvents, paint removers, fuels, insect sprays, and fumes cannot be excluded. Any chemical capable of inducing damage to bone marrow is potentially leukemogenic [leukemia causing].

Yet, in both humans and animals, spontaneous cures have been noted even in chemically caused cancers. John A. Osmundsen, reporting in the *New York Times* the proceedings of the American Society for Microbiology (May 7, 1964), says, ". . . cancer cells arise constantly in the body but are usually killed by defense mechanisms . . . [thus] reinforcement in a general way [of] the body's natural defenses . . . might prevent the development of malignancies. . . .

"Exposure of animals to antigens from chemically caused cancers thus called forth the production of antibodies against the tumors, which prevented their growth in animals. . . . Leukemia cells were [also] killed with ultraviolet radiation. . . ."

Vitamin E has proved helpful in leukemia. Adelle Davis, in a speech, "Your Health Is in Your Hands," presented to the American Nutrition Society, stated, "In one case, the bone marrow was examined and disclosed leukemia. After treatment for several weeks with 300 units of vitamin E daily, a recheck of the bone marrow showed it to be normal."

To sum up the cause and treatment of cancer:

"The concept of malignancy as a systemic disease, before tumor development is recognizable, has gained world-wide support from many research specialists. . . .

"Often repeated research would seem to indicate that malignancy is *first* a mild infectious disease involving the whole body. Out of this mild systemic disease a malignant tumor may or may not develop.

"Whether the systemic disease can be cured would seem to depend upon the number of immunity factors the animal has, or can generate, to fight the virus attacking his body. . . . Steadily mounting data suggest that viruses contribute to the cause of most, if not all, types of cancer. . . .

"In searching for cases of systemic malignancy one finds hints that the cancer-causing virus infection exists with, or perhaps because of, imbalances and deficiencies. . . . It is also to be noted that malignant tumors develop in apparently healthy animals in response to repeated small doses of certain chemicals found in man's environment. . . .

"Both research and clinical experience provide bases for the following clinical concept: even if it were possible to surgically remove every bit of tumor mass and every cancer cell in a patient, he would continue to develop new cancer cells and would eventually die of malignancy, unless there were a simultaneous removal of those systemic malignancy conditions which *caused* the . . . tumor mass formation.

"It would seem that surgical removal of a tumor mass should never be followed by a blissful period of 'wait and see what happens—because all the cancer cells have been removed.' Instead there should be a close cooperation between physician and patient in a vigorous effort to rid the body of contributing viruses . . . [and] to rebuild immunity factors in the patient. . . ." (From a documented report, "Is the Answer to Cancer Just Around the Corner?" Independent Citizens Research Foundation, Inc., 1964.)

29 Some little-known cancer treatments

I wish to make it clear that I am not endorsing any of the following as a treatment for cancer. But neither do I take the position that many treatments which have been condemned are worthless. There are reports of documented cases that such treatments have been of help to some people in some situations. In terminal cases, no treatment, no matter how potent, with the possible exception of prayer and spiritual healing (and this has happened), can be relied upon, although some dramatic recoveries have been reported even in terminal cases.

If you have questions about *any* treatment which you may have read about anywhere, I suggest you write to the International Association of Cancer Victims and Friends, 4742 63rd Street, San Diego, California.

In addition to the following "unorthodox" or "unaccepted" treatments, I am including some natural folk remedies for one reason only: to call them to your attention. They carry no guarantee.

They have been used throughout past and present centuries by various tribes or groups of people. I merely wonder why some of the huge grants of money already allotted for research on drugs and synthetic medicines are not more often used to test these natural substances.

Richard Harris in his illuminating articles on the Kefauver investigation (*New Yorker*, March 1964) reported the Senator's opinion of the part the drug industry has played in the problem of cancer: "Despite the urgency of the struggle to find cures for cancer, research in this field has been seriously delayed by disputes with the government over patent rights."

SHOULD THESE REMEDIES BE IGNORED?

Dr. Ann Wigmore, D.D., N.D., has been conducting experiments, under medical scrutiny, on human cases of leukemia. She has been testing the effect of the drink made of fresh wheatgrass, which she calls "Wheatgrass Manna." She says, "More than a dozen victims of this dreadful ailment have had health miracles blossom on their bodies."

You may write to Dr. Ann Wigmore, Box 189, Astor Station. Boston 23, Massachusetts, for information and instruction on how to grow and use the wheatgrass. Dr. Wigmore is quick to point out that wheatgrass should not be construed as a cure for any disease. But by furnishing the body with live minerals, vitamins, trace elements, and chlorophyll, it may be able to repair itself. Judging by the many testimonials which are coming to Dr. Wigmore from all over the United States, this type of nutrition is apparently producing a protective effect in some people.

Iscador the name for a remedy said to be derived from mistletoe. This remedy is being studied by the Society for Cancer Research in Switzerland. The society seeks no material gain, is directed by practicing physicians, and may be contacted by writing to: Society for Cancer Research, Kirschweg 9, Arlsheim, Switzerland. Please include international postage for reply.

Calvacin, an antitumor agent extracted from the giant puffball mushroom (*Calvatia giganteum*). It has been found active against

14 types of animal cancer, as reported in *Science*, by 13 investigators from Armour and Company, Sloan-Kettering Institute, and Michigan State University. According to the science page of the *New York Times*, January 8, 1961, which called attention to this discovery, "The substance is not available for treating malignant tumors in humans but may go on clinical trial by mid-1961." Where is this remedy and why is it not available?

LAETRILE

In his book, *A New Approach to the Conquest of Cancer, Rheumatic and Heart Diseases*, Howard Beard, Ph.D., one of the discoverers of Laetrile writes, "Every now and then we read of 'spontaneous cures' of even terminal cases of cancer in humans, and we are apt to discredit such incredible phenomena. We believe that such unusual cures are due to 'natural' cyanogenic glucosides that have, in some manner, been ingested by the patient. . . . Be that as it may, it is a fact that in Kentucky and neighboring southern states, folks believe that by eating almonds, which like the apricot kernel are rich in cyanogenic glucosides, they can both ward off and 'cure' cancer! The first Laetrile we used some three years ago was . . . the cynaogenic glucosides of the apricot kernel . . . that was followed by prunasin . . . as a starting material."

Information about almonds crops up again in the readings (see p. 94) of the late Edgar Cayce, formerly of Virginia Beach, Virginia, which advocated eating a few almonds a day to thwart a tendency toward cancer. This is reported in the book, *There Is a River* by Thomas Sugrue (New York; Henry Holt, 1942).

In his book, *Laetrile, Control for Cancer* (New York: Paperback Library, 1963), Glenn D. Kittler asks, "Does Laetrile work as predicted? . . . Over the past years quite extensive data have been accumulated by highly competent clinicians in various parts of the world on the use of Laetrile in hundreds of cases of terminal cancers. . . . in these terminal cases significant results have been obtained with the Laetrile which cannot be fully explained as spontaneous remissions, as due to psychological factors or as the delayed effects of the previous radiation or surgery. [Laetrile therapy in such terminal cases is often made difficult by prior surgery and radiation.]"

Laetrile has been tested in Canada for the past five years by the McNaughton Foundation in Montreal. It is used in many of the largest and finest hospitals in Canada, including the University of Montreal Hospital, McGill, and the Royal Victoria hospitals. The treatment has been used by its founders for the past 35 years and nothing in its formula or method of administration has been kept secret. Like the other "unorthodox" cancer treatments, it has been banned in California, where all cancer treatments have been outlawed except radiation, surgery, and prayer.

Yet, E. T. Krebs, M.D., the proponent of Laetrile, says, "I have never refused it to any doctor (M.D. or D.O.) in California who has requested it for the treatment of a case if he is equipped to use it and signs this request on his professional stationery."

Laetrile is not supplied to patients.

Write Krebs Laboratory, 642 Capp Street, San Francisco 10, California.

THE FROST METHOD

I. N. Frost, M.D., has also not yet been silenced. In a letter addressed to the House of Representatives, Washington, D.C., dated 1961, he says, "Within the past eight years I have not treated a single case of cancer that has not had surgery or radiation, and has not advanced to the state of having to be placed on narcotics and tranquilizers before coming to me that has not entirely recovered —this means all types of cancer. My treatment is harmless! . . . I will not operate on a cancer patient other than for a biopsy report, in order that I may prove that it is cancer. I believe that by getting the patient before he has had other treatment, it will be possible to cure approximately 800 out of 1,000 cases of cancer. Also, I believe that some patients who are not entirely cured will be greatly relieved of their suffering and will live in comfort for a longer period of time."

Dr. Frost makes a vaccine from the patient's own fluids and supplements it with other treatments, including Mucorhicin and other natural treatments. His address: Dr. I. N. Frost, P. O. Box 12, Raymondsville, Texas.

ANTINEOL

Dr. Henry K. Wachtel, Scientific Director of the Chemical Hormone Corporation, is the discoverer and sponsor of Antineol, a hormonal substance. Dr. Wachtel explains the function of Antineol as follows: "Today the only hope for checking cancer is to find a procedure which will increase the resistance of the body to such a degree that the body itself gets rid of the cancer. This is the aim of Atineol therapy.

"The action of Antineol is two-fold: It acts on the size and growth of the tumors and it improves the general health of the patient. This improvement includes increase of body weight of the emaciated patient, regained appetite, regeneration of the shrunken muscles, arresting of anemia, and heightened morale. The patient loses his characteristic cancer 'look.'

"Tumors usually start to decrease after the first few Antineol injections. . . . pain caused by the pressure of tumors on nerves disappears. . . . The effect of Antineol injections depends on the general condition of the patient. . . . if the vitality of the patient is so low that he is unable to live at least one month more, the injections cannot revive him. If a vital body organ, especially the liver, is already destroyed by cancer, the injections are ineffective. . . .

"The improvement lasts as long as the lacking hormone is supplied to the body. . . . Every experienced physician is able to note the improvement if it occurs. . . . It can be stated that most cancer patients profit from the treatment. This is especially important for cases where all other treatments failed to succeed and the patient was abandoned in his pain and despair. . . . Antineol has been found beneficial in most kinds of cancer. Antineol has never been used in Leukemia . . . [and it has been] found to be inactive in Hodgkins Disease. . . .

"Antineol is a crystalline chemical substance derived from the pituitary gland of cattle. . . . It has been thoroughly studied in pharmacological tests and found to be non-toxic. . . . Upon requests by doctors, Antineol is sent to doctors for investigational studies. Requests for details of the procedure should be addressed to Dr. Henry K. Wachtel, Chemical Hormone Corporation, 670 Lexington Avenue, New York 22, New York. (From Bulletin No. 4, "The Hormonal Approach in Treatment of Cancer," published by the Independent Citizens Research Foundation, 71 West 23rd Street, New York 10, New York.)

KREBIOZEN

There has been tempestuous argument over Krebiozen. Those who have reported success with its use feel that its purpose has been misunderstood; that it has never been intended as a cure, but as a factor in *immunity*. A 1962 report from the Krebiozen Research Foundation explains that Krebiozen is "considered to be a local tissue hormone or 'autocoid,' . . . is believed to be the natural cell growth controlling substance responsible for the natural immunity and defense of an organism against cancer."

OTHER THERAPIES

The late Max Gerson, M.D., in his book, A *Cancer Therapy: Results of Fifty Cases*, based on the nutritional approach to treating cancer, mentioned the old remedy used by Italian women suffering from breast cancer—fenugreek tea. Fenugreek seeds are obtainable wherever other herbs are supplied.

Johannes Kuhl, M.D., in Germany has used a unique type of nutritional approach. E. L. David, commenting on the treatment writes, "For the last 10 years Kuhl observed promising results with his diet system, which is simple and inexpensive. He gives patients suffering from chronic diseases fermented vegetables and fruits and also leavened bread, rich in natural lactic acid." Information on equipment for fermenting foods in the Kuhl manner is available from E. L. David, 6 Redcliff Close, Old Brompton Rd., London S.W.S., England. It is necessary to enclose international postage if you wish a reply. A full description of the process appears in reprint form in an article in *Fitness* magazine, Pasture Road, Letchworth, Herts., England. (Enclose international postage.)

Another cancer treatment, known as Mucorhicin, is based on this same principle: a ferment or mold (not unlike the penicillin idea) which is used as an antibiotic approach to cancer. However, according to the Drosnes-Lazenby Clinic which produces it, "Mucorhicin is a *natural growth* as distinct from *synthetic antibiotics*. It is administered orally."

A description of it and its use with various patients is available from the Independent Citizens Research Foundation, Inc., or inquiries may be addressed directly to J. W. Wilson, M.D., medical supervisor of the clinic, 4774 Liberty Avenue, Pittsburgh 24, Pennsylvania.

The North American Newspaper Alliance, reporting from Washington, D.C. (February 22, 1964), said, "Magnetic fields, it has been found, inhibit rapidly dividing cells. This has raised the prospect of an entirely new method of treating cancers.

"Mice kept for weeks between the poles of an electromagnet showed a greatly increased rejection of any transplants of malignant cells and almost complete inhibition of spontaneous breast tumors. . . . When the magnetic field was stopped, however, the cancer started to grow again."

Dr. Harold S. Alexander of North American Aviation Corporation's missile division reported that mice live up to 45 per cent longer after they have been subjected to certain types of magnetic fields, and cancerous mice lost their malignancies. He displayed photographs of two mice from the same litter. . . . The one which had lived for a while in a magnetic field appeared only about one-third as old as the other.

"Aside from the effect on malignancies, we don't yet know why the mice live so much longer after four to six weeks in a magnetic field," Dr. Alexander said. "But we think the experiments have some effect on the rate of cellular reproduction."

"A New York City gynecologist and cytologist, Dr. K. E. MacLean," (in *Fate* magazine, July, 1964,) "is the first M.D. to use an electromagnetic activator in the treatment of advanced cases of cancer. So far, though he has confined his treatment strictly to cases which are considered 'hopeless' the results have been remarkable.

" 'Cancer cannot exist,' " MacLean claims, " 'in a strong magnetic field.'

"The interesting side effect of repeated exposures to magnetism, on human beings aside from its beneficial effect as a cancer treatment, is the restoration of pigmentation in the hair of many of his patients—in most cases from a silvery white to its former natural color.

"Dr. MacLean's full head of hair is dark brown; he has exposed himself to a 3600 Gauss Magnetic field daily for about five years. He is tall and athletic appearing and looks to be about 45 years old. He is 64. . . .

"MacLean's application of a magnetic field seems to relieve pain from *any* cause and to help speed the human organism's return to normalcy. He has shown it to be equally effective in treating most kinds of arthritis, rheumatism and bursitis. After five years he has not discovered a single adverse side-effect from exposure to a *straight* line magnetic field." (For further information see "Human Electronics—Radiesthesia," ch. 12.)

NATURAL REMEDIES

An herb used by Indian tribes for cancer is reported by them as being helpful. This is the Mallow plant (also known as Malva). One species is a dwarf type; the other a large variety. Both grow wild in Europe and in the United States, particularly near trash piles. A picture of the plant for identification purposes appears in the book, *Eat the Weeds*, by Ben Charles Harris, registered pharmacist and herbalist, and curator of Economic Botany of the Museum of Science and Industry, Worcester, Massachusetts. (The book is published by Natura Publications, 237 May Street, Worcester.) Borrowing the Indian method, American housewives who have prepared this plant as a home remedy, pulled the plant from the ground, washed it in eight waters, dried it and stored it until it was ready for use. They then ground it, cooked it in a stainless steel pressure cooker, extracted the juice with a juice press, bottled the juice and took a teaspoonful four times a day. (Please note: I am making no claims for its use.)

The following is a home remedy passed on to me by a man who collected simple remedies which he claimed were effective. He had great faith in one remedy for cancer—even serious cases. He wrote about this home remedy, "It is the easiest to obtain, the simplest to apply, and pleasant to take. It is used widely in the South and we all swear by it. I did not discover this remedy," he said. "I simply rescued it from smothered obscurity after two doctors brought it from Europe, demonstrated its effectiveness and were promptly persecuted for announcing it. This formula has already been published in a large daily newspaper as follows: 'It is a half-day diet. Eat nothing during the forenoon. Begin early in the morning sipping slowly a 24-ounce (or a 12-ounce if stomach is weak) bottle of unsweetened Concord grape juice. Finish the bottle by 10 o'clock A.M., wait until noon to eat lunch. No pork. The stomach must be in a healthy condition to digest the juice properly or no benefits result. In this case, use a smaller amount of the juice and dilute it with half water. Gradually increase and in about three weeks the stomach can probably take the juice straight. If it physicks, reduce the quantity, but continue. Many people notice good results from this half-day diet within six weeks, but it may take longer.'"

H. E. Kirschner, M.D., writes of an ancient folk remedy which was used in past centuries and which he had used for certain cancerous conditions, including skin areas. This remedy is a plant, known as Comfrey. It is said to contain a certain healing ingredient. Dr. Kirschner writes,

"In cases of obstinate ulcers, gangrene, tumors, burns, open wounds, skin cancer or inflammation caused by insect bites, the Comfrey leaves can be prepared for a poultice by putting them through a juicer (or crushed with mortar and pestle). However, as the Comfrey leaves contain no juice, but a thick mucilaginous substance—like okra—the macerated leaves are gathered from the basket of the juicer following the operation, and not from the spout. The mass of triturated Comfrey leaves can then be spread on a cloth and applied to the infected area. . . .

"To make Comfrey tea, I take four small fresh leaves, cut them up and steep them as I would tea. In using the roots of Comfrey, according to Potters Cyclopedia of Botanical Drugs, a decoction is made by boiling one-half to one ounce of crushed root in one quart of water. Dose: one wine-glassful (four to six ounces). In cases of gastric ulcer, internal tumors or lung ailments, this tea should be used in liberal quantities every day. . . . As a blood purifier Comfrey has been widely used in European countries for centuries. . . . Pure blood builds healthy tissue and if Comfrey were used for no other reason than to keep the blood stream pure, it is well worth the effort to grow and use this plant in the diet.

"I have found Comfrey very easy to grow. Planted in rich soil, surrounded by a heavy straw mulch and given plenty of water, you will find Comfrey an all year round source of the same vital elements that we have in alfalfa, parsley and other medicinal herbs." *

Dr. Kirschner also incorporated Comfrey raw in his "green drink," the formula of which appears in his book, *Nature's Healing Grasses* (Yucaipa, California: H.C. White, 1960).

In addition to Comfrey Leaf poultices, natural folk remedies for skin cancer are: rubbing the area every day with castor oil, or taping a split grape (dark) over it.

May Bethel, writing in *Herald of Health* (December, 1963), says, "I have seen a case of skin cancer healed by the application of a preparation made from red clover blossoms. A strong tea was made. After straining the tea, the liquid was allowed to simmer until it became black and of the consistency of tar. After several applications the skin cancer was gone and has not returned. There will be some who will say that it was not skin cancer, but it was diagnosed as skin cancer."

In nearly every report on cancer where good results were obtained, there appears a common denominator—raw food. Cyril Scott cites a case of a Dr. Kuhne's method of treatment of a woman for whom doctors had recommended an immediate operation. Cyril Scott writes, "She ignored this advice, however, took hip and friction bath sitz-baths instead, lived on unfired natural food, and soon began to get well."

Cyril Scott also writes, "Dr. Bremdini, of Florence, discovered that lemon juice would relieve the intolerable pain of cancer . . .

* For sources of Comfrey plants, see Bibliography.

(for relief of mouth cancer). In his torment he begged for a lemon to suck which immediately diminished the pain, next day he begged for another lemon which gave him still more marked relief. . . . The doctor next tried it (elsewhere upon the body). A piece of lint soaked in lemon juice, and then applied, produced immediate relief. . . . In a number of cases of similar nature the results were the same."

The use of fresh garlic for cancer in mice is summarized in *Science* (November 29, 1957) as follows:

"Extracts of garlic (*Allium sativum*) have been shown to contain a powerful bactericidal agent . . . studies have been made of the effect of these substances on the growth of sarcoma 180 ascites tumor in CFW Swiss mice. The mice were inoculated with a dilute suspension of tumor cells freshly drawn from donor mice. . . . Pre-incubation of the inoculum with saline (control) results in rapid growth and death of all animals within 16 days. . . . When the enzyme was allowed to react with the substrate and the inoculum was pre-incubated with the reaction mixture (garlic), no tumor growth occurred, and the animals remained alive during a six-month observation period."

Beet juice is another natural remedy. E. L. David, Biological Researcher, London, England, writes, "Studies by Dr. A. Ferenczi (Nobel Prize-winner) concerning the anti-tumor effect of beetroot juice were published in 1955, 1959, and 1961. . . .

"It has been determined that beetroots are rich in kalium [potassium], phosphorus, calcium, sulfur, iodine, iron and copper, and that they also contain traces of the rare rubidium and caesium. In addition to protein, carbohydrates, and fat, the vitamins B-1, B-2, B-6, C, P and niacin are present in this remarkable root.

"The anti-tumor effect of the beetroot juice may be explained by its high iron content, which acts as a regenerator and activator on red blood corpuscles. By their regeneration, these corpuscles supply cancer cells with more oxygen, thus improving the impaired cell respiration and also activating respiratory ferments (Warburg theory). As a result of these happenings, hypertrophies break down and tissues take up their natural structures, if the disease is not too far advanced.

"Medical science has not examined the healing properties of

beetroot juice against leukemia, but there are cases known in folk medicine where the body succeeded in defeating this incurable disease. . . .

"The juice of the fresh beetroot may cause belching and it has a rather musty, beet-like taste which can be repulsive to patients who have to drink a tumblerful or more daily." (It can be made more palatable by fermenting it according to the Kuhl method mentioned elsewhere in this section. Directions are available from Mr. David, see p. 239.)

"According to Dr. Ferenczi, the *raw* beet juice has the anti-tumor effect. . . ."

Another natural remedy-turned-drug is extracted from the garden shrub, periwinkle. The discovery of the plant's effect was made almost simultaneously by scientists of the Collip Research Laboratories in Canada and the Eli Lilly Research Laboratories in the United States. The trade name is Velban or VLB. According to Margaret Kreig, who reports its discovery in an article which took her one year to research, and which appears in *This Week* magazine (August 11, 1962), there are "dramatic effects. . . . tumor tissue seemed to melt away."

She writes, "When administered with care, they slow or halt various kinds of malignancies without damaging normal cells. Many clinicians are impressed by the fact that Vinca drugs are working where others have failed and that side-effects are controllable. 'The activity in carcinoma of the cervix is worthy of particular attention,' one cancer specialist reports, 'because this form of cancer has always resisted chemical treatment.' "

The source of the drug is *Vinca rosea*, also known as "Little Pinkie" or "Bright Eyes." The current major source of supply is India, where the wild plant is cultivated, though it is now being planted for laboratory use in this country. The company which has done much research on the value of the plant doubts that it will become a profitable crop for farmers in the United States. It grows as a perennial in warm climates, but in this country it must be replaced annually and labor costs are high.

HOMEOPATHY

Fraser Mackenzie, C.I.E. of England, says, "If a homeopathically trained physician sees a case of cancer when the stage of tumor formation is established he generally regards it as being late for cure. Nevertheless he will try to find the constitutional remedy and although it would be wrong to make extravagant claims, there are on record, *thousands of successful results* from homeopathic treatment which are, to say the least, encouraging." (From *Commonsense about Cancer* by Fraser Mackenzie; Homeopathic Publishing Co., George Street. Hanover Square, London, W. 1.)

A RECENT DISCOVERY

Just before this book went to press, I discovered a book by an English physician, which seems to take some of the fear and mystery out of cancer. Maud Tresillian Fere, M.D., in her little book (112 pages), called *Cancer—Its Dietetic Cause and Cure*, wraps up much that one needs to know to prevent or possibly cure cancer. Dr. Fere is a licensed physician of the Royal College of Physicians and Surgeons, in Scotland; has earned a diploma of public health in London; and is a tuberculosis Medical Officer of the Royal Institute of Public Health, also in London.

Dr. Fere has eliminated the agonizing pain of cancer without the use of drugs and has brought about complete cures, not only in her patients but in herself, since she, too was a victim. In her book, she not only presents basic causes of cancer, but she outlines the step-by-step method she uses for its reversal.

Armed with the background information I have given you in this chapter, if you know of anyone who is already stricken with this dread disease, or if you want to be free of fear of cancer yourself, for the rest of your life, I recommend that you obtain Dr. Fere's book.

Cancer, Its Dietetic Cause and Cure, is available for $2.00 from Gateway Book Company, Gateway House, Bedford Park, Croydon, Surrey, England.

I have presented this long list of medically used and natural cancer treatments to show you that there *is* hope that cancer can be prevented, controlled, and in some cases eliminated. If you wish further information about cancer, please do not write me. I can only repeat what I have already said in these pages. Instead, write to the addresses given. If you are blocked in receiving treatment, then write to your Congressman or see him personally when he is in your home state. Demand action! Congressmen are the bridge between the people and a government that *should* serve the wishes and the needs of the people.

Finally, for your protection, join the National Health Federation, which is dedicated to help fight your health battles. This group is an honest, sincere organization with expert lawyers and can apply pressure where it is needed. Membership is only $5.00 per year; write them at P. O. Box 686, Monrovia, California. It may be one of the best expenditures you will ever make, both for your own as well as for your country's welfare.

30 Constipation

I am told, on good authority, that in one southern city, where retired people congregate, every morning many of them gather on park or street benches to discuss their No. 1 favorite subject: constipation. They worry aloud about whether they have or have not had their daily trip to the bathroom. The topic becomes almost a fixation. I have news for them: constipation can be so easily controlled that I am afraid they are going to have to find a new topic of conversation. First I will tell what the remedies are. Then I will give you the authorities and the reasons why they work.*

Remedy 1: One cup of yogurt a day (1 glass of acidophilus buttermilk works for some people).

Remedy 2: Blackstrap molasses—begin with 1 teaspoon and work upward gently until you find the amount best for you. (Rinse mouth with water after taking.)*

Remedy 3: Chew 1 tablespoon of flaxseed three or four times a day: or pulverize them fresh each day in your blender or little electric nut-grinding mill available at health centers. Sprinkle the ground flaxseed over salads, cereals, or in beverages. If you do add it to liquid, drink it quickly before it gets too thick. Flaxseeds are available at health and drug stores.

Boris Sokoloff, M.D., in *Middle Age Is What You Make It,* tells of the famous scientist Metchnikoff who noticed that healthy persons with normal, regular bowel movements always maintained a good supply of a particular kind of friendly bacteria in their colon. These bacteria, Metchnikoff named *Lactobacillus acidophilus.*

"Without reservation," says Dr. Sokoloff, "we may call this microbe friend, since it protects the colon from hostile microbes. It fights them, it destroys them by means of lactic acid which it produces in abundance. A normal, healthy colon houses a number of these benign microbes which do not allow any hostile or dangerous germ to gain the upper hand. But if for any reason our friend disappears from the colon or is decreased in numbers, the hostile germs immediately infiltrate the colon and constipation appears."

Laxatives wash these friendly bacteria out of the colon and if continued, the bacteria are nearly all lost. Constipation may then become chronic. Antibiotics also destroy helpful bacteria, according to Dr. Jesse D. Rising of the University of Kansas. Fortunately, these friendly bacteria never completely disappear from the colon. There are always a few remaining, ready to come to the aid of the sufferer if given a chance. To increase them, Dr. Sokoloff advises taking "plenty of cultured milk."

Metchnikoff found that the bacillus is necessary for human

---

* See also, Clark, *Stay Young Longer.*

health and the preservation of youth and vitality. Inhabitants of the Caucasus and Bulgaria, known for their vitality and longevity, consume soured or cultured milk containing this bacillus regularly. Yogurt is a cultured milk and encourages friendly bacteria. Europeans have eaten this type of food for centuries.

Lancet (February 2, 1957), says, "There is considerable evidence that for some complaints (e.g., gastro-enteritis, colitis, constipation, biliary disorders, flatulence, migraine, nervous fatigue) cultured milks and especially acidophilus milk can be extremely valuable."

John G. Davis, Ph.D., D.Sc., of London, says that yogurt is beneficial in reducing putrefaction in the intestinal tract and bowel function. Stomach rumbling and flatulence as well as belching are also remedied.

I have known people, who have "tried everything," to eliminate constipation by the use of yogurt.

The *Journal of the American Medical Association* for November 11, 1955, reports a study in which yogurt-plus-prune-whip was given to 194 patients. No laxatives were required for 95.8 per cent of the patients. For most people the added prunes are not necessary. Plain yogurt is usually sufficient.

Yogurt—or any of the cultured milks—is made by adding the desired type of bacillus to milk and allowing it to incubate. Too high a temperature kills the bacillus. In a few rare cases of constipation, greater help than that provided by the cultured milks may be necessary. If so, the bacillus may be taken straight. It is available at health stores, under various trade names. It is composed of live strains of *Lactobacilli acidophilus* and *bulgaricus*. The label usually explains that the product is alive with millions and millions of friendly organisms which assist in re-establishing or reinforcing the favorable intestinal flora. The substance is taken by the tablespoonful after meals.

A Chinese woman living in America wrote me that though she had used yogurt for years, she decided that she needed something stronger. She found the bottled bacilli extremely beneficial. Her letter says, "It worked on me within two days. I doubled my energy, my eyes feel cooler, my body lighter. My husband has also noticed great improvement."

Since antibiotics kill the friendly bacteria, many doctors, if they prescribe an antibiotic, also prescribe yogurt or the live bacillus in some form. In foreign countries it is used to control diarrhea as well. In Chile, small bottles of the combined bacilli—*acidophilus* and *bulgaricus*—are available without prescription at drugstores. Those who are troubled with constipation (or diarrhea) buy the bottles, take the contents on an empty stomach one-half hour before breakfast or before drinking hot liquids. They continue for as many days as necessary to produce the desired results.

Yogurt not only contains friendly bacteria, but B vitamins, necessary for smooth digestion. There is evidence that it helps you to manufacture some of your own B vitamins in your intestinal tract. It also supplies calcium which is better assimilated in acid than in sweet milk, thus soothing the stomach and digestion. It has been used for nervous, spastic stomachs as well as for more serious colitis. After yogurt has been successfully started, brewer's yeast, the cheapest available source of the B vitamins, may be added for further help.

I have heard people say, "But I can't take brewer's yeast. It produces gas." Let me assure you this is only temporary. When the friendly bacteria are introduced, first through yogurt, and later by brewer's yeast, the unfriendly bacteria already present in the intestines will resent the intrusion and put up a fight. Gas is the result. But as soon as the friendly bacilli have sufficiently multiplied, the battle should end. Nutritionists feel that the more gas the greater the need for these friendly microbes!

If you dislike the tart flavor of commercial yogurt, make your own.* The too-tart flavor is a result of the overmultiplying culture, which grows exactly like yeast when it is added to bread dough. It multiplies in a warm, not hot, temperature. If you take it from a 100° oven the minute it sets like custard and whisk it to the refrigerator, it will retain its milk flavor and discourage further growth. Multiplication in the intestine is, of course, desirable. Dr. Sokoloff recommends a daily intake of at least 100 billion bacilli—the amount approximately found in one or two cups of yogurt—or 1 tablespoon of the bottled bacilli. After you have grown accustomed to yogurt, begin gingerly on brewer's yeast. Start with a tea-

* See Clark, *Stay Young Longer.*

spoon daily in water or juice and work upward. Dr. Tom Spies recommended at least one-fourth cup daily for his patients. I personally take brewer's yeast powder or flakes, added to water or juice. It is available at health food stores. Do *not* take live baker's yeast! *

Catharyn Elwood in *Feel Like a Million*, writes, "The muscles of the intestinal tract may become flaccid and prolapsed if the B complex vitamins, especially B-1, are not plentiful in the diet. These water soluble vitamins are not stored but are lost in the urine and perspiration. So play safe by including the rich B vitamins found in brewer's yeast, sprouted grains, wheat germ, molasses, rice polishing, liver, and yogurt every day. . . . Remember, *your nerves move your bowels* and they can and will do the job if your B-complex intake is adequate."

SOME "DON'TS"

Do not take mineral oil! It robs the body of vitamins A, D, and E, calcium and phosphorus, and may cause rectal itching and even pneumonia. (*American Journal of Digestive Diseases*, 19:344.)

Dr. Royal Lee warns against the use of milk of magnesia because, he says, it may cause nose bleed.

Do not take cathartics or laxatives. This makes the condition worse and only creates a vicious cycle.

HELP FOR HEMORRHOIDS

Catharyn Elwood says, "If you are troubled with a tenderness, soreness, or hemorrhaging of the anus, a peeled garlic bud, oiled and inserted as a suppository and allowed to stay over night, has been found most healing.

Journal of Natural Living (Vol. 2, No. 9) adds, "A correspondent writes that suppositories whittled out of raw potato, together with a poultice of grated raw potato, will dissolve piles and afford amazing relief from discomfort. Also, we have personally

* See Clark, *Stay Young Longer*.

known a case where huge clusters of external hemorrhoids, protruding like bunches of grapes, disappeared in a matter of hours when kept moist with fresh raw lemon juice."

Exercises, either those involving the abdominal muscles, or a mile-a-day walk can help, too.

Above all, don't worry about your "innards." Tension inteferes with elimination by tensing up the very muscles you want to relax.

31 Eyes—how to see better

CAN EYESIGHT BE HELPED BY NUTRITION?

Medical studies say Yes.

The blood stream carries away waste matter and brings a fresh supply of necessary nutrients to every cell in the body, including the eyes. If the blood is nutritionally deficient, it cannot adequately "feed" the eyes. The only way the blood can receive the building or rebuilding material is from the absorption of the substances you eat through the walls of the intestines. The eyes need feeding as well as any other organ of the body—perhaps more so, since they are subjected to such continuous strain. If eyes are undernourished, the structure of the eye suffers damage; they get tired quicker from less work; sharpness of vision lessens; and the accommodation to near or far objects takes longer. Resting them does not always restore their efficiency.

Adelle Davis says, "I have had many persons report that after their nutrition was improved, their glasses seemed no longer suited to their needs. On going to an oculist, they have been told that their eyes were much stronger than formerly. . . . Good nutrition, however, cannot correct conditions for which glasses are needed. . . . Among elderly persons, visual difficulties caused by multiple nutritional deficiencies are almost the rule rather than the exception. In all probability, such deficiencies are often responsible for failing vision so frequently accepted as an inevitable part of growing older."

Carlton Fredericks, Ph.D., in his leaflet, "You See with What You Eat," says, "Visual acuity—the actual level of the ability to *see*—can be improved with proper nutrition. And some cataracts —whether or not originating with faulty diet—can be checked but not reversed with vitamins. Such conditions as sensitivity to bright light, a twilight blindness, and night blindness are known definitely to originate with vitamin deficiencies."

DO YOU LACK VITAMIN A?

According to the *American Journal of Surgery*, Dr. Jacob Jacobson of New York found that vitamin A increased blood supply to the eyes and improved vision in patients whose vision was impaired by arteriosclerosis or diabetes. These patients had not responded to other types of therapy.

People deficient in vitamin A complain of inability to see well at night or in bright light. This is because bright light actually destroys vitamin A in the eyes. People who work in bright light use more vitamin A than others. Those who spend much time on the beach, desert, in snow, or driving against the glare of headlights, are using and losing vitamin A. Typists who face bright light on white paper, or people who continuously read, sew, or watch television often have more need for vitamin A.

RAF flyers in England were required to take capsules of vitamin A during the war, and American parachutists, because the Japanese could see our night-landing soldiers before they could see the Japanese, were finally required to take vitamin A. Vitamin A is now an accepted preventive for night blindness. Early Egyptians recommended liver (rich in vitamin A) for bad eyesight.

ARE YOU DEFICIENT IN VITAMIN B-2?

Those who suffer from watering eyes, a feeling of "sand" under the eyelids, or inability to adjust from darkness to sudden illumination are admitting to a deficiency of riboflavin (vitamin B-2). A deficiency of this vitamin makes it hard for people to drive in twilight—that dim gray hour when it is too early to turn on headlights, yet too dark to see comfortably without them. Riboflavin shortage shows up in irritation of the white surfaces, reddening of the tiny blood vessels, itching or granulation of eyelids. A B-2 deficient person often rubs or wipes his eyes.

Such a need for these vitamins, A and B-2, is not imaginary. Light is believed to enter the eye through a screen made of riboflavin, which is orange in color, before striking the purple rods of the eyes. This "visual purple" is sensitive to light and is bleached by it, therefore partially destroying the vitamins stored there. "The dye must be replaced if you are to see again. That is why staring at a bright light might bring a temporary period of total blindness afterward. The body is busy bringing up its reserves of vitamins to replace those destroyed by the light ray," says Carlton Fredericks. These are the same light-sensitive vitamins destroyed in food when subjected to light. Leaving bottled milk sitting on a sunny doorstep destroys these vitamins.

B vitamins apparently affect the optic nerve. In pernicious anemia, especially, loss of vision and changes in the optic nerve take place. A study at Frederiksborg Hospital, in Copenhagen, revealed that such vision can be restored by early and adequate treatment with vitamin B-12.

Another type of "dim vision" is associated with excessive smoking and alcohol consumption. New information indicates this type of dim vision is due to B vitamin deficiency, particularly vitamins B-1 and B-12. The retina or optic nerve has been found to be extremely sensitive to tobacco. (*Lancet*, August 9, 1958.) Still another source of dim vision is related to contamination from everyday fallout. (See "Fallout—How to Bypass It," ch. 32.)

OTHER NUTRIENTS ALSO HELP

Vitamin E assists the muscles and circulation to the eye, according to three Italian researchers. Dr. C. Malatesta found that a deficiency of vitamin E causes severe degeneration in the retina and lens. Dr. R. Seidenari discovered that patients who were beginning to need spectacles for close reading were able to focus better after being given vitamin E. And Dr. E. Raverdino supplied his patients who had developed a blind spot, 600 I.U. of vitamin E a day. In the majority of cases, except where central vision was completely destroyed, vision improved and the blind spot was reduced.

Vitamin C is necessary for good vision, too. Catharyn Elwood says, "Blood and urine tests have confirmed the theory that if oldsters have cataracts, vitamin C is not found in their lens, where it is concentrated in normal eyes." Rutin can be added to vitamin C to strengthen capillaries.

Here is a summary of the nutrients found helpful to eyes:

Vitamin A: 5,000 units daily is supposed to be sufficient, but Carlton Fredericks suggests at least 15,000 in light of recent research. Water-soluble A is better assimilated by many people who are unable to utilize fat-soluble A.

Riboflavin: (Vitamin B-2) found in brewer's yeast. B-2 is available separately for therapeutic purposes but should be taken together with the full B complex.

Calcium: Plus vitamin D and vitamin F (found in unsaturated fats) and acid for assimilation.

Vitamin C: Bioflavonoids (vitamin C complex) and rutin.

Vitamin E

Protein

Vitamins B-6 and E and protein have been known to help strengthen eye muscles.

I used to consider it an old wives' tale that sunflower seeds were supposed to help vision. Since talking to people whose word I respect, I have changed my mind. Those who eat a handful of raw sunflower seeds daily, report they no longer need dark glasses and many discover that their eyes are changing for the better. If you will look at the analysis of sunflower seeds in *Stay Young Longer*, you will see that they are actually a high vitamin food, especially rich in vitamins needed by the eyes.

Speaking of dark glasses, do read about John Ott and the effect of darkness on vision, as discussed in the section on "Arthritis." Experiments with monkeys are now under way at the University of California, Riverside, to confirm the theory that weakness of vision can result from lack of use as well as overexposure to darkness.

CAN NEARSIGHTEDNESS BE HELPED?

Nearsightedness often begins in childhood. *Lancet* (May, 1958) reports a study in which myopia, or nearsightedness, was more common in children who did not eat animal protein (meat, fish, eggs). Protein supplements arrested progressive nearsightedness in children over 12. The vision of those under 12 continued to deteriorate somewhat, but less rapidly if they were given added protein. Protein not only arrested but improved nearsightedness in some children over 12.

The *American Journal of Opthalmology* (May, 1950), suggests that nearsightedness is due to a lack of calcium and vitamin A.

Dr. Hunter J. Turner in the May, 1944, issue of the *Pennsylvania Medical Journal* blames nearsightedness on soda pop, because of its carbonic acid (the stuff that makes pop fizz).

WHAT ABOUT CATARACTS?

Medical Press (June 4, 1952) states that in cases of cataract the lens shows a diminished amount of vitamin C.

Animals denied B-2 (riboflavin) develop cataracts. If the vitamin is given early enough, the cataracts disappear. After studying cataracts and opacities, Dr. Sydenstricker of the University of Alabama Medical School gave generous amounts of B-2 plus an adequate diet to people exhibiting symptoms of vitamin B deficiencies. The eyes became normal in about two weeks. Other authorities believe, however, that cataract damage, if severe, can be arrested but not repaired.

Dr. A. Cantarow* considers that a lack of calcium allows cataracts to form. Vitamin C is necessary to help calcium function properly. (*Physiological Review*, 23:76; 1943.)

Dr. D. T. Atkinson, writing in *Eye, Ear, Nose and Throat Monthly,* believes cataracts develop because the lens of the eye is undernourished. He reports that he has been able to prevent cataracts from developing in 450 patients who showed beginnings of cataract, by a diet including 8 to 10 glasses of water, greens such as the tops of garden vegetables, a minimum of a pint of milk, two eggs, and vitamins A and C—all daily.

Optical Development (February-March, 1957) says, "Proper nutrition is of major importance in the process of vision. It is evident that the full quota of vitamins, minerals and amino acids is to be featured as essential factors in the prevention of visual defects at all stages of life, and in the correction of various dysfunctions, if they have not passed the reversible stages."

Further confirmation that there is a relationship between cataracts and nutrition comes from *Nutrition Reviews* (August, 1962). "Cataracts have been observed in a variety of animal species fed a number of nutritionally deficient diets."

A deficiency of riboflavin (B-2) produces cataracts in rats and swine, but not in monkeys. In horses some types of cataracts have been presumably cured by supplementary riboflavin.

A deficiency of vitamin E produces lens opacities in fowl.

A dietary deficiency of tryptopan (an amino acid) has produced cataracts in rats. A deficiency of other amino acids, phenylalanine, valine, histidine and possibly threonine and isoleucine produces cataracts in rats. Cataracts have been observed in pigs maintained on a low protein diet for more than one year. (Protein contains amino acids.)

* *Calcium Metabolism and Calcium Therapy* (Lea and Febiger, 1931).

According to this report (*Nutrition Reviews*) it has been known for a long time that rats fed a ration of large amounts of galactose or xylose (types of sugar) develop cataracts. It has also been known for some time that a galactose ration increases intestinal absorption and urinary excretion of calcium, sodium, and potassium, thus creating deficiencies of these minerals.

Cataracts are often associated with diabetes in humans. Diabetics, of course, have a disturbed sugar level.

CATARACT IMPROVEMENT WITHOUT SURGERY

One school of thought believes that a cataract is not a disease in itself, but an end-result of impaired circulation to the eyes. Sometimes this is caused by congestion in the cervical and dorsal vertebrae area, which may be relieved by chiropractic or osteopathic adjustment and massage. Circulation may be encouraged to the eyes by other means, too. Lying with the head lower than the feet; "palming" as explained by Dr. Bates (see p. 267), may provide relief.

An exciting new approach to treatment of cataract and other eye disturbances is visible-ray therapy. Research by R. Brooks Simpkins, of England, has revealed that the use of wavebands of the visible color spectrum provide natural energy and medicinal treatment for eyes and vision.

Mr. Simpkins says, "In this field the medicinal properties of the rays have proved to be efficacious in the treatment of affections such as senile cataract, chronic glaucoma, choroiditis, retinitis, and conjunctivitis . . . the visible rays have proved also to be of great value in the complementary treatment of refractive errors such as farsightedness, nearsightedness, astigmatism, old-age sight and nystagmus. . . .

"Visible ray therapy gives suitable electrical stimulation of the motor nerves of the eye muscles and of the complicated visual processes generally. . . . My own case records provide substantial and extensive evidence that in the eyes of otherwise healthy adult people senile cataract can largely be prevented from developing

—and that different stages of development of this feared, and rather widespread, disease can be arrested and dispersed and the transparency of the crystalline lens restored."

Mr. Simpkins' method of treating the eyes is with colored glass filters, such as red, green, blue, yellow and orange. Patients peer into a device, which is somewhat like a lighted stereoscope. Between the light and the patient's eyes, the colored filters allow the rays to reach and stimulate the eyes. Mr. Simpkins, who has done 25 years of research on this technique, says, ". . . large numbers of people have been astonished by the improvement in their unaided vision after a single treatment . . . the mechanical energic properties of the visible rays give us a remedial therapy which no other method of treatment could be expected to achieve. My own long experience has proved that this is indeed the case, however variable the benefit obtained for individual patients, many of whom had previously been told that nothing more could be done for their eyes, either as regards their pathological or their refractive conditions."

Mr. Simpkins describes his method for the average person in his book, *Visible Ray Therapy of the Eyes* (Health Science Press, Rustington, Sussex, England, 1963; available from Harmony Book Store, Box 115 New Castle, Pennsylvania; price $4.00). For the profession, R. Brooks Simpson has written a highly technical book on the same technique, called *Oculopathy*, also available from the same source.

Infrared and ultraviolet rays should not be applied to the eyes, according to Mr. Simpkins. It has long been known that some cataracts have been traced to continued exposure to heat from open fires, when people sit too close to them and look directly into them. Dogs have frequently acquired cataracts from sleeping on the open hearth.

Early investigators have found that vitamin A liquefies necrotic (dead) tissue when applied locally to a wound. Other vitamins applied to various types of scar tissue or wounds have proved healing. This may explain why certain natural remedies have proved useful to some people in treatment of cataracts. Here are a few of these folk remedies collected from various places.

A drop of U.S.P. raw linseed oil in eye daily (available from druggist).
A drop of fresh lemon juice or diluted apple cider vinegar in the eye at
   night; a drop of filtered sea water in the morning.
A drop of Eucalyptus honey (warmed) in eye.

One simple remedy was given to me by a relative who learned
it from a hospital orderly. It consists of putting 1 drop of castor oil
in each eye once a day for nine days. Wait 10 days. Repeat the
treatment. Folklore has reported good results of the use of castor
oil with warts, corns, and brown spots on the hands, all considered by some to be forms of scar tissue. I have personally witnessed
warts dropping off after being loosened by castor oil.

An herbal solution, used by homeopathic physicians, is reported
to be helpful in many cases. This liquid, known as *Cineraria mari-
tima*, is available from Erhart and Karl, Manufacturing Homeopathic Pharmacists, 17 N. Wabash Avenue, Chicago 21, Illinois.
When a drop is put in the eye, it smarts slightly. Oral homeopathic remedies can be prescribed by homeopathic physicians. Excellent success has been noted in some cases.

There is one homeopathic treatment, a combination of several
homeopathic substances which is being used by a hundred or
more doctors for treatment of cataracts, with a report of 90 per
cent good results. It is also used by some veterinarians for removal
of cataracts in animals. This remedy is said to have originated in
the early 1920's with a Dr. Garduno of Mexico. He used the medicine with advanced cases of cataract in elderly people. I have seen
the documents which list each type of cataract and the length of
time it had existed. In every case reported treated by this homeopathic combination, either complete cure or definite improvement
was reported.

The medication is dispensed through physicians only, usually
opthalmologists. It is necessary to take the medication for six
months. It is pleasant to taste and somewhat expensive, but certainly less expensive than surgery. If it helps sight to return, it is, of
course, invaluable. Ask your doctor to write for literature and to
consider the product known as "Afaco." Address: International
Afaco, Ltd., Pharmaceutics, 5443 Broadway, Chicago 40, Illinois.

Charles Pflueger, M.D., reports that he uses an inexpensive homeopathic medication with excellent success for many of his cataract patients. This medication, which is taken orally, contains about eleven different ingredients. It is called Cineraria Compound, available from homeopathic pharmacies. In other patients, Dr. Pflueger finds the oral administration of sulphur helpful. In addition to medication and a good diet, he also recommends eye exercises based on the Bates Method to aid in removing tension and increasing circulation to the eyes. As a result, many cataract victims have been helped to see again without surgery.

Tension may cause cataracts. Some tension-relieving exercises have brought dramatic results in cataracts which had not reached the irreversible stage. (See p. 266.)

If cataracts have progressed too far, surgery may be necessary. Professional therapists urge the use of natural remedies as early as possible in this condition and suggest that surgery be used only as a last resort.

GLAUCOMA

Glaucoma is considered a "stress" disease of the eye and there is also, in the opinion of various researchers, a relationship to nutrition, perhaps characterizing it as a deficiency disease. Ethel Maslansky, nutritionist of New York City, has found that in glaucoma, patients usually exhibit deficiencies of vitamins A, B, C, calcium and other minerals. Dr. Rolf Ulrich reports a connection between coffee and glaucoma. He forbids his glaucoma patients to drink coffee.

Glaucoma has, according to *Clinical Physiology* (Autumn, 1962), been caused also by certain antispasmodic drugs. Cataracts, too, have been caused by various drugs.

"There is one type of glaucoma which can be prevented," *Health Bulletin* (February 15, 1964) states, quoting the opinion of Dr. L. K. Sarin, Wills Eye Hospital, Philadelphia. "This type is one that accounts for a very small percentage of cases. It is caused by the doctors themselves, when they use steroid drugs injudiciously. Steroids are sometimes put into the eye by practitioners, who are not specialists, to treat eye inflammations."

WHAT ABOUT CONTACT LENSES?

Consumers Bulletin (March, 1963) writes: "Hundreds of dollars and untold nervous energy have been wasted by the beguiled contact lens wearers. . . . Seldom have any contact lens wearers recounted their eye injuries. Yet damage has occurred, ranging from a slight corneal scratch to loss of an eye. Instances are on medical file of permanently handicapped vision.

"Contact lenses are still one of the greatest helps for vision with an eye that has a conical shape. . . . In this condition, because the cornea may be sharply pointed, satisfactory vision may be obtained only by the use of a contact lens. . . . Contact lenses for a person who has had a cataract removed from one eye and where the other eye has excellent vision, are remarkably helpful sometimes. Although since the eye (with cataract removed) can no longer accommodate or focus from near to far vision . . . two pairs of glasses are necessary, one for far vision and one for near."

Dr. Harvey M. Rosenwasser, a Philadelphia optometrist, reports that certain drugs can change the shape of the eyes, making the fitting of contact lenses difficult. These drugs include tranquilizers and diuretics, used for treating obesity and high blood pressure. Dr. Rosenwasser states that tranquilizers can also cause other eye difficulties: pupil contraction or dilation, light sensitivity, nearsightedness, farsightedness, itching, dryness, blurred vision and "tunnel vision." (*Health Bulletin*, Vol. 1, No. 41, 1963.)

NATURAL EYE REMEDIES

Fate magazine (November, 1963) reports, "There is an old legend that a sty can be cured by rubbing a gold wedding ring over it. Researchers at the Mayo Clinic tried the treatment on hundreds of patients and staff members suffering from sties. About 92 per cent of the sties disappeared." I have not been able to check this report further.

OTHER REMEDIES

Rubbing a beginning sty with a small piece of whole nutmeg.

For swollen eyes, warm or cold compresses combined with eye gymnastics; drink a small glass of cucumber juice every morning.

For red or irritated eyes put your hands in hot or ice-cold water and apply the palms to the eyes several times.

For pockets under the eyes; eye exercises, application of pads soaked either in witch hazel, or an infusion of rosemary leaves, 20 to 40 grams per quart of water. (The above remedies by Diane Rashey, *Herald of Health*, April, 1962.)

For excessive eye blinking and watering, Dr. A. Huber advises taking calcium.

For bloodshot eyes, Royal Lee, D.D.S. suggests the following: B vitamins, niacin and riboflavin; foods—carrots, brewer's yeast, sprouted grains, liver and kidney.

Floaters are fuzzy specks and hairlike objects you see floating before your eyes. Dr. Lee believes that they are due to a failing pancreas which is not secreting the enzyme chymotrypsin, necessary for the digestion of certain proteins. If these proteins are undigested, according to Dr. Lee, they may float in the fluid of the eye. Dr. Harvey E. White has another explanation. He considers floaters stray red blood cells. Some doctors believe they are due to toxicity in the liver.

Dark circles have been explained by various causes: toxicity or infection in the body, too little sleep, or intestinal parasites.*

Bags under the eyes: Adelle Davis in *Let's Eat Right to Keep Fit*, says, "When the diet is so inadequate that sufficient albumin cannot be formed, waste materials are not completely removed from the tissues. Many weeks or months of mild protein deficiency may occur. . . . If the deficiency becomes more severe, the tissues are noticeably puffy, and the entire body waterlogged. The ankles swell, especially toward the end of the day; swollen face and hands and puffy bags under the eyes are evident in the morning."

Another cause of water retention is a deficiency of unsaturated fatty acids or vegetable oils in the diet. Magnesium also plays a part.

* See "Anemia," pp. 162-164.

Dr. Ann Wigmore, D.D., N.D., has devised a drink made from fresh grown wheatgrass (see p. 235). A doctor wrote Dr. Wigmore: "On the simple menu and 2 wheatgrass mannas a day, my improvement has been truly amazing. One eye had been ruined by surgery, the other from glaucoma and cataracts was too dim for reading. In two weeks my bad eye could tell day from night—my dim eye could read my wrist watch."

ARE EYE EXERCISES HELPFUL?

Eyestrain, according to Dr. J. M. Weber, can result from nervous tension. One of our problems these days is staring. We stare at the television, at the blackboard; we stare at a page or a book. This tires the eyes and prevents the muscles from adapting easily from close to distant objects. A little-used muscle becomes weak. Hence, exercise and relaxation can be helpful. Studies of children with myopia have reported improvement through exercise. *The International Record of Medicine* (September, 1957) says, "A specific course in visual training may improve acuity, size of visual field for form, refracted error and reading speed in selected individuals."

Conrad Berens, M.D., professor of clinical opthalmology, New York University Post-Graduate Medical School, adds, "The shape of the eye does change with growth, and the necessity for glasses may be eliminated merely because of the natural development of the eye.

"Eye exercises in relation to vision should be considered in the same light as physical exercise in relation to the general health of the body. . . . No miraculous cures should be attributed merely to eye exercises but their value as an aid to treatment should not be ignored. In some cases of actual eye muscle defects or eye fatigue, exercises have helped improve the nerve and muscular control of the inside and outside muscles of the eye."

There are many helpful eye-exercise books but most people who start out with enthusiasm fall by the wayside after a time, because there is no one to make them keep up the exercise.

From *Secrets of Better Sight*, written by the Niagara School of Speech in Cleveland, Ohio, come some helpful suggestions:

Blink slowly and often to "oil" the eyes, whenever your vision is not as clear as you would like.

Squeeze your eyes tight, tighter, tightest, then open slowly. This acts as a quick refresher. Do it during driving—at the stop lights. Do it when you wake in the morning if your vision seems a little misty.

Don't always sit or read the same distance from your television, movie, or book. Change intervening distances to avoid eye muscles becoming too independent upon that one distance.

Another decidedly impressive self-help book is *Relax and See*, by Clara A. Hackett, with Lawrence Galton (published by Harper, 1955). Miss Hackett has worked with 2,800 persons with eye troubles ranging from middle-aged sight to glaucoma and cataract. She says that the techniques, based on the original concepts of W. H. Bates, M.D., but with important modifications, have been responsible for improving vision in 90 per cent of her students, sometimes within a few weeks. William Gutman, M.D., of the staff of Flower Fifth Avenue Hospital, New York, who wrote the Foreword, says, "I have seen excellent results of this system of eyesight training in a great number of cases, even where severe pathology was present." Easy-to-follow directions appear in this excellent and helpful book.

Tension appears to be a major problem in vision. Irving A. Kurinsky, has noted, for instance, that in every case where cataract has occurred, tension has preceded it. Often the victim is a sensitive individual and has been through a particularly difficult period, perhaps involving the loss of a loved one or some similar crisis. This, of course, has contributed to tension which can choke off circulation and prevent any organ from receiving proper nourishment. As a result, an ailment can develop anywhere in the body. The eye is no exception. Hans Selye, M.D., has pioneered in this concept in body illnesses; W. H. Bates, M.D., in eye ailments.

Dr. Bates arrived at his conclusions after examining thousands of pairs of eyes a year at the New York Eye and Ear Infirmary. He examined tens of thousands of school children, hundreds of babies, and thousands of animals. He says:

"It has been demonstrated that for every error of refraction there is a different kind of strain. Primarily the strain to see is the strain of the mind. . . . The remedy is not to avoid either near work or distant vision, but to get rid of the mental strain which underlies the imperfect functioning of the eye. . . .

"While it is true that eyeglasses have brought to some people improved vision and relief from pain and discomfort . . . they always do more or less harm, and at their best they never improved the vision to normal. That the human eye resents glasses is a fact which no one would attempt to deny. . . . It is fortunate that many people for whom glasses have been prescribed refuse to wear them, thus escaping not only much discomfort but also much injury to the eyes. As refractive abnormalities are continually changing from day to day, from hour to hour, and minute to minute . . . the accurate fitting of glasses is, of course, impossible. At their best it cannot be maintained that glasses are anything more than a satisfactory substitute for normal vision.

"It has been demonstrated in thousands of cases that all abnormal action of the external muscles of the eyeball is accompanied by a strain or an effort to see, and that with the relief of this strain the action of the muscles becomes normal and all errors of refraction disappear. This fact furnished us with the means by which conditions, long held to be incurable, may be corrected.

"These facts appear to explain sufficiently why vision declines as civilization advances. Under the conditions of civilized life, men's minds are under a constant strain.

"Most people when told that rest or relaxation will cure their eye troubles ask why sleep does not do so. The eyes are rarely, if ever, completely relaxed in sleep. . . . The idea that it rests the eyes not to use them is also erroneous. The eyes are made to see with, and if when they are open they do not see, it is because they are under such strain . . . that they cannot see. . . . Very seldom is the impairment or destruction of vision due to any fault in the construction of the eye. . . . The eye with normal vision does not *try* to see. Whenever the eye tries to see, it at once ceases to have normal vision."

Dr. Bates has devised various relaxing exercises to relieve strain —both in the body and in the eye. They include:

Swaying! Stand with your feet apart, facing one side of an open window or door. Rock from side to side. As you rock so that you can look beyond the door or window, let your glance take in some far distant object; as you swing to the other foot, let your glance fall on the inside of the wall by the door or window frame, upon some near spot. This helps the accommodation of vision from far to near.

Swinging! Face the wall. Stand with feet slightly apart. As you turn toward one foot, let the entire body, shoulders—arms hanging limply—swing as far as comfortable to the right, then swing as far as comfortable to the left. Let the whole body "go" as you pivot from one foot to the other, with one heel rising as you go.

Palming! Cover the closed eyes with your palms without putting pressure on the eyeballs. Try to imagine a field of perfect black. The longer the period of palming, the greater the relaxation.

Sunning! Expose the closed eyes to the morning sun. You may move your head from side to side. Dr. Bates adds, "When you have become used to the strong light, raise the upper lid of one eye and look downward as the sun shines on the sclera (membrane of the eyeball). Blink when the desire to comes, or when you lose the power of relaxation. One cannot get too much sun treatment."

According to the Bates theory, when tension is replaced by relaxation, blood flow increases, the lens receives better nourishment, scar tissue (such as cataracts) may loosen and be carried away as waste material; tissues are rebuilt and sight improves.

One man I know who was afflicted with cataracts followed these exercises faithfully. His stress, following the death of his wife, resulted in cataracts of both eyes. When the cause of his trouble was later explained to him and he applied the Bates relaxation system, his cataracts were reversed and his vision returned. Except for very light glasses during periods of intensive reading necessitated by his work, he does not need to use glasses. He keeps up with his relaxing eye exercises daily to maintain his improved vision.

Frederick Lardent in, *Are Your Glasses Really Necessary?*, says that deep massage of the back of the neck-spinal region often helps vision due to tension. He also suggests clasping fingers behind neck, pressing your neck firmly against your clasped hands, then moving your head from left to right.

Here is a quickie exercise. O. Everett Hughes, N.D., writing in *Natural Health Guardian* (February, 1958) said, "I wore glasses for years, but after taking these exercises for a year, optometrists told me I did not need glasses.

"Close one eye tight. Put more power to it, trying to shut it tighter. In other words, squeeze the eye hard, while shut. Go easy the first few times. Now change to the other eye and do the same with it. Then with both eyes, look hard at some object straight ahead. Look at the object very hard. Put power behind the look. Then look hard to one corner, but keep facing ahead. Just turn the eyes. Put pressure behind that look. Now change and look to the other corner. Remember, don't turn the head. Do this 'hard look' exercise to all corners of the eye. If you notice any soreness, you can put a little more pressure in that direction."

Another system of sight improvement has been attracting attention. Captain Robert B. Hagmann, while instructing pilots in the Air Force, made some startling discoveries about vision. As a result, he now specializes in helping people to achieve better sight. He has helped many a person to overcome difficulty in getting a driver's license. He has also devised a system of retraining eyes. He agrees with one of Dr. Bates's theories: that glasses are a crutch and should be made gradually weaker instead of stronger as vision improves and should be discarded as soon as better vision makes it possible. He has had success with vision improvement in about 1,000 people. Captain Hagmann has done much research on vision and has learned that seeing has a connection with the brain. He believes it is necessary to train the brain as well as the eyes. For example, he finds that most people use one eye more than the other; one ear (for telephoning) and thus possibly only one area of the brain. His goal is to correct this imbalance.

Confirmation of his theory has recently come to light in a 10-year animal study conducted by three scientists at the University of California, Berkeley. In this study the fact that there is a correlation of vision and brain was proved conclusively.

Captain Hagmann uses his unique "mental calisthenics," as he calls his eye-training system, with people of all ages, in all types of work. A few have discarded glasses in as little as two weeks. Others have taken longer. Still others are wearing progressively weaker lenses. Testimonies of reversal of cataracts with this treatment are not uncommon. For those who cannot go to San Francisco for personal treatment, Captain Hagmann has made a home course available. Address: The Hagmann System, 165 O'Farrell St., San Francisco 2, Calif.

I have tried various types of exercises and I have achieved the best results under the Hagmann system. But I must be honest. The results are entirely up to each individual. No one can do the work but *you*. If you are faithful and persevere, you will undoubtedly get results. If you are lazy and procrastinate, as I often do, you will not advance as rapidly. (I conjure up all sorts of alibis for skipping my exercises, and improvement slows down when I backslide.)

So do not start on any system of eye-improvement exercise unless you have the determination to follow through. Otherwise you will be disappointed, not in the system, but in yourself.

32 Fallout—how to bypass it

When open nuclear testing ceased in this country most people sighed with relief and said, "Now we don't have to worry about *that* problem anymore."

I wish it were true, but it isn't. Even though new fallout is now greatly reduced, we are still stuck with the old! And Russia and China evidently are still at it.

After a nuclear test thousands of tons of these particles were sucked up into the air. Some fell to earth immediately; some were carried by winds around the earth before being spilled out; others were blown thousands of miles before being captured by rain, snow, and fog and eventually returned to earth. Dr. Edward Teller reports that some particles rose as high as the stratosphere and may take from 1 to 10 years to sift downward. Meanwhile the radioactive debris attached to these minute dust particles continues to give off radioactivity until it eventually decays.

Underground testing was once assumed to be safe, providing there was no vent in the earth. But Dr. E. A. Martell, of the Cambridge Air Force Research Center, says, "I think in connection with the iodine 131 problem we should look to our underground tests quite carefully as a possible contributing and conceivably the important source."

The escape of radiation was detected from a Nevada underground test site as recently as March, 1964, according to the Atomic Energy Commission.

IS IT DANGEROUS?

Nuclear physicists disagree on the subject of fallout danger. Dr. Hermann J. Muller, who received the Nobel Prize for the discovery of the effect of radiation upon heredity, says, "From 35 years of laboratory experience with radiation, damage results. The damage either hurts our own bodies or those of succeeding generations. Contrary to what you may have heard or read, there is no such thing as a 'safe' or 'harmless' dose. . . . effects are concealed or delayed." He adds, "Fallout from a 100-megaton bomb would be likely to induce more than 100,000 cases of leukemia, bone cancer, and other fatal ills in the present population with each explosion."

Dr. Muller, often called the father of modern genetics, was the first to crusade against overuse of medical, dental, and shoe-fitting X rays.

The National Academy of Science report of 1956 says, ". . . the best index of genetic damage [includes] mental defects, epilepsy, congenital malformations, neuromuscular defects, gland and blood defects, defects in vision and hearing, and in the gastrointestinal and genitourinary tracts."

Most experts agree that fallout causes premature aging.

If you have noticed recent mental fuzziness or peculiar physical symptoms without explanation, you might very well charge them up to fallout.

WHAT ARE THE SYMPTOMS?

Mira Louise, naturopathic nutritionist of Australia, writes, "In recent years, it has been my practise to make a biochemic analysis for a large number of my patients . . . to determine the deficiencies in the blood in order that the various biochemic cell-salts could be administered in correct proportion. Until May 1957, it was comparatively a simple matter . . . but in June of that year, a dramatic change took place. From the analysis, it was obvious that something was robbing the people of potassium, calcium, fluorine, sodium, iron, magnesium, sulphur, copper, silica and iodine. The cause was finally traced to strontium 90 and other chemicals in nuclear fallout. Undeniable symptoms of radiation sickness were apparent in many instances. Where the deficiency in calcium had averaged about 25, the average deficiency 'count' was now in the vicinity of 200 and over. The other minerals showed a proportionate or even greater deficiency.

"Of the reactions to contamination, one of the most distressing is the disturbance of the fluids in the body. This is called dehydration, that is, a drying up of the body, and it accounts for the hot, parched skin, the falling hair, acute head pains, burning eyelids, lightheadedness with 'the whole world going round in circles.' There is also a type of weeping sinus trouble, inflamed roof of mouth with swelling, buzzing in the ears, loss of appetite, distended or bloated abdomen, appendicitis and acute constipation. . . . Unfortunately, neither the human being nor animal can replace this fluid by drinking large quantites of water or any other fluids. . . . Small alkalinising drinks of dilute orange juice, grapefruit, grape, apple, carrot, celery, cabbage, or lettuce juice with a biochemic tablet dissolved in it will help the body to manufacture its own fluids. . . ."

Many other unsuspected disturbances, according to Miss

Louise, result from fallout contamination: anemia, boring pains in the bones, bone disorders, cystic conditions, warts that become sore or swollen, recurring attacks of what appears to be "Asian flu," gastro-enteritis, headaches, perpetual tiredness or exhaustion not relieved by rest, numb hands and feet, boils, carbuncles, skin rashes, breathlessness, weakness, confused mental states, vagueness, and inability to remember, are but a few of the symptoms she ascribes to this type of contamination.

She concludes, "Strictly speaking, the radioactive particles do not contaminate the body. They merely absorb the minerals, *the working elements*, from the bones and the blood, thus leaving the body more or less powerless to carry on the normal functions such as digestion, assimilation, the elimination of waste matter, and the reproduction of new blood cells. Thus we see that the body, having no means of nourishing itself or of repairing its cells and eliminating the waste *contaminates itself*."

As a result, new diseases are cropping up, the causes of which resist the usual treatment.

WHY THE PRESENT DANGER?

If nuclear testing is banned, why is fallout *still* a problem?

Radiation from fallout has a delayed reaction, and everyone in the world has already been highly exposed.

Alaskan Eskimos have levels of body radiation 3 to 80 times higher than people in the mainland United States. Eskimos eat caribou and other animals which feed on radioactive lichens contaminated in fallout from nuclear bomb tests.

The year 1963 was considered a record fallout period. Furthermore, the effect is considered cumulative and even without further testing, we will continue to be exposed to fallout hazard for at least a decade or more. Normally, after a nuclear test, fallout is washed to the earth by rains and snow. It is also stored in the soil where it remains for years. In 27 years, strontium 90 will be half as potent as when it first fell. Foods raised on this soil can be contaminated. Animals feeding on pasture can pick up the contamination.

I assure you, that in spite of reassurances to the contrary which you may read in the newspapers, this information is not fiction. I have been doing research on the effect of fallout for more than a year, have already published a thoroughly documented article on the subject, and have conferred with health departments on the dangers involved. With the exception of insecticides, it is our greatest problem today. Do not make the mistake of shrugging it off and discounting it. Everyone should take immediate action.

To show you how some of the delayed reaction works, Dr. Teller, in his book, *Legacy of Hiroshima*, noted that hair of cows exposed to the early Alamogordo tests fell out in patches, but the animals apparently suffered no other damage. The hair grew in again and the cows appeared to be unharmed. Recently, however, the *Journal of the American Medical Association* reported that at least one of these cows later developed cancer of the right eye and had to be sacrificed.

Safety in animal tests is not always a criterion. Dr. Harry Kornberg, of the Hanford Atomic Energy Commission, found radioactive iodine given to sheep and pigs in doses 500 times the amount considered safe for humans, and strontium 90 in doses 100 times the "safe" amount for humans apparently produced no harmful results, even in 10 generations of these animals. Higher doses *did* cause bone damage and tumors.

Radioactive iodine produces the same effects as X rays. It is 18 times more dangerous to babies than to adults. Children whose thyroids were exposed to X rays during treatment for enlarged thymus glands have developed thyroid cancer as much as 12 years later.

HOW DOES FALLOUT ENTER THE BODY?

Some fallout is inhaled from the air. Much of it is absorbed from eating foods affected directly, or from meat and milk of animals which have eaten contaminated products.

Once fallout is inside the body it can attack *unprotected* cells.

The Civil Defense Department tells us that the amount of radiation a person can stand depends on such variables as age and general health and vigor.

Apparently, if a body is well fortified with the proper nutritional substances, it will be less likely to absorb detrimental elements. People on a calcium-poor diet can absorb up to five times as much strontium 90 as those on a calcium-rich diet. Also, because of the affinity of the two elements, the more calcium expelled, the more strontium 90 is excreted with it. Presumably this works with iodine, too.

Dr. Russell Morgan, chief radiologist, Johns Hopkins University, says, "The addition of stable iodine has shown by studies that 1 mg. for children and 5 mg. for adults daily will induce gradually over a few days a reduction of about 80 per cent of radioactive iodine collected in the thyroid gland, and more reduction can be achieved by larger doses. . . ."

Natural iodine products include kelp and dulse and other food from the ocean.

As to the amount of calcium necessary, one report advises, "The addition of calcium compounds to the diet can greatly reduce the amount of strontium 90 deposited in the bones. Six tablets (half a gram) of strontium-free dicalcium phosphate (made from decontaminated limestone) daily would cut the strontium intake by 50 per cent." One manufacturer now provides a deep-mined limestone calcium supplement, presumably safe.

Since strontium 90 is known to affect the bone marrow, taking bone marrow in some form has been found helpful. Bone marrow injections helped the survival of four Yugoslavian scientists who had been exposed to a dangerously high radiation dose. The National Cancer Institute found bone marrow a source of radiation protection for animals. Oral bone marrow products can be purchased at drug or health food stores, as can most of the other special foods mentioned here.

Other substances which laboratory tests have proved helpful are olive oil (it counteracts radiation and aids bone marrow), cod-liver oil, vegetable oils, lecithin, bioflavonoids (vitamin C complex), and pectin.

Willard E. Baier, chemical engineer and director of Sunkist Grower's research and development program, reports that the entire United States fruit and vegetable industry has been following the Russian research with sunflower seeds. The Russians are convinced that the pectin in the seeds can help counteract the effect of strontium in the body. The theory is that pectin can force the strontium through the body without its being absorbed. Very little pectin is needed to do the job, according to Mr. Baier. About 10 to 50 grams a day would take care of it. An additional source is found in apples, lemons, grapes, etc.

Pyridoxine (vitamin B-6) helps to prevent ill effects.

Dr. Joseph D. Walters recommends the sprouting of nonchemically treated seeds, rich in many protective nutrients. Seeds for sprouting include alfalfa, lettuce, radish, mustard, safflower, kohlrabi, cabbage, celery, soy beans, and garbanzos.

Hansgeorg Weidner writing in German scientific publications, recommends millet and buckwheat as preventives against radiation. Both buckwheat seeds and the whole plant with the blossoms are helpful. Buckwheat also contains rutin helpful in capillaries.

Protein has been found protective against radiation. Since they are protected by their shell, eggs are considered safe. Poultry meat is said to be less susceptible than animal meat (according to the Poultry and Egg Board). Because the ocean dilutes fallout, fish are considered safe. Liver protects against X ray, hence it presumably helps with fallout.

At McGill University, a study with rats revealed that kelp acts as a binding agent in the intestines when it encounters strontium. In test animals the strontium absorption dropped markedly. (*Medical World News*, July 3, 1964.)

One of the most dramatic radiation aids is brewer's yeast, a rich source of protein, minerals, and vitamin B complex. In studies on 90 mice fed years before radiation, 20 per cent survived, whereas of another group not fed yeast, all died. In two groups of 40 and 80 people, those fed yeast *after* irradiation revealed a hemoglobin drop to 85 per cent of its original value, followed by a recovery to 95 per cent. Those unprotected by yeast exhibited a hemoglobin drop to 66 per cent. Brewer's yeast restored it to 95 per cent. Giving the dried yeast to people *prior* to irradiation prevented hemoglobin fall in many cases.

RECOMMENDED SAFETY MEASURES

Leafy greens seem to be especially fallout prone. Remove outer leaves and wash carefully. Washing removes up to 60 per cent of the fallout. If you grow your own vegetables, lime your garden to help plants use the calcium to resist the uptake of strontium 90. One report indicates that lettuce may be the only leafy green able to distinguish between calcium and strontium 90 and therefore may be safest, but this has not been proved.

A skin or shell apparently protects the interior of fruits, nuts or vegetables. More fallout tends to lodge in rough skins than on smooth surfaces. Even so, most fruit should be peeled. In apples, contamination is found on skins and in cores. According to the Public Health Service, potatoes should be baked and the skins discarded. Corn left in the husk until milling is safe.

WHAT ABOUT BEVERAGES?

If fallout has been high in your area, bottled water is recommended. The Public Health Service finds Asian tea leaves more contaminated than those from the Southern Hemisphere. About 20 per cent of the contamination remains in the tea after brewing. In soluble teas, there is even less. Herb teas are a good substitute if derived from uncontaminated sources. Instant coffee has been found to be more highly contaminated than brewed coffee.

Milk has stirred up the greatest controversy of all! All dairies should install strontium decontaminating plants.

According to *Nature* magazine, consumers can remove the strontium 90 from milk by adding calcium phosphate, stirring and then straining out the grains of calcium to which the strontium adheres.

Professor Humberto Aviles, of Mexico writes (English translation): "Investigators of atomic energy, have informed recently

[1953] of the qualities of the 'F' vitamin of making resistant to atomic radiations, the animals of experimentation." . . . . "The 'F' vitamin . . . has the big advantage that it can be of daily use adding it to the food diet and in emergency cases it can be swallowed and the skin rubbed with it for more protection. To all of these advantages of the 'F' vitamin add the safety of protection it offers to those who work in investigations, atomic installations and to all those who are employed near a source of radioactivity."

Vitamin "F," another name for unsaturated fatty acids, is found in vegetable oils. An especially rich source occurs in whole flaxseed, linseed oil, or fresh-ground flaxseed.

Fred R. Klenner, M.D., reports, "Guinea pigs saturated with vitamin C lived after being exposed to double the known lethal radiation dose."

E. L. David, biological researcher, London, England, writes, "At the Eighth International Congress for Prophylactic Medicine, September 6, 1961, Dr. S. Smith reported that the red beetroot juice (raw) proved to be an important therapy against X-ray and radioactive damage. This could be an epoch-making announcement to humanity, which has reason to be worried and frightened."

There is a search all over the world for plants to protect the human body against radiation. Moss, ferns, and healing fungi are some of these. Native tribes in some Latin American countries are using various plants but we do not yet know their names. Meanwhile, we can apply the nutritional knowledge already discovered.

Some researchers find that radioactivity, besides lodging in bones, is absorbed through the skin. So exercise and bathing may help.

Making changes in your family's diet is not as difficult as it sounds. Make a list of tested protective foods and include them gradually in your everyday eating. When you shop, keep the general principles of how fallout works in mind to guide you in your choices. Better health—even survival—may be your reward.

SUMMARY OF PROTECTIVE FOODS

Calcium supplements (plus vitamins C and D, for assimilation).
Natural iodine products—kelp, dulse, Japanese "nori."
Bone marrow.
Olive oil; cod-liver oil; vegetable oils; flaxseed.
Lecithin granules.
Vitamin C; bioflavonoids plus rutin.
Pectin—in fruits and sunflower seeds.
Sprouted seeds and grains.
Millet, buckwheat, as cereals.
Proteins, including sea food.
Brewer's yeast.
Raw-beet juice.
Wash leafy greens.
Discard peelings of rough fruits and vegetables.
Choose beverages carefully.

33 Fatigue

Fatigue can stem from a multitide of causes.

Here is a checklist to help you find the possible source of your fatigue:

IS IT PHYSICAL?

Do you push yourself relentlessly? Experts maintain that if you take a 10-minute rest break every hour you will achieve more in the long run.

During a rest break, have you tried lying down with your feet higher than your head to stimulate circulation to your brain?

Do you get enough outdoor activity? Exercise in fresh air, breathing more deeply, using a fresh set of muscles—all help to relieve tension and fatigue.

Do your feet get tired? If so, read the next chapter.

Does your back get tired? Read "Backache," Chapter 26.

Are you overweight? Read "Overweight and fasting," Chapter 42.

Are you constipated? Read "Constipation," Chapter 30.

Have you checked these possible disturbances with your nutritionally oriented physician?

 Anemia?

 Toxicity?

 Infections? Also, read "Infections," Chapter 39.

 Low blood pressure? It is often correctable by extra protein and optimum nutrition.

 Sluggish thyroid? Iodine in kelp and optimum nutrition, including brewer's yeast, often help.

Do you skimp on sleep, or do you have trouble sleeping? Read "Insomnia," Chapter 40.

Do you rest or relax *before* you get tired?

IS IT EMOTIONAL?

Do you resent your situation, your environment, even a person near you? First, try to analyze the situation honestly by yourself. If your problem involves an adult, try talking the situation over and clearing up misunderstandings. Remember, stored resentment contributes to fatigue. It is better to express your emotions as you feel them than to dam them up until they—and you—explode. If you need further help, seek professional counseling, perhaps from a family service organization listed in the yellow pages of your telephone book. Sometimes just talking out your problems with a trained and sympathetic listener helps.

Do you worry too much? Prayer is an excellent safety valve.

Are you bored? Try to find a new and stimulating interest, preferably something that will cheer others as well as yourself. Too often we expect the universe to revolve around us, personally.

Are you compulsive? Some people grit their teeth with determination to finish a job at a specified time, even if it kills them. They usually finish triumphantly, but dead tired. Fatigue often arises not from the work itself, but from sheer monotony. Change your activity often. Shift your attention to some other task—preferably an enjoyable one, and then return to your original chore. It will appear easier. Don't work too long at one job.

Is your work pure drudgery? Change it permanently as soon as you can, if you can. If you can't, punctuate it often with things you do enjoy. Escape whenever possible in little ways: a walk, a book, listening to a record. It will lighten the load.

Do you feel defeated? Do something nice for yourself. Allow yourself a few luxuries. Try a warm, lazy bath or a massage. Indulge yourself in some activity you *love*.

Try being alone at certain intervals. Get away from your family regularly, even for a little while. You will be more agreeable, a better parent, a better companion. Nerves can stand only so much. Pamper them. Do not resort to pep pills or tranquilizers. They are a crutch, make things progressively worse and, according to experts, can cause narcotic addiction—even death. Higher and higher doses are necessary to produce the initial effect of one pill.

A book, *Karin Roon's New Way to Relax* (New York: Greystone Press, 1949) presents a practical system of common-sense techniques for releasing tension and increasing energy. It is excellent and helpful.

IS IT NUTRITIONAL?

Don't be too quick to say No! I have known more people to reverse fatigue through certain nutritional measures than by any other means. Those who have scoffed the hardest were the most enthusiastic when their fatigue disappeared.

Do you overdrink coffee for a pick-up? Or oversmoke? Or eat sugar or sweet foods? If so, you may experience a false pick-up and soon be more tired than ever. These pepper-uppers are only temporary. Irritability, the constant need for a pick-up of some kind, even shakiness, can come from a common disturbance called low blood sugar, or hyperinsulinism. It is not corrected by sugar, alcohol, coffee, or smoking. Such props give you a quick lift followed by a sudden energy nosedive.*

* Two books explain more fully how to correct this disturbance: Abrahamson and Pezet, *Body, Mind and Sugar* and Clark, *Stay Young Longer*.

Tests at Tokushima University School of Medicine, Japan, show that fatigue arises less from diets rich in protein or fat, than in carbohydrates; and that animal protein lessens fatigue more than vegetable protein. So fortify your coffee or smoke with a few bites of protein or fat—it will not cause you to gain weight. (*Nutrition Reviews*, October, 1962.) Try cheese, or nuts, or natural peanut butter spread on crackers or stuffed into celery. Such snacks will shore up your energy for hours.

Do you take vitamins? A recent study (*General Practice*, May, 1963) found vitamin B complex and vitamin C a specific help with fatigue and general debility.

Have you tried liver or desiccated liver tablets? The Office of Naval Research discovered in animal studies that liver prevents fatigue.

A little apple cider vinegar in water may help.

Did you know that overwhelming fatigue can result from pesticide poisoning? It can be reversed. Did you know fatigue can also be a consequence of fallout? Read previous chapter.

Do you overeat at any one meal? Studies reveal that nibbling, or eating four smaller meals, produces less fatigue than eating fewer but larger meals. If your total daily calories remain the same, you will not gain weight.

On the basis of research for *Stay Young Longer* and this book, I have adopted three formulas for outwitting my own fatigue. One is to alternate unpleasant chores with pleasant tasks. I also try to do the hardest or most unpleasant chore first, to get it over with.

The second is an emergency remedy. When I need a quick burst of energy, instead of pep pills, I take 1,000 mg. of ascorbic acid (vitamin C) plus a calcium tablet (read "Infections," ch. 39). I use calcium tablets instead of tranquilizers.

I consider the next suggestion the best. I swear by it and so do my family and friends. It is almost magic. I have seen it eliminate housewife fatigue, executive fatigue (male), pregnancy fatigue, and nervous fatigue. Whenever I feel an energy let-down, I stir a tablespoon or more of brewer's yeast in a glass of juice or water. Within ten minutes energy returns. It produces a quicker pick-up than a cup of coffee and lasts hours longer.

Fatigue treatment should not be limited to a gimmick, however. Even single factors, such as I have just mentioned, are not the whole story. The only wise approach is through an all-around nutritional program. Not one food, nor one vitamin, but everything is necessary. I have found a little book, *Prescription for Energy*, by Charles De Coti Marsh, of London, England, extremely useful (see Bibliography). The author tells exactly what to eat to relieve fatigue and gain unlimited energy. To begin the day he recommends uncooked cereals, but not the packaged variety widely advertised in the United States.

He says, "Re-energizing must begin with foods . . . which create energy, maintain energy, and prolong energy. They must be taken in their natural state. These cereals are: corn seeds, wheat seeds, rye seeds, maize seeds, barley seeds, and oat seeds. These must be freshly milled. In *uncooked* cereals we do have one perfect food for perfect health which contains the essential vitamins and energy creators."

In addition to cereal seeds, Mr. Marsh recommends fresh raw nuts taken directly from the shell.

He also approves of root vegetables. He says, "Any seed or root vegetable that will grow again will renew human vitality."

This is his breakfast formula:

½ cup Brazil nuts, walnuts, or almonds.
½ cup wheat, barley, or oats.
½ chopped apple.

These seeds and nuts are to be milled in a little electric nut mill (available at health food centers) *immediately* before eating. The fruit is added after milling. The mixture can be moistened with fruit juice or milk.

He advises, "Take two tablespoons of nuts, two tablespoons of grains, mill as suggested and take this mixture for breakfast with no other foods. Now go through the day until feeling hungry and note the time. It is amazing but the average person used to a cooked breakfast will not feel actual hunger until 12 to 16 hours have passed."

The rest of his book is devoted to suggestions for nutritive foods, menus, and recipes for the other two meals. It also includes the analysis of the high vitamin-mineral-enzyme content of the raw-cereal-nut-fruit breakfast, showing that it is not accidental that such a breakfast combination can contribute so much "high octane fuel" to human energy. Be sure, when buying the cereal seeds, to get the untreated varieties. Those coated with fungicides and other chemicals have produced dangerous and disturbing after-effects.

34 Feet

A pained-looking face often results from painful feet. As I watch women hobble around shopping in tight-fitting, uncomfortable shoes and see them sit down at every opportunity, slipping off their shoes and rubbing their feet when they think no one is looking, I often wonder why they punish themselves. It is one thing to dress smartly for a social event where looks are important and where sitting is allowed at least part of the time. But when you walk or stand for long distances in dress shoes, your comfort, your disposition and your very health are threatened. Women should have the courage to ignore high fashion and sales pressure. As a reward, they would feel healthier, more comfortable, and more agreeable.

Elizabeth, Queen of England, who must stand for many hours, pampers her feet to minimize her fatigue. According to news reports, she wears toeless shoes. Other dignitaries wear flats under cover of long ball gowns. Some courageous women even go bare- or stocking-footed. More power to them! They will live longer, look younger, and feel better, while their fashion-bound sisters will be aging and ailing.

IS YOUR FOOT NORMAL?

"Wet the bottoms of your feet and then step on the floor or a piece of paper which will show the imprint of the foot. If the imprint shows only the front ball of the foot and the heel, then your foot is normal," says C. O. Benson, formerly instructor of physical education at Washington University, St. Louis, Missouri.

HEELS

Try walking without shoes, with your weight on your toes. In due time you'll become exhausted. High-heeled shoes produce exactly the same effect. According to Mr. Benson, "The habitual wearer of high-heeled shoes cannot possibly possess good calf development, but on the contrary will lose all symmetry of her legs in time. . . . The constant wearing of high heels will result in the muscles at the back of the leg becoming shorter from lack of use. Low heels will be worn only with pain. With a normal foot, however, there is no reason why high heels cannot be indulged in infrequently."

Dudley J. Morton, a New York orthopedic surgeon and associate professor of anatomy at Columbia University for 20 years, says, "Women should take care of their feet during the day. If they do, they can safely abuse them for social purposes at night."

SPACE SHOES

Alan E. Murray has provided a solution, following the advice of Howorth's *Textbook of Orthopedics*, which says, "Most of the foot complaints of the present day are directly attributable to faulty shoes. The foot should not be required to conform to the shape of the shoe, but the shoe should be constructed to fit the foot." In making shoes which fit each individual, Mr. Murray provides body and foot comfort. By word-of-mouth advertising only, the Murray space-shoe business has grown to five buildings in Bridgeport, Connecticut, a factory in Delaware, New Jersey, two salons in New

York City and 100 representatives throughout the United States. Imitations have sprung up everywhere, but they are unable to copy the original because it is protected by 40 patents.

Mr. Murray has designed his shoes for comfort and not for correction. Nevertheless, I have seen progressive plaster casts made of feet which have lived in the Murray "space or glove-mold shoe" for a period of years and the improvement in the same pair of feet is amazing. A few of the people in the public eye who swear by the Murray space shoe are: Arthur Godfrey, Danny Kaye, Joe DiMaggio, Martha Graham, Beatrice Lillie, and Robert Cummings. Add to the list innumerable dancers, postmen, waitresses, sales girls, dentists, and housewives. They all cheerfully admit that the space shoe is the ugliest shoe in the world and probably one of the most expensive, but pure bliss to walk in. Yet, somehow these shoes look "smart." Perhaps it is because they are worn by smart people.

On the wall of the Murray laboratories, where the shoes are molded to the exact contour of the customer, hangs a cartoon. Scene One: Women are hobbling painfully down the street on spike heels. Their faces, old before their time, are lined with the strain which comes from aching feet. Only one lone passerby looks fresh, young, and rested. She is wearing the space shoes, but everyone is glaring at her because she dares to be different.

Scene Two: Time has passed. Everyone is now sauntering down the street wearing space shoes. Their faces are fresh, relaxed, youthful. Only one woman is hobbling painfully on spike heels and everyone is staring at her incredulously because she is out of style!

Alan Murray originally developed the space shoes for himself, when, as a skater, his feet just went to pot. Those who have gratefully joined him in wearing the shoes claim they have had relief, even cures, for their fallen arches, corns, bunions, mosaic warts, heels spurs, and hammer toes.

Space shoes are "grounded" so that the wearer does not accumulate static electricity.

Mr. Murray believes that it isn't necessary to wear molded shoes all the time. You can wear dress shoes more comfortably when the occasion warrants because, meanwhile, your feet have had a rest. The shoes are expensive. It also takes two months from the time the plaster cast of your feet is made until you receive your shoes—if you're lucky and the waiting list isn't too long. But Mr. Murray feels that a good pair of shoes can take 10 years off a person's age. The shoes last at least five years and can be repaired.

The price obviously frightens many people away. Yet I know any number of foot sufferers who have a closetful of unused shoes which cost a total of four times the price of one pair of space shoes. As one woman who is on her feet all day in business told me, "I got space shoes after trying everything else. I cried every night with foot pain until I did."

A space shoe cradles the foot. "Space shoe" means a shoe with room for your foot to move around in, not one to wear to Mars. But for those who can't afford them, it is possible to make your own for around $15. A do-it-yourself kit is available. Dominican nuns at North Guilford, Connecticut, who spend long hours at prayer and their other occupations, are now using these kits as a means of self-sufficiency, economy, and comfort.

Long ago, I made a pair from a kit with the help of my jittery husband. (We were afraid they wouldn't come out all right, but they did.) For walking and gardening, they are excellent and when I get around to making my next pair, I am going to try something a little fancier. If you don't find a Murray space-shoe representative in your classified phone book, write for information to Murray Space Shoe Corporation, 616 Fairfield Avenue, Bridgeport 3, Connecticut.

HOW TO WALK

A sure way to find out if you are walking correctly is to look at your worn-out shoes. If heels are worn evenly across, under the ball of the foot and at the base of the big toe, you are doing fine. But if wear is greater on one part of the heel or sole than another, then trouble lies ahead. C. O. Benson suggest simple walking and exercise procedure to correct foot troubles.

To walk correctly:

Don't pound the heels. It jars the body.
Put the heel down first—slightly on the outside of the foot.

Continue weight on the outside of the foot to the little toe then across the foot to the big toe.

Walk slightly pigeon-toed. It will help to correct fallen arches, flat and lengthening feet, and cause the least possible strain on all arches.

For exercise:

Rise slowly on your toes and back down again.

Stand on a thick book. Reach the toes over the edge, trying to reach the floor.

Pick up marbles with your toes.

Flex and rotate your ankles. Bathe the feet in warm water to help circulation.

Massage your feet at every opportunity. There is a theory that there are nerve endings on the bottom of the feet and toes which correspond to various organs of the body. By constricting an area in the foot—or the toes—you may be interfering with circulation to some part of the body. (See "Pressure Therapy—Acupuncture," ch. 10.) This may be the explanation of the remark we hear so often, "When your feet hurt, you hurt all over."

Meanwhile, I hope those of you who "pound the pavement" or the hard floor, have discovered foam-rubber inner soles, available at drug and notion counters, to cushion the shock of walking or standing on a hard surface.

Simon J. Wikler, a chiropodist and author of that excellent little book *Take Off Your Shoes and Walk* (Devin-Adair), says, "Most Americans have poor feet and are unaware of it. Because of poor feet, they have posture distortions, are easily fatigued and become prone to degenerative illness. I have discovered that it is possible to have strong healthy feet." And Dr. Wikler's book tells how. He also gives suggestions for relief of bunions, corns, and many other foot miseries.

Dr. Wikler spent many years trying to find out what causes foot trouble so that he could help people to prevent it. In school, he had been taught that a foot should be supported in order to be healthy. Yet, wherever he traveled and found people wearing loose-fitting shoes, or no shoes at all, there he found straight, undeformed toes. Those who constantly went barefoot did not have fallen arches, did have good posture, and never complained of feeling tired.

It was a little boy who finally supplied the answer. He was only two and one-half, yet he tired easily, often fell while walking, and begged to be carried. He already tended toward fallen arches. When Dr. Wikler asked his mother why she bought shoes which pinched the child's toes together, she answered that she had bought the widest pair available.

Later, at Dr. Wikler's suggestion, the child was allowed to go barefoot. His toes spread out, his fallen arches were eventually cured. He acquired better balance and soon appeared tireless. Since that time, Dr. Wikler has examined thousands of feet in both adults and children. His conclusion: The major cause of foot troubles is due to the type of shoes we wear. And this affects the whole body. He says, "If strain on the body is excessive and lasts for long periods, . . . the body becomes exhausted and breaks down, and chronic diseases are often the result. Postural stress from distorted feet can cause such strain."

Dr. Wikler spent his savings trying to get a shoe company to market his special shoe for children. Time after time, he was turned down. Finally, after he had written his book, a major company decided to manufacture the shoe. Today there is a remarkable shoe for children under three, designed to avoid a lifetime of foot troubles. It is called the "Wikler shoe by Buster Brown." Now, will Dr. Wikler please prevail on a shoe company to make a similar shoe for adults?

Except for the molded space shoe, the closest thing to it is a pair of moccasins. Clement G. Martin, M.D., says you can wiggle your toes in moccasins. Otherwise, many people walk all day with toes in a cramped position in their pinched-toed shoes.

Dr. George A. Schroeder, chiropodist and podiatrist, says, "Our feet have to carry the entire weight of the body structure in a precarious position. . . . This is an immense amount of work which, unfortunately, we do not appreciate, and are hardly even aware of.

"The feet are truly the foundation of health. Any misalignment of the foot bones throws the entire system out of plumb, affecting the nerves, veins, muscles and heart."

Dr. Schroeder feels that improperly designed shoes, including pointed toes and spike heels can cause back ailments, arthritis, poor circulation, fatigue, and many other disturbances. His book, *The*

Miracle Healing Power of Body Mechanics Therapy (Prentice-Hall) is full of self-help. Case histories of sufferers from many ailments, who are completely relieved after needlessly suffering for years, testify to the success of Dr. Schroeder's methods. Men as well as women have followed the complete and explicit directions in his book, obtaining freedom from pain in back and feet.

Pinched toes and high heels are not the only hazards of shoes. At the National Association of Chiropodists, Dr. A. L. Shapiro announced, "Inflammations of the skin of the feet are often due to irritation from toxic chemicals in shoes. Modern footwear contains a wide variety of adhesives, dyes and materials which can come in intimate contact with the feet and allergic reactions may develop."

I have found that massaging gently with a lava stone, available at most drug counters, helps do away with callouses and corns.

Bonnie Prudden advises, "Go shoeless as much as you can. Stiff and aging feet are caused by the press of shoes, not years."

Anyone who has heard me lecture knows I always take off my shoes before I begin to speak. Now you know why!

35 Migraine headache

SYMPTOMS

If you are a sufferer from migraine, or know someone who is, you already know that it is an excruciating pain. To date, little help has been available. Most chronic sufferers call migraines "sick headaches" because nausea and vomiting often accompany the almost unbearable pain, which may last for three days. Aspirin has little or no effect, probably because a migraine is not due to superficial causes. *Yet migraine headaches are preventable.*

If you have ever had a migraine, you do not need to be told that it gives its warning before it strikes: black spots or a brilliant zig-zag line appear before your eyes, or you suddenly have fuzzy vision, or experience only half-vision. I call this visual distortion a "razzle-dazzle."

When the headache arrives it is on one side only, often centered around one eye. Any sound seems overloud. Normal light makes you flinch. Irritability is overwhelming. Many go to bed with a migraine, others can't bear the thought of eating. Days later after the migraine mercifully wears off, you arise weak and shaken, try to get back to normal and within a surprisingly short time, feel more energetic than usual—until your next attack.

I can recite these symptoms with my eyes shut because I used to be a migraine victim. I suffered from them during my childhood, although in those days they were known as "bilious spells." Not until I met my husband, who had also been a victim, did I learn how to avoid them. He had learned how to handle them from Thomas H. Holmes, M.D., who with Harold G. Wolff, M.D., did extensive research on migraines. Thank goodness!

THE MIGRAINE PERSONALITY

If it will comfort you, Walter C. Alvarez, M.D., recently of the Mayo Clinic, says, "A migraine is so clearly correlated with a keen, eager personality that it has been called the disease of the alert mind. It is like a Phi Beta Kappa key, awarded to only the best students at college."

Migraine sufferers have a migrainous personality. They are perfectionists. They feel compelled to drive themselves until they finish something and then they drop with exhaustion and a mixture of triumph, relief, and a feeling of being extremely virtuous. In no time the headache starts up. Sometimes it takes a special trigger, such as excitement or fright, to start the headache.

Dr. Alvarez adds, "Common triggers are sight-seeing or shopping trips; getting into a crowd; hurrying or being hurried by someone; dreading some event; seeing flickering lights; looking at checked or striped designs, glimpse of reflected light, a poorly functioning television set; waiting for a late breakfast; eating a food to which one is allergic; encountering certain smells or noises; getting angry; feeling let down after hard work; suffering from boredom. Occasionally menstruation is the main cause."

It is not uncommon to find smoldering resentment against a person or a situation a key to migraine. One woman who dreaded visits from her dominating mother-in-law discovered her migraines were connected with her arrival. Other people, unhappy in their marriage, become migraine victims. A migraine follows a clear-cut pattern, though often unsuspected until the owner has had his attention called to it.

Before my husband (a Phi Beta Kappa) met the migraine expert, he couldn't understand why he had a migraine every Friday evening. By Monday morning he seemed to recover sufficiently to return to work where he drove himself relentlessly day and night, without let-up, until Friday night again and the next attack. On Fridays he felt he had earned the luxury of a let-down for having worked so hard. Yet the headache always ruined the long-awaited rest.

Dr. Harold G. Wolff, with a team of researchers at Cornell Medical College, working on 10,000 cases, came up with some answers; a migrainous personality feels he *must* finish the job, no matter what the effort. His favorite response is, "I'll rest—as soon as I get a chance." And when he finally stops he slumps with a vengeance.

Mistake one: Such a person pushes himself beyond his endurance before letting himself slump. Just before the attack begins, blood vessels in the head shrink. This cuts down the brain's blood supply, and accounts for the visual disturbances.

Mistake two: When the person lets down—and it is usually a sudden let-down—the blood pressure rises, the blood vessels dilate, their walls swell, an enzyme produced in the brain by stress is released, and the head begins to throb and pain cruelly. Digestive upsets follow, and the migraine is in its fury.

"So don't push yourself so far in the first place," Dr. Holmes told my husband. "Relax a little each evening. A cocktail may help. Do your slumping gradually, not all at once. It is the extreme tension followed by extreme let-down which causes first the ebb and then the flow, abnormally dilating the brain's blood vessels.

"But if you have already approached the initial stages of the migraine, you can still save yourself. *Don't give in to it. Don't go to bed. Let down gradually, not suddenly.* Keep moving, keep doing something, no matter how slight, to keep those blood vessels from overrelaxing. Getting out into the fresh air will help. Coffee is excellent because it constricts your blood vessels again. A heat lamp and massage on the back of your neck may restore circulation and relieve pain. Keeping active instead of giving in and going to bed will be the hardest thing you have ever done, but it's worth the effort."

Let me give you an example. One summer, we were due to leave for our vacation in Maine. I, like all women, had a million things to do beforehand. The house had to be cleaned, the refrigerator emptied. I always like a "clean sweep," during which I get a lot of extracurricular jobs done, although they don't have to be done *then*. Of course, I could have bypassed a last-minute desk cleaning, weeding in the garden, and straightening out some drawers, but I didn't. At last in the car, I sank into the seat exhausted and said, as usual, "There, that's over!" This happens every time I go on a vacation, but I never seem to learn.

The drive to Maine took nearly eight hours and our destination was a motel close to a lighthouse on Maine's craggy coast. About half-way there, the warning migraine symptoms made their first appearance but a few minor emergencies along the way kept me alert until bedtime when I really slumped. In the middle of the night I woke up with a dilly of a migraine. I was groaning so loud it woke my husband.

"Okay," he said grimly, "get up and get dressed."

"I can't," I wailed. "I'm too miserable."

But he made me do it anyway and, bless him, gave up his own sleep to do it. First he made a cup of coffee for me. Then he took me out in the cold gray dawn by the lighthouse and walked me back and forth, with me protesting at every step, while the big light flickered on and off, until dawn. It was the first time in years I had seen the sun come up. But suddenly my headache stopped!

We found a fisherman's diner open, and still unable to face food, I sat in the car waiting for my husband to bring me more coffee and a piece of toast. In the diner, he explained I couldn't get close to food that morning. The cook, jumping to the conclusion that I was pregnant, winked knowingly. But no matter. Although my head was still a little groggy, it remained pain-free, and as I avoided slumping again, my digestion began to clear up. By keeping reasonably active and letting down gradually, I completely recovered in a matter of hours.

A dozen questions naturally arise. Why do children get migraines? Why do they often occur in adults with menstruation? Why do they often stop with menopause? Why are they generally periodic?

One reason they occur in childhood is because they can be caused by allergies. I realize now that my childhood headaches might have been triggered by chocolate, to which I later discovered an allergy. How I wish I had known about Dr. Coca's pulse test then. (See "Allergies," p. 155.)

But Sol Hirsch, M.D., offers the most comprehensive explanation for the previously unsolved mysteries of migraines. He says, after treating them successfully for many years, "The patient gets an attack for two reasons: (1) an inherited predisposition, built in and lying in wait for the suitable moment to erupt, and (2) depletion of energy, from any cause beyond the body's ability to spring back, which provides the suitable moment."

Dr. Hirsch considers these *unavoidable* depletions:

Menstruation.
Lactation.
Endocrine disorders.
Low blood sugar.
Faulty vision.
Allergy.
Infection.
Inborn weakness of constitution.
Higher requirement for essential nutrients.

He considers these causes avoidable depletions:

Disregard of limitation.
Consistent overwork or overplay.
Speeding in all activities.
Poor sleep and rest habits.
Poor eating habits and poor nutrition.
Disregard for individual needs for rhythm between work, rest, and play.
Excesses in sex, smoking, and drinking.

"Avoidable or unavoidable, depletion to the level of energy expenditure is a signal for nature's protective mechanism to step in. The resulting migraine attack, therefore, may be likened to the popping of a safety valve." The migraine draws upon the body's reserve energy.

The reason for the periodic returns of the migraine, he says, is that different people have different levels of energy reserve. Dr. Hirsch cites cases in which an attack occurs regularly in some people every six weeks, or every four weeks, or whenever their energy eventually runs out. The final depletion, whether overwork, or menstruation, or whatever, is simply the "last straw" and pulls the switch for the migraine for the poor victim who has no more surface energy to cope with the situation.

Dr. Hirsch's successful treatment is aimed at permanently raising the energy level in addition to educating the patient to recognize his own migraine pattern. In general, treatment includes tonic injections, desiccated liver, doses of thyroid extract (kelp and B complex could help, too) and a highly fortified diet with *all* supplements. Extra energy thus protects the migrainous person from becoming a victim of that final stress, avoidable or unavoidable, when it comes along.

NUTRITIONAL APPROACHES

I hope you will ask your physician to write to Sol Hirsch, M.D., 910 Grand Concourse, Bronx, New York, for a reprint of his excellent and helpful article from the *New York State Journal of Medi-*

cine, entitled, "Clinical Observations on Migraine and Its Treatment," from which this information was reported.

A drug, ergotamine, sold under various trade names, is sometimes prescribed but it, as well as other drugs, may cause disturbing side effects.

Dr. D. T. Quigley considers migraine a deficiency disease. He tells of a case of a 29-year-old girl who was forced to give up her career as a schoolteacher, because of migraines. One by one, to obtain relief, she had a right ovary, gall bladder, appendix, tonsils, and teeth removed. No relief. A brain surgeon performed an exploratory operation. Still no relief. Finally, she submitted to a hysterectomy. The migraines persisted. As a last resort she sought Dr. Quigley's advice.

After listening to her story, he asked, "Did any of the many doctors ever ask you about your diet?"

"No," she said, "not one."

The woman was placed on a high vitamin, high mineral, high protein diet with every known supplement. Her attacks dropped from one a day to one a week; then to one only, in the second month; and finally to none at all. ("Diet Deficiency in Everyday Life," Reprint No. 63, Lee Foundation for Nutritional Research, Milwaukee 3, Wisconsin.)

The important thing to remember about migraines, whether they are of physical, emotional, allergic, or nutritional origin, is not to wait until you get the next one. Prevent it! There is no doubt that improved nutrition has helped me to eliminate regular migraine. I no longer have them except on rare occasions when I push myself too far.

Analyzing your behavior can also be a definite help. Dr. Wolff tells all migraine patients who come to New York Hospital:

Everything doesn't have to be perfect. Make reasonable changes. This does not mean failure, but being more intelligent.

There is more than one way of doing a thing. Sometimes another way is more human, more rewarding. Be tolerant of others and their ways.

Relax. People are not as critical of you as you are of yourself.

Marriage fills a human need to escape loneliness. It is giving comfort as well as gaining it.

Cut down on your day's work. Don't set impossible goals for yourself. Change things which worry you and then avoid the worry.

Dr. Wachtel, in his book *Your Mind Can Make You Sick or Well*, tells of a woman who was alienating her family as well as suffering from migraines because of her perfectionism. Her grown children avoided coming home because Mama wouldn't let them relax. A little device finally solved her problem. She made a list every morning of everything she felt she had to do. Then she crossed off anything she decided wasn't absolutely necessary to do that day. Finally, she tore up the list with the remaining items and threw it away. This became a symbol of tearing up her old habits. It brought double dividends: her headaches vanished and her children returned more often because of the relaxed atmosphere.

Nevil Layton, M.D., finds that migraine responds to vitamin B-2 (riboflavin), particularly in less severe cases. Although he gives it by injection, he states that 10 mg. three times a day taken orally has been reported by other investigators as being useful. (*Medical Press*, December 2, 1959.) Dr. Layton uses a combination of vitamins by injection: B vitamins nicotinamide, riboflavin, pyridoxine, plus 800 mg. of vitamin C.

John E. Eichenlaub, M.D., says, "Migraine or any other types of throbbing headaches usually stem from engorged blood vessels. Strong coffee helps to shrink those vessels. One or two cups of strong coffee usually do enough good . . . to make up for their jitter-spurring action."

Dr. Eichenlaub also recommends ice bags. He says, "Ice also helps to shrink engorged blood vessels. If you do not have an ice bag, a plastic refrigerator bag works fairly well. Apply the ice twenty minutes at a time, allowing the skin to rest for at least ten minutes between applications. (Ice bags should be padded with a dry towel to prevent ice burns.)"

Dr. Eichenlaub suggests that if the pain gets too bad, taking aspirin along with the coffee will help. If you don't drink coffee, Anacin now contains aspirin *and* caffeine.

It is true, as you will see in Chapter 3, "Why Drugs?" that aspirin can be dangerous. Phenacetin, which appears in A.P.C. combination tablets, has been reported as causing dangerous blood changes. (*Consumers Bulletin Annual,* 1963-1964.) The only time I have ever allowed myself to take aspirin is to get relief from a migraine, and then I have taken the minimum dose. Nor do I feel guilty in drinking coffee at such a time, since it acts as a medicine. At least this makes a wonderful alibi for a coffee lover!

The final remedy I will mention I have only recently discovered. It is, in my case at least, a better preventive than cure, but if I take it immediately at the first symptom, it works like a charm. I have checked with two other people who report equal success. It is a homeopathic remedy known as "Iris 6x" and is available from homeopathic pharmacies. (See "Homeopathy," ch. 7.) Usually homeopathic remedies are not considered "specifics," meaning that only certain remedies fit certain people. But since it is harmless and without side effects, it is certainly worth a try.

36 Hearing

Loss of hearing may be due to many causes. It may be congenital, or it may result from a childhood disease, chronic illness, an injury, infection, allergy, poor circulation, prolonged or very loud noise, or even a poor bite. The two basic types of hearing loss are conduction and nerve (perception) loss. A pure conduction loss means that the hearing nerve is normal but that there is an obstruction to the passage of sound waves before they reach the inner ear where the hearing nerve is located. The obstruction usually occurs in the ear canal, ear ossicles, or eustachian tubes.

An abnormal growth of spongy bone causes one common type of obstruction. Sound waves cannot get past the barrier. Fenestration, a type of surgery which cuts a window in the bone, may give relief for this type of deafness. Another type of surgery is known as mobilizing the stapes, a tiny bone of the middle ear. This quick and helpful operation for people who are candidates for such help was originated by Dr. Samuel Rosen of New York City.

Radium has been used in types of conduction deafness where lymphoid tissue obstructs the openings of the eustachian tubes. Tympanoplasty is used to clean out diseased tissue and restore the eardrum by means of a free skin graft, if the drum has been ruptured.

Nerve (perception) loss indicates damage to the nerve of hearing somewhere between the inner ear and the brain. It is by far the greater cause of hearing impairment and affects persons of all ages for various reasons.

Some other types of hearing loss go hand in hand with hardening of the arteries or with catarrhal trouble.

Dr. Samuel Rosen says, "Narrowed arteries to the inner ear might dull hearing by impeding blood flow to the cochlea—the shell-shaped organ within the skull which houses auditory nerve endings."

Dr. Bernard J. Ronis, a Temple University medical professor, claims that allergy has caused more than half of all hearing losses in children. And, although unnecessary tonsillectomies are being discouraged by many physicians, occasionally it is indicated for impaired hearing. Children who have greatly enlarged tonsils and adenoid tissue, and suffer from impaired hearing, have been helped by a tonsillectomy. A St. Louis University physician reports 26 out of 37 such children were helped. (*Laryngoscope*, Vol. 29, p. 1017.)

Since this book is dedicated to natural treatment, I am inclined to deplore surgery unless it is the last resort. I have, however, witnessed one case of a child's immediate hearing improvement by removal of enlarged tonsils and adenoids. This does not mean that every child should have his tonsils out! It is wise to consult an otologist and get a second opinion before making such a decision.

I have seen some types of tonsil infection respond to the natural treatment of vitamin C therapy. (See "Infections," ch. 39.)

NUTRITIONAL TREATMENTS

In case of sudden deafness, Dr. Woodrow D. Schlosser, consultant to the Pennsylvania Academy of Opthalmology and Otolaryngology in Philadelphia, has found that hearing can be restored to 50 per cent, if the patient seeks help within the first six weeks. The treatment is simple. In most instances it is based on the assumption that a blood vessel leading to the inner ear has become spastic. Histamine and nicotinic acid, a B vitamin, have been used with success.

Sudden deafness has also been helped by injection of B-12.

Those with nerve deafness cannot expect help from medical or surgical means, but because in some cases the disturbance is associated with nutritional deficiencies, if nerve deafness has not progressed too far, nutritional therapy may help.

Nicotinic acid, a B vitamin, which stimulates circulation, has been helpful where hearing loss accompanies artery hardening. (*Journal of the American Medical Association*, November 30, 1957.) Lecithin and unsaturated oils may also help in case of cholesterol deposits, according to Lester M. Morrison, M.D.

Large doses of vitamin C have helped hearing, particularly if infection of the middle ear is involved. (*Journal of Laryngology and Otology*, Vol. 54 [1939], p. 256.)

Dr. M. Joseph Lobel of New York City has done considerable work with nutrition and deafness. He recommends injections of large amounts of vitamin A to bypass poor digestive absorption. Of 300 patients, 259 reported an average gain in hearing of 18 per cent. The others failed to benefit from the treatment. Tinnitus or ringing in the ears was helped or eliminated entirely. (*Archives of Otolaryngology*, May, 1951.)

From Italy comes a report that people with various types of deafness were given by injection: 30,000 I.U. vitamin A, 50 I.U. vitamin E, and organic iodine, either daily for 2 weeks followed by alternate days for 3 weeks, or three times a week for 8 to 10 weeks. Patients with slight or medium hearing loss attained normal hearing.

Drs. Hans Hirschfeld, Max Jacobson, and Augusta Jellinek, of New York City, developed a nutritional treatment for deafness which they tried on 78 cases. Some of the patients showed hearing gains of 40 per cent to 50 per cent, particularly in high tones which usually disappear first when hearing is afflicted. The treatment was given in capsules three times daily or by injection. It combined vitamins A, C, and B complex, with amino acids, glutamic acid, histidine, and methionine, plus urea. In the report issued by the American Medical Association, the doctors state, "The special significance of the new compound lies in its direct influence on the stimulation and the restitution of the function of the auditory nerve itself." The substance used for injection is called Amvitol.

Fifteen years' experience with nutritional treatment using amino acids and vitamins have been reported in the *Bulletin of the Academy of National Medicine* (France [1961], 145:16-20). The substances included: thiamin (vitamin B-1) 10 mg.; riboflavin (B-2) 2 mg.; pyridoxine (B-6) 5 mg.; nicotinamide (another B vitamin) 40 mg.; methionine 15 mg.; histidine 20 mg.; tryptophan 10 mg.; and choline citrate, 10 mg. The course of treatment consisted of 12 intramuscular injections on alternate days, repeated with intervals of 15 days until four courses had been given in about five months. In hard-of-hearing subjects, an immediate improvement of auditory acuity was often produced within 15 to 30 minutes after injection. Children showed improvement in three to four weeks. Perception of conversational frequencies was noted, but a very great gain was noted in high-pitched tones. Of 2,840 patients treated, 1,646 improved rapidly and considerably, both subjectively and by audiometric tests; 457 more were subjectively improved; and 737 showed no improvement.

OTHER TREATMENTS

Bernard Welt, M.D., has pioneered in a unique treatment for hearing disorders. I first learned of him through a lawyer who had taken his wife to Dr. Welt for treatment. The lawyer's letter, including another which follows, tells the story.

The lawyer writes, "Dr. Welt is an ear, nose and throat specialist who, after long and tedious experiments, has developed a technique which improves the hearing in many patients. Some cases he cannot help; with others he seems to be extremely successful. To give you an idea of what happens to those he does help, I am enclosing the letter from a boyhood friend of his, a writer in Hollywood. I was in Dr. Welt's office when his friend first came in and I saw him improve under the treatment."

Here are excerpts from the friend's letter: "My arrival home without a hearing aid caused reverberations in this community. My secretary is still half convinced that I am wearing the little button in some mysterious place. My wife is completely delighted to reestablish oral communication with me again after twenty long years.

"Hardly a day goes by without a new sound being added to my expanding aural palate. I hear the wind sighing through our tall Eucalyptus trees, and the humming of the humming birds when they come to the feeder outside our window. . . . Today I attended a concert and heard without any amplification my son perform a sonata, and noted the brilliance of the piano. And when I play myself, the notes are audible, not distant, fugitive or imaginary. . . ."

Dr. Welt, who is director of the eye, nose, and throat sections at Greenpoint Hospital, Brooklyn, New York, and surgeon at the Brooklyn Ear and Eye Hospital, developed his treatment for deafness as a result of many years of research. He first noticed, in agreement with other researchers, that hearing acuity often varied with the time of day. Some investigators had already reported that certain patients heard better in the morning; others heard better at night. No explanation was given by these investigators and no effort was made to establish the validity of the observations by means of repeated audiograms. Dr. Welt did conduct thorough and repetitive audiogram testing, and rediscovered these variations of hearing occurring at different times of the day in both adults and children. His hypothesis is that there is a relationship between the varying hearing acuity and the variation of the urinary pH in a patient with normal kidney function. He developed a type of therapy, a group of medicinal compounds in solution, to attempt to reverse the condition he had noted.

Acting upon this hypothesis, which originated with Dr. Emanuel Revici, Dr. Welt then examined all cases of deafness brought to him from five years of age upward. Only cases with intact eardrums were accepted for investigation. Cases suspected of having intercranial lesions were rejected. If after a therapy lasting three months no improvement was obtained (a decrease of 10 decibels or more on the audiogram), therapy was discontinued and the case classed as unimproved.

Following treatment, he saw and tested each case every week for a three-month period. The intervals between testing were then gradually lengthened from one week to two weeks until a maximum improvement was noted. Meanwhile, the patient was receiving continuous medication. If a regression in hearing was noted, the patient was instructed to return sooner for retesting, a change of dosage for the medication, or a complete change of medication with another group of compounds. If no result was obtained in a three-month period, the patient was advised to discontinue therapy, but could continue if he so wished. Occasionally, this proved worthwhile.

Treatment is extremely simple and consists in taking by mouth, three or four times a day, a prescribed dose of one or perhaps two of the solutions. The results in the change of audiogram of 118 patients (236 ears) suffering from varying degrees of impaired hearing, have been measured and tabulated. Out of 236 ears, 93 ears (39 per cent) attained normal hearing as judged by the audiogram only; 37 per cent of the cases were unimproved in air-conduction response and 44 per cent in bone-conduction response. Dr. Welt found good response greater in the earlier decades of life. In the younger age group (under 30) 59 ears out of 86 attained a normal audiogram, whereas in the older age group (over 30) only 25 out of 150 did so.

All told, in addition to those who acquired completely normal hearing, 97 ears out of 236 were improved to within normal audiogram range. The average duration of impaired hearing prior to treatment in these cases had existed just over four years. The av erage duration of treatment required to bring about restoration of these cases was a little over seven months.

Dr. Welt stresses the point that up to the present time, there has been no truly systematic medical approach to the problem of chronic progressive deafness. He cannot promise how long a result might last. He keeps a case under observation for a two- or three-year period. He has seen cases of improved hearing maintained with little loss after three years, even with no treatment given during the year prior to the check-up. Some cases have experienced regressions in hearing as often as two or three times. Each time the downward course has been halted and reversed. Dr. Welt found that virus infections, asthma, pregnancy, and especially childbirth are apt to cause regressions, but these states may be overcome by continuing the therapy or changing to another group of compounds.

Dr. Welt points out that there are differences in the results, depending on whether the case is one of neurosensory or conductive hearing loss. In nerve cases, response is not as successful as it is in conductive groups (as judged by the speech-reception threshold and the discrimination scores). Occasionally, the bone conduction only is improved, or only the low tones. However, this adds to the hearing comfort of the patient so that he can tolerate a hearing aid, whereas he could not tolerate one before. In Dr. Welt's group of cases, ranging in age from under 5 to 30 years of age, some patients were not obliged to wear aids at all and some patients have given them up after hearing has improved.

Dr. Welt does not offer his method as a cure. Rather, he proposes it as a form of therapy which in some measure may alleviate the handicap associated with chronic progressive deafness and the tremendous burden to the individual as well as to public health authorities in dealing with these problems.

Your doctor may write directly to Dr. Welt for his formulas and instructions for treatment. (See Bibliography for address.)

A "natural" method of restoring hearing was reported in *Mercury* magazine, February, 1957. The article was called "Hearing Can Be Restored." Father Charles Carty, editorial manager of Radio Replies Press, writes that as a result of reading the article, he obtained treatment from Dr. Curtis H. Muncie (now deceased), of New York City, and from his son Dr. Curtis J. Muncie, of Miami, Florida. The improvement was obtained by finger manipulations, called finger surgery (no instruments are used), and immediately restored the hearing in one ear to 81 per cent and hearing in the other ear to 70 per cent. As a result, he could hear whispered confessions without a hearing aid.

Both doctors, father and son, according to Father Carty, have treated collectively 15,000 deaf persons. They have restored hearing in many, though not all, with improvement ranging from 20 to 60 per cent. They have even helped deaf mutes. They were not able to help anyone suffering from complete nerve degeneration.

The technique is designed to establish reconstruction of the eustachian tubes by use of the surgeon's finger and thus hope to re-establish hearing. A report of the types of deafness which have been successfully treated by this method include catarrhal deafness, hereditary and progressive deafness, nerve deafness, congenital deafness, Meniere's Disease (vertigo), tinnitus (ringing in the ears), aviation deafness, deafness following fenestration surgery and stapes mobilization. The method has been introduced in London, Glasgow, and Paris. Individuals or otologists may write directly to Dr. Muncie for further information. (See Bibliography for address.)

HEARING AIDS

If surgery or nutritional treatment have not solved your hearing problem, or if special treatments just mentioned are unavailable to you, a hearing aid can make the difference between success and failure in leading a normal life.

The hearing aid industry is making giant strides in perfecting instruments to provide better hearing. They have come a long distance from the large unwieldy box carried in one's pocket accompanied by a dangling cord leading to the ear. Now eyeglasses, behind-the-ear aids, aids concealed in earrings for women, and tiny in-the-ear aids are available. There are even aids for *both* ears for those who really need them. No one with a hearing difficulty (and at last count 18 million Americans do suffer from some sort of deafness) need be embarrassed about advertising the fact. For some reason, the average person is not self-conscious about wearing glasses, but most people are sensitive about wearing a hearing aid. Thanks to today's aid, it can be scarcely noticeable in men, and completely hidden in a woman's hair-do.

When a person decides to do something about his hard-of-hearing problem and wonders which dealer to approach, he should be forearmed with the following information from a top authority.

Beatrice Henderer, director of Audiological Services of the New York League for the Hard of Hearing, makes several suggestions to those who are considering a new hearing aid:

Do try more than one kind of hearing aid. Be sure it is made by a reliable manufacturer.

Don't believe all you read in advertisements. What is good for one person may not be good for another.

Do get a hearing aid which has sufficient power for your particular hearing loss and which will give you needed reserve power.

Don't be influenced by the appearance of an aid, if it is inadequate for your hearing loss. A poor-fitting aid is money wasted.

Don't get a hearing aid that does not have fitting flexibility. You may require a boost in certain speech frequencies, particularly in the high-pitch range.

Do get an aid worn directly at the ear. It provides better reception. Don't buy a behind-the-ear aid with the microphone placed at the rear. Otherwise, you will pick up sounds behind you, not in front of you!

Do get accustomed to the use of your aid. Wear it around the house, then to a friend's house, to the neighborhood stores.

Don't delay returning your aid for checking, if necessary. A slight adjustment may make a great difference in your hearing.

Do study lip reading and auditory training, if your aid does not give you expected results.

Don't get discouraged if you do not hear as well as you would like with your aid. Remember that it is an "aid" to hearing and that no mechanical device will be the same as normal hearing.

But there are still more facts you should know before selecting a hearing aid. Naturally, the first need seems to be to intensify sound. So the average person makes an appointment with a dealer, usually chosen at random from the yellow pages of the telephone book. The dealer gives the customer a test with the only device available—until recently—called an audiometer. This instrument, in general, tests pure tone, both as to range (high or low tone) and intensity (loud or soft) to determine the amount of hearing loss. An aid, either the only one or one of several which that dealer sells, is then chosen according to the audiometer tests, and an earmold is made to fit the hearing aid and the customer's ear canal. The hearing aid usually has a volume control which can be turned up or down as necessary.

When the new wearer of the aid first tries it, several things may happen. At first he is delighted that soft sounds which formerly escaped him are now audible. They are so audible, in fact, that when he gets out on the street the traffic noises become so deafening that he has to turn down the volume control, or turn the aid off altogether in order to be comfortable. At home, he can now hear the radio and television at a normal volume level, as long as he is looking straight at it. And people no longer have to shout.

Then two things become apparent. He finds that although he hears a voice more loudly, he doesn't always understand the words. If his back is turned, if he is in a large circle and some distance from the speaker, or if he is in another room, the words become fuzzy and unintelligible. If someone speaks to him when the radio or television or conversation is under way, he is even more handicapped, becomes irritable and nervous, and extremely disappointed with his aid.

There is one explanation for these experiences. The world is a noisy place. People who have normal hearing have trained themselves to ignore what they don't want to hear, and to pay attention to what they do want to hear. When a person first dons a new hearing aid, all sorts of sounds become audible. Rushing sounds of a passing car, heel clicks on the pavement, barks of dogs or crinkling paper become noticeable. Some noises are pleasant, some are disturbing.

Donkeys working in coal mines lose their sight because there isn't enough light for their eyes to use. In a similar manner, the auditory nerve has become weak and lazy while it had less work to do; the brain center has become dull or has forgotten how to hear accurately or to understand. As a result, those who have had a hearing loss over a period of years, have lost the ability to use their ears fully. This condition usually improves by using a hearing aid. In due time you will learn to ignore disturbing sounds, just as you did with normal hearing. At first you may need to concentrate more on listening to conversation to compensate for your long period of lazy hearing. But hearing rehabilitation can take place with practice and use of the aid.

However, there is another explanation for these difficulties encountered in wearing an aid. Because the hearing aid industry has progressed so fast, it has not been possible for many representatives to help the hard-of-hearing customer get the best fitting for his particular predicament. It is true, as most dealers will tell you, that you will grow accustomed to those disturbing noises, and that you must face the fact that a hearing aid can never be as good as normal hearing. Even so, there are some people who, after a fair trial and a great deal of money spent, become completely disillusioned with their aid. They dip into their savings or acquire on time payments another aid, thinking that surely this one will give greater clarity and less distracting noises. I have known people who have tried four or more different types of aid and still could not hear distinctly under some circumstances. This need not happen, unless extremely severe ear damage has occurred.

People are beginning to choose a hearing aid as they would clothes. Many people go to a clothing store, take a suit or dress off the rack and try it on. On some, the choice fits perfectly. They are the lucky ones. Others, who have certain figure problems, either need alterations, or if they can afford it, custom-made clothes. Those who cannot afford custom makes get along the best they can with store-bought clothes. And so it is with hearing aids. It is true there are differences in premade aids, not only in appearance but in performance. The dealer can choose a commercial brand to approximate the needs of the individual. He can even make a few alterations.

But for those people who have specific problems, a custom fitting is preferable and is no more expensive than some of the better aids. It would be to the advantage of the person who is dissatisfied with his aid, or even for those who have not yet acquired an aid, to find a special consultant, trained in otometry, to provide accurate fitting.

There is now a new type of measuring device (available to all dealers) which can provide a more accurate fitting and the closest-to-normal hearing yet made available by a mechanical aid. I talked with a consultant who offers this newer type of custom-fitting service. This is what he told me:

"Each person is different, thus his hearing problem is different. An aid should be chosen not only to correct loss of high or low tones, or on the basis of greater volume, but to suit the needs of the whole individual. The earliest instrument used for testing, the audiometer, analyzes only these problems. But new equipment, of which few people are aware, has become available within the last two years. It is called sound-pressure equipment. It helps to pinpoint other problems. For example, if a person is obliged to turn the volume control down in order to be able to tolerate street noise, it is an indication of a poorly fitted aid. Such inconvenience is not necessary for most people. If a door slams, a book drops, or someone is talking against background noises, or the din of a cocktail party, of radio, television, there should be no distortion of sound to the average well-fitted listener. If a person is talking to you from another room, or when your back is turned, your aid should compensate. The sound-pressure equipment makes this possible. It is far more accurate in determining your special problems and finding the correct solution for you than trying on a dozen aids, hoping you will get the right one. The sound-pressure equipment can spot these troubles before you choose your aid and usually within thirty minutes.

"A special consultant (it is possible for a layman to be trained in otometry to qualify for this work) can determine the maximum enhancement of hearing for each individual by using the audiometer *plus* the sound-pressure equipment. On the basis of these measurements he can, and does, then order a custom-made hearing aid built to exact specifications and adapted to any style preferred. As a result, the individual's hearing will be corrected to the point where it will approximate normal hearing. He should not have to turn it down on the street or up when someone across the room—or even on the lecture platform—speaks."

HOME REMEDIES

Telephones with volume controls are now available at only a slightly higher price than regular instruments.

Here are some home remedies you might try:

To open portals to the ear, say *You, Air, Yee,* making a face as you overemphasize the sounds in a long, loud tone, several times daily.

Dr. Eleanor Amend offers the following four suggestions to improve hearing in her book, *Health Can Be Yours Naturally:*

Squeeze upon the joints of the ring finger and the corresponding (fourth) toe, covering all sides thoroughly, a few minutes daily. (She says that this method has often worked after every other scientifically accredited method has failed.)

Tuck a wad of cotton or clean compress in the space behind the last tooth; bite down hard for several minutes; repeat two or three times daily.

Place fat pads of middle fingers in ears and hum something—anything of your choice—for a few minutes every day.

To help impeded circulation, *regularly* bend the head forward three times, backward three times, and to each side three times; do it twice daily.

Clinics are available throughout the United States to teach lip reading and to help re-educate the hard-of-hearing. Ask your doctor about them.

A book which is helpful but little known is *The New Way to Better Hearing,* through hearing re-education, by Victor L. Browd, M.D. It presents a technique of overcoming hearing disabilities and learning to hear well with or without professional instruction or hearing aids. This hearing re-education involves no surgery, drugs, or medication. It requires just a few minutes a day at home. The method is based on results of government tests at Harvard University and often brings improvement within weeks.

37 Heart

Someone dies of heart disease in the United States almost every two minutes.

At a testimonial dinner some time ago for two television personalities, a comedian, Parkyakarkas, died of a heart attack. The almost unbelievable incident in connection with his death was that the master of ceremonies, after calling for a doctor, asked if anyone in the audience had nitroglycerine pills (used by persons with serious heart conditions). *More than a dozen men in that relatively small audience came forward with such medication!* What is America coming to?

Melvin E. Page, D.D.S., of the Page Biochemical Foundation, St. Petersburg, Florida, states, "People do not have to be subject to coronary disease! Their chemistry can be changed for the better.

"All people are unique in that there is only one of a kind. Each person has his own chemical make-up. He was born with it. Some have good chemical make-ups and some not so good. It is our work to supplement glands that are weak so that his chemistry is nearly as good as the one more fortunate in his chemical inheritance. He then has the chemical efficiency that these glands control to enable him to protect himself against disease. This is real preventive medicine.

"A cardiogram does not tell when an attack is imminent; it only tells of a condition that has already happened. It is important that a patient should see his doctor once a year, but this is not enough. Coronaries often occur in people who have been in perfect health, insofar as they know, all their lives."

As you may recall, President Dwight D. Eisenhower had an

"all clear" physical examination within a month prior to his coronary accident.

All other organs of the body can rest when tired. The heart must work continuously.

A single procedure to prevent—or treat—heart disease is not enough. The rage over cholesterol is beginning to wane. It did not supply the hoped-for explanation for heart attacks in all people. The excitement over unsaturated versus saturated fats is also diminishing. While important, saturated fats are also not the only cause of heart attacks in everyone. There are reports from various places scattered over the world that certain groups eat liberal amounts of animal fat and thrive!

There is further support for this theory. Two scientists, a physician, and two nutritionists, reporting in the *American Journal of Clinical Nutrition* (March, 1964), suggest that it is the sugars in the American diet, not the fats, which may be responsible for the increase of heart disease; countries with the best records of heart health, consume the least amount of sugars. The authors have also found that there is a greater consumption of unsaturated fats (considered acceptable) today than seventy years ago when heart disease was much less of a problem.

Stress, and the executive heart, still attract a great deal of attention, judging by the millions of tranquilizers taken daily. But, again, avoiding stress does not alone solve the problem. The truth seems to be that *not one factor, substance, or procedure is to blame for heart attacks.* There is an interrelationship among many factors. *Not one but all should be considered.*

To prevent a heart attack, or even to alleviate it, where should you begin?

Proper "fuel" is necessary to keep your hard-working heart in order. Many researchers have learned that certain nutritional substances provide better fuel than others and seem to protect the heart. Such nutritional substances have also been found to keep other organs and glands, which are the heart's co-workers, in optimum condition. This correct nutritional program can help promote good over-all body chemistry. So let us look first at the scientific information we have.

WHAT NUTRIENTS PROVIDE PROTECTION?

A study at the Minnesota Agricultural Experiment Station reported that cattle deprived of vitamin E rations appeared to be in perfect health, but suddenly dropped dead of heart disease. When the wheat germ was restored, the deaths from heart disease ceased. (*Science*, 104:312-313; 1946.)

The brothers Shute, Dr. Evan and Dr. Wilfred, both M.D.'s of Canada, together with Dr. Arthur Vogelsang, have been using massive doses of vitamin E (alpha tocopherol) on heart disturbances for many years. By 1955 they had treated over 10,000 patients successfully, including angina, rheumatic heart, and hypertension (high blood pressure).

Among their cases was one man, a wheelchair angina invalid, who experienced excruciating pains just in carrying on a conversation. Massive doses of vitamin E freed him from his wheelchair so that he could fish all day, play bridge until midnight, and enjoy nine holes of golf. Another angina patient, 71, suffered from extreme pain after the slightest exertion. Vitamin E made it possible for him to do heavy work at a tannery. A 26-year-old man, stricken with rheumatic fever during childhood was able, with the help of vitamin E, to work in a foundry. A 52-year-old musician, with recurrent attacks of coronary thrombosis over a period of five years, after taking vitamin E did not spend another day in bed. ("For Heart Disease, Vitamin E," by J. D. Ratcliff, *Coronet*, October, 1948.)

The therapeutic explanation for vitamin E is that it apparently increases oxygen to the heart and other muscles. It also, according to the Drs. Shute, dissolves clots if they are fresh, or bypasses sites of older clots or vascular blocking, thus increasing the circulation. As they put it, "Alpha tocopherol is uniquely valuable in the treatment and prophylaxis of coronary occlusion. It is simple, cheap, can be self-administered indefinitely and rarely requires even initial hospitalization. It has no rivals. Even the anti-coagulants in common use are not comparable in any sense, whether in safety, price or effectiveness. The mortality rate achieved by its use is perhaps the best argument for it—a rate only a fraction of that attainable by the best modern treatment of any other type. The de-

gree of clinical improvement is also dramatic in many instances."
(W. E. Shute, E. V. Shute, *et al., Alpha Tocopherol (Vitamin E)
in Cardiovascular Disease,* The Shute Foundation, 1954.)

Lancet, the British medical journal, also reports that vitamin E is
effective in coronary occlusions and arteriosclerosis.

Although vitamin E is now used with success in most major
countries in the world, it is still a controversial vitamin in America.
There are two possible reasons for this: Physicians who report *successful* results *employ massive amounts of vitamin E* until relief
takes place, whereas doctors in this country use small doses. According to the Drs. Shute, this does not produce the same effect.
The other reason for probable lack of success in this country is that
the vitamin E used here is largely synthetic and in high doses can
be as dangerous as an excessive intake of vitamin D.

How much vitamin E do the Canadian physicians recommend?
"As our experience has increased, our doses of alpha tocopherol
have risen in parallel," says Dr. Shute. "There exists in the body a
'physiological dam' and a large enough dosage must be given to
raise the level of the vitamin E in the body until it over-runs the
dam. Our success with this procedure has been marked, notably, in
persistent anginas, arteriosclerotic conditions, chronic leg ulcers,
and chronic phlebitis. Patients who did not receive help from 300
to 400 units have been helped by 600 to 2,400 units daily.

"Half a dose of alpha tocopherol," says Dr. Shute, "does not do
half a job, as we pointed out years ago. One either uses the proper
dose for that patient and his particular condition, or one is not
using anything. Too small a dose is equivalent to half-treating a
diabetic. Half the dose of insulin the latter needs leaves him still
an untreated diabetic. . . . When one is treating, and no obvious
improvement occurs promptly, one should raise the dose to a level
which proves helpful. If one is in doubt, it is safer and wiser to
overtreat than to undertreat."

According to Dr. Shute, the only people who should exercise
caution in taking large doses of vitamin E are those with high
blood pressure. Suddenly administered large doses may temporarily
increase the blood pressure. It is safer for high blood pressure patients to start with small doses and work up very gradually—hand
in hand with a sympathetic physician.

An easily understood book on the values of vitamin E is *Your Heart and Vitamin E*, by the Drs. Shute. The medical text for physicians is *Alpha Tocopherol in Cardiovascular Disease*, by the same authors. (Currently out of print.)

W. J. McCormick, M.D., of Toronto, reminds us that vitamin C is necessary, too. It strengthens the blood vessels and connective tissue; it prevents or attacks infections; helps supply oxygen to the heart; and it helps to regulate the deposition of cholesterol by protecting the liver, which detoxifies poisons and manufactures lecithin. (*Clinical Medicine*, July, 1952.)

Vitamin C complex (bioflavonoids) have been found helpful in treating and preventing cardiovascular diseases. Drs. Bale and Thewlis give the reasons why:

1. Older people often have a deficiency of vitamin C in their diets.

2. Bioflavonoids (including rutin) have been found to prevent capillary fragility, thus helping to prevent strokes. (*Geriatrics*, January, 1953.)

Vitamin C has also been found helpful in reducing the cholesterol level. (*Nutrition Reviews*, July, 1964.)

Vitamin B-1 (thiamin) has long been used for heart problems, particularly for slow heartbeat, murmurs, palpitations, enlarged or nervous hearts. B-6 (pyridoxine) is a newcomer. Studies indicate that it is helpful in preventing atherosclerosis, or artery hardening. (*Journal of Chronic Diseases*, July, 1955.)

These two B vitamins are not the only ones necessary, however. Drs. H. A. Levy, M. G. Wohl, and C. Alpert say, in connection with heart problems, "It now appears that all of the major members of the B-vitamin complex are in short supply." (*Clinical Research*, 7:18; 1959.)

Dr. M. M. Gertler agrees. Speaking at the New York Academy of Sciences, he emphasized that vitamin B complex supplements should be an integral part of the treatment of every patient with congestive heart disease. (Vitamin B complex is found abundantly in brewer's yeast and liver.)

Edward Podolsky, M.D., has reported that calcium supplements have a digitalislike action on the heart. He also reports studies of the good effect of calcium lactate on high blood pressure. (*Illinois Medical Journal*, August, 1939.)

Rolled oats have been found to lower cholesterol. When 21 healthy men, aged 30 to 50 ate bread made of rolled oats everyday for three weeks, the average cholesterol drop was 25 points. It rose again, somewhat, after the rolled oats were discontinued, (*Lancet* [1963:ii], 303-304.)

Animal studies conducted in Italy showed that pantothenic acid (a B vitamin) aids the heart, as established by electrocardiogram. A similar study disclosed that rats deprived of pantothenic acid exhibited a reduced heart rate. When pantothenic acid was restored, the hearts became normal in ten days.

Perhaps the most dramatic discoveries in heart management, with the exception of vitamin E, are two nutritional substances reported by Hans Selye, M.D. He found that serious heart disease appeared in all of his animals subjected to stress, *except those which had been given potassium or magnesium.* He noticed that sodium speeded up heart damage in animals but when he gave potassium and magnesium to counteract the sodium, it saved the animals' lives.

Potassium is found in whole grains, blackstrap molasses, potatoes, green vegetables, almonds, figs, and other fruits. Refining of grains for cereals or white flour produces about a three-quarter loss of potassium.

Magnesium is found in nuts, egg yolk, milk, and citrus fruits. Unmilled grain products contain about 500 per cent more magnesium than refined cereals and flour.

A diet is often a fad, a current interest of the moment, tried for a specific purpose. Good nutrition, on the other hand, is a well-rounded method of eating to provide a plan on which you can live the rest of your life. Sol Hirsch, M.D., warns that most people judge their daily diet on their one main meal, which they consider good. He warns that it is necessary to study the entire 24-hour-a-day intake. Is it diluted with coffee, cigarettes, sugars, refined foods and nonessentials, making the over-all nutritional intake not so good? *Not one, but all nutritive elements just mentioned* are needed to restore and maintain heart health. They work together to promote good body chemistry.

SMOKING AND THE HEART

Smoking, according to Dr. McCormick, is the "greatest despoiler of vitamin C, depletes the body of the vitamin by the adrenal reaction, and the toxins of the smoke which have a destructive action on the stored chemical. . . . Over ten years ago, in laboratory and clinical tests, it was found that the smoking of one cigarette, as ordinarily inhaled, destroyed the vitamin C content of an average orange. This observation was confirmed by researchers in the United States and in Poland."

Dr. Lester M. Morrison cites his experience with the effect of tobacco on the heart:

"Like many other physicians, in my twenty-five years of practice I must have treated literally thousands of patients who at one time or another suffered from symptoms of some degree of tobacco poisoning. Some were dramatic, some resistant, some funny and some tragic.

"Usually the toxic effects on the heart will be noticed by the patient from 'skipped' heartbeats or palpitations of the heart, nervousness, or a rapid heart rate, often producing dizziness, shortness of breath, especially on exertion, headaches from rises of blood pressure, or pains and distress over the front portion of the chest.

"One male patient of mine . . . had a mild case of coronary artery disease. This showed itself by chest pain after exertion or excitement. A habitual smoker, he improved so greatly under treatment, which included his abstaining from tobacco, that he was now itching to get back on the 'weed.' In order to demonstrate to him the effects of smoking on his own heart, I asked him to resume smoking for one test period. . . . After smoking and delightedly inhaling two and one-half cigarettes, he developed severe anginal pains over the chest which reflected itself in striking abnormalities in his electrocardiogram. . . . This experience has been reduplicated in countless patients.

"And in patients with high blood pressure, tobacco smoking in moderate to heavy amounts has a strong tendency to send the blood pressure even higher. . . . It is thoroughly established (as a result of exhaustive studies) that tobacco causes a marked interference with the circulation to the hands, the feet and the legs. In the conditions of the peripheral arteriosclerosis and atherosclerosis, especially of the legs, nicotine has been shown to aggravate and increase the constriction already present in the peripheral blood vessels of human subjects."

THE HEART AND LOW BLOOD SUGAR

Benjamin P. Sandler, M.D., not only agrees thoroughly with Drs. Morrison and McCormick on the effect of tobacco on the heart, but he introduces a completely new and previously unexplored cause of heart attacks: low blood sugar. (See Bibliography.)

He says, "When the blood sugar falls (even slightly) . . . symptoms are usually mild and may consist of light headache, faintness, muscular weakness, hunger, irritability, and perhaps feeling of nervousness or tension.

"When the blood sugar falls [still lower] . . . the symptoms will consist of headache, dizziness, unsteady gait, faintness, weakness, marked irritability, pallor, sweating, tremors, palpitation and general nervousness. If the blood sugar falls to [an extreme low] . . . unconsciousness usually occurs."

Dr. Sandler believes that cardiac symptoms are caused by abnormal blood sugar fluctuations, and that a *rapid*, rather than a gradual blood sugar drop can cause a heart attack. He believes these symptoms, both cardiac and neurologic, may be prevented by a low carbohydrate diet, which elevates and stabilizes the blood sugar levels, supplying the optimum blood sugar (and oxygen) continuously to the heart. He recommends a high protein, a low carbohydrate, sugar-free diet, which is the diet for the low blood sugar (hyperinsulinism) problem. (This is explained more fully in "Fatigue," p. 280.)

WHAT ABOUT CHOLESTEROL AND FAT?

There have been many dire warnings against eating fat, particularly the wrong kind. But at the annual conference of the American Heart Association in Cleveland, Ohio, October, 1962, Dr. Paul Oglesby, University of Illinois, former president, American Heart Association, announced some surprising results of a long-term study on coronary heart disease. The study, carried out on 1,989 men between 40 and 55 for four and one-half years, showed no significant differences between those who did consume animal fat, vegetable fat, cholesterol, saturated or unsaturated fats, and those who did not.

The study thus suggests that there may be no direct relation between a high level of cholesterol in the blood, a high intake of cholesterol-producing and other fatty foods in the diet.

As early as 1955, Dr. L. W. Kinsell insisted that low-fat diets so commonly prescribed, do not necessarily lower blood cholesterol. He put his patients on a very high-fat diet, but he gave them *natural* oils.

In the battle, two important factors have apparently been overlooked. For instance, milk and dairy products have been condemned. Dr. H. Martland, chief medical examiner of Essex County, New Jersey, said in a 1934 address before the New York State Medical Society that he believed that large numbers of cases of sudden death of men between the ages of 45 and 60 were the result of overeating dairy fats. Dr. H. M. Sinclair, noted British nutrition researcher, also refers to the inferiority of cow's milk. On the other hand, unsaturated fats or vegetable oils have been widely recommended.

In both instances, a crucial point has gone unnoticed. One needs to ask *what kind* of milk can cause trouble. And does a certain characteristic of unsaturated oils create danger?

First, let's answer the milk question. You will see evidence in *Stay Young Longer* that pasteurizing milk destroys lecithin, which has been found to dissolve cholesterol in the body. However, in whole certified raw milk, the protective lecithin is still present.

Dr. Lester M. Morrison finds that lecithin not only reduces the amount of cholesterol in the blood, but in proper dosage dissolves the fatty plaques which have already piled up in the arteries. This is important news since physicians used to believe that once these fatty or cholesterol deposits became imbedded in the artery walls, the condition was irreversible; and as the passageway narrowed, a clot (thrombosis) could lead to a coronary attack or stroke.

Francis Pottenger, Jr., M.D., famous for his animal experiments with raw milk, tested both raw and pasteurized milk on babies. He found that those fed raw certified milk tended to be healthy, whereas those given pasteurized, boiled, powdered, or canned milk developed various ailments.

Dr. G. Kirkpatrick considers the development of enlarged hearts with valvular involvement a result of pasteurized milk. He found that some children with this defect recovered rapidly if raw milk were substituted for pasteurized milk.

Dr. Kirkpatrick states, "Without raw milk, recovery does not take place, and those who reach the age of 10 or 15 will, upon examination, show chronic heart diseases which are usually diagnosed as rheumatic fever; so the patient goes through life a semi-invalid. I personally know of many children who were suffering from heart complications, who have made complete recovery in a few months by drinking raw milk along with other wholesome food, and with no direct treatment for the heart." (*Raw Milk Versus Pasteurized Milk*, Seattle, National Nutrition League, 1950.)

Certified raw milk is medically approved and considered perfectly safe.

Now, what is wrong with those vegetable oils that everyone is gulping down? Let me repeat what I reported in *Stay Young Longer*. Most commercial oils are *processed* and refined. Processing is a commercial attempt to convert a natural dark oil into a lighter, more attractive oil for sales appeal. In refining, the valuable substances which have the property of lowering the cholesterol are removed. (Among these vitamin E, the very vitamin we have mentioned which, when removed from cattle feed, caused them to drop dead of heart attacks!)

Dr. M. K. Horwitt reported that diets high in *refined* corn oil or cottonseed oil, *without* the addition of vitamin E to the diet, caused brain damage in chickens. He cited at least one human case.

For this reason, I use *only unrefined or cold-pressed oils*, so that the valuable vitamin E and other protective substances are not removed.

HOW MUCH FAT SHOULD YOU EAT?

A study conducted in India with over 1,000 men recommend that:

In normal people 20 to 25 per cent of the diet should be fat.
About one-third of this fat should be from polyunsaturated oils.
In people with actual or potential heart disease, one-half to two-thirds of the fat should be polyunsaturated. (*Indian Journal of Medical Science* [1960], 14: 489-500.)

The Canadian Heart Foundation considers that 50 per cent of the intake of animal fats should be replaced by unsaturated fats of vegetable origin. (*Borden's Review of Nutrition Research*, Vol. 24, No. 4; 1963.)

Many people are afraid to eat eggs because they contain cholesterol. A Russian study revealed that the majority of 225 Russian poultry farm workers who ate large amounts of eggs were found to have a normal, or below normal, cholesterol level. They also had normal arterial pressure and were apparently healthy. (*Vrach Delo*, April, 1964.)

Some physicians actually prescribe eggs as part of a cholesterol-lowering program. One of these, Joseph D. Walters, M.D., says, "I recommend two eggs a day, often raw, to reduce cholesterol in my patients. But the eggs must be fertile and the chicken-feed of the hens uncontaminated with insecticides. People who are allergic to raw egg white usually have no trouble with raw *fertile* egg white. The fertile egg white makes cystine, an amino acid, available to the body. Most people are deficient in cystine. Furthermore, a fertile egg (one which could hatch), because it contains both the embryo as well as food for the developing chick, is nutritionally superior to the infertile egg."

For added heart protection, Dr. Lester M. Morrison (see Bibliography) suggests the following five-step plan:

Take daily as a food supplement, preferably 2 to 4 tablespoons of lecithin granules.
Add vitamin B complex in its most potent form. (Dr. Morrison ad-

vises brewer's yeast. Liver also contains a rich supply of B complex.)

Add daily 25,000 units of vitamin A and 150 mg. of vitamin C.

Take 2 tablespoons of soy, corn, or safflower oil daily. [Be sure it is cold pressed.]

Include 2 to 4 tablespoons of wheat germ.

I, personally, add several hundred units of a vitamin E supplement each day.

There is some other assurance that a heart attack may be prevented. Dr. Paul Ohren and his associates recently reported that studies conducted at the Institute of Thrombosis Research, Oslo University, Norway, revealed that soybean and linseed oil—both rich in linolenic acid—were effective in reducing blood clots.

Dr. Ohren rejects most polyunsaturated oils because they are very low in linolenic acid. But, even a small amount (about 1 tablespoon daily) of linolenic acid was effective in reducing clots and may be a definite dietary method of preventing heart attacks. Soybean oil is the only oil commonly used which is rich in linolenic acid. (*Lancet* Nov. 7, 1964.)

WHAT ELSE AFFECTS THE HEART?

Prolonged stress is known to cause atherosclerosis (artery hardening). Emotions constrict the veins. Investigators at the University of North Carolina proved this by studying the effect of students doing mental arithmetic. They applied pressure to two points in the arm, isolated a length of vein, and asked the students to begin their mental calculations. To increase tension, money awards were offered for correct answers. Everybody worked hard on the mathematical problems. The resulting emotional tension did increase constriction in the vein and it increased blood pressure as well.

Dr. Meyer Friedman and Dr. Ray H. Roseman at Mt. Zion Medical Center, San Francisco, have been studying the effect of emotion on the heart for more than eight years. They found higher fat levels in the blood of aggressive men and women because they are hard drivers, worriers, and never-let-uppers; they are strongly competitive; they want to work alone and conquer new fields; and they do not rest between chores. Calmer men in quieter jobs and mousey women had lower blood fat levels.

Dr. Frank G. Nolan, noted heart specialist, believes that nagging wives may be responsible for some husbands' heart disturbances. He tells the story of a male patient of whom he was taking a cardiogram. His wife happened to walk into the room and the needle jumped! Dr. Nolan admits that not all wives are responsible for their husbands' heart disease, but he warns that you'd better watch it, wives!

A friend of ours was an angina patient in a hospital. While he was left alone in his room, he was pain-free. But the minute there was a knock on the door and a visitor or relative came in, the man's pain appeared.

So try to analyze what situations bother you. Then try to see if you can eliminate or bypass them. It may take some effort to make over your job or your life, but it will be well worth it.

WHAT ABOUT EXERCISE?

Dr. Paul Dudley White, the well-known heart specialist, is a firm believer in exercise for both prevention and cure of heart disease. He feels that regular, not sudden violent exercise, can be helpful. In rehabilitating heart patients, he advocates the rocking chair as the first exercise, with gradual increase to other types of exercise, including slow stair climbing. He, in his late 70's, bicycles and often climbs thirteen stories rather than wait for an elevator.

Some people are afraid that exertion will bring on a heart attack. Experiments show otherwise. Dr. T. G. Klumpp says, "It is a demonstrated fact that tissues and functions atrophy if they are not used."

Dr. Arthur M. Master, of New York, tested nearly 2,600 patients. He found that most heart attacks came during sleep or rest. Only 2 per cent had a heart attack during severe exertion. Other studies found that exercise reduced cholesterol in those who had high levels but had no effect on those with normal blood cholesterol levels. (*American Journal of Clinical Nutrition*, 7:139; March-April, 1959.)

Research has found that a regularly exercised heart can take more emotional as well as physical stress. Isometric exercises, very popular today, are excellent for strengthening many body muscles. They cannot, however, reach the heart or the lungs. This indicates that other types of exercise are needed to exercise the heart muscle (and the lungs). Walking, swimming, golfing (without using a cart) are the easiest. It is important to choose the type of exercise which appeals to *you*, though. If you adopt one which you hate, you will unconsciously remain tense, with a do-or-die attitude, which defeats the tranquillity you seek, and the relaxed boost to your circulation, which feeds the heart.

It is amazing how regular exercise can recondition the heart. I lived for several years in a New York suburb. The steps leading up from the train platform to the station were so high that they were called "heart attack heights." When I first climbed those stairs, I huffed and puffed like all the newcomers. Yet all the regular commuters seemed to take them in their stride with no effort. Several months later I heard some other newcomers complaining about the height of the stairs, and I suddenly realized they no longer bothered me. For about six years I watched people strengthen their heart muscles by taking those stairs daily without a second thought, or any effort. Yet whenever I met a weekend guest, unaccustomed to the climb, the response was always the same: he, or she, arrived at the top of the steps panting and saying, "How do you people manage these stairs day after day?"

Actually, those stairs were probably a life-saver to those who used them daily. They provided excellent exercise similar to that recommended by Dr. Paul Dudley White.

The heart, like any other muscle, can be strained by too much exercise, too soon. Conversely, it can be strengthened by regular daily exercise so that if sudden strain is experienced, it can take it.

In a special report, *How to Postpone Your Heart Attack*, H. W. Holderby, M.D., recommends a nutritional program including natural organic food, vitamin E capsules daily, lecithin granules, liquid cold-pressed oils, and eggs—all daily.

Dr. Holderby adds three more suggestions: cut down on stress; don't use tobacco; and do take more exercise. He concludes, "We should have twenty minutes of perspiring exercise daily to burn the sludge out of our blood vessels."

STROKES

There are big strokes and little strokes. There is evidence that little strokes may be followed by serious strokes. There is also evidence that both may be prevented. A serious stroke usually results in relatively fixed paralysis and/or loss of vision or speech lasting for long periods of time.

A small stroke occurs when the blood supply to the brain is cut off for only a very short while. It is not uncommon. A fall caused by blacking-out may be the result of a little stroke. The symptoms may include difficulty in thinking correctly, blurred vision, slurred speech, loss of memory, dizziness, inability to concentrate, feeling of confusion, irritability, weakness or numbness of a hand or leg or facial distortion. (It may pull up to one side.) Sudden spells of crying plus a feeling of sadness, changes in handwriting or sudden arthritic changes in a hip or wrist may possibly take place.

Dr. Walter C. Alvarez, formerly of the Mayo Clinic, states that during a period of 10 to 20 years, a person may gradually be pulled down by dozens or more little strokes and never give them a second thought. Dr. Alvarez tells of a woman whose husband became confused one morning for 20 minutes and was unable to talk. He had always been kind and understanding. But after that episode, he became irritable, irascible, and unreasonable. He was so changed that his wife hardly knew him. Dr. Alvarez believes that the man suffered a small stroke which was responsible for the symptoms which followed. (*Journal of American Medical Association*, April 2, 1955.)

Robert P. Goldman tells of a minister who suffered loss of memory often and became increasingly irritable. He was moved from parish to parish by his superiors who hoped that he would snap out of it. Finally, a doctor diagnosed his trouble as a series of small strokes, prescribed medication, and the minister has been free of symptoms for three years. (*Parade*, July 9, 1961.)

The supposition is that tense, harried persons over 40 are more susceptible to small strokes than younger, calmer people. The drugs usually prescribed for such conditions include anticoagulants, dicoumarol and coumadin and other prescription drugs. But possible side effects accompany these drugs.

"A fair number of emergency patients," writes Morton M. Hunt, "nowadays arrive at hospitals bleeding from the bowel or urinary tract and prove to be heart patients taking anti-coagulant drugs to prevent further heart attacks. The drugs unfortunately, have also prevented normal clot formation when tiny breaks occurred in internal membranes." (From "Side Effects: A New Worry for Doctors," *Look*, December 31, 1963.)

It may be that some physicians do not know that there are other natural and safer anticlotters.

The usual treatment of heart conditions is a combination of diuretic drugs and low-sodium diets for edema, but this may cause a washing out of the water-soluble vitamins and thus result in further harm to the heart. This is the opinion of Dr. M. M. Gertler at a conference at the New York Academy of Sciences. Drs. Levy, Wohl, and Alpert, also previously mentioned, agree. Dr. Arthur J. Seaman, who conducted a six-year study at the University of Oregon Medical School, reported that drugs used to prevent blood clotting (a factor in strokes and heart attacks) were no more effective than taking no drug at all.

What, then, can be used safely to prevent small (or large) strokes? Vitamin E has been shown to produce anticlotting functions. (*Clinical Physiology*, Vol. 3, No. 1. Also, *Nagoya Journal of Medical Science* [Japan], 22:341; 1960.)

At a government testimony in Washington, D.C., Dr. E. V. Shute, of Canada, testified: "The point I would like to make is that everybody, including ourselves, who has studied the incidence of embolism in cases of thrombosis treated with alpha tocopherol [vitamin E] has noted the unusual fact embolism [clot] almost never occurs. In our studies we have never had a case.

"The reason why anti-coagulants are so generally used nowadays in the treatment of heart disease is that they were first found useful in preventing thrombosis in vessels of the extremities (feet and legs). The line of reasoning making dicoumarol useful in coronary disease automatically makes alpha tocopherol more useful still and, of course, it is infinitely safer, because with anti-coagulants the incidence of thromboembolism is reduced only by half to a quarter."

In addition to vitamin E, another preventive natural substance has proved useful. Eighty-nine cases of patients who had had one to four little strokes were treated with CVP, a water-soluble citrus bioflavonoid compound (vitamin C complex) containing 100 mg. bioflavonoids and 100 mg. ascorbic acid in capsule form. Patients were followed up for from one to five years. Treatment reduced the incidence of little strokes to 17 per cent. Of the group which was treated by CVP, three had another little stroke. Of a matched, untreated group, 18 had 12 little strokes, and 18 severe strokes, of which five were fatal. (*Journal of American Geriatrics* [1961], 9:110-118.)

More impressive, still, is the fact that if bioflavonoids also include added rutin, protection is still greater. Rutin is a natural ingredient of buckwheat and tends to strengthen fragile capillaries. The *Encyclopedia of Chemical Technology* by Kirk and Othmer says, "Rutin has been proved effective in certain hemorrhagic conditions in which capillary fragility or permeability is involved, and it may be important in preventing vascular accidents (strokes) which occur in people of high blood pressure."

In the book, *Vitamins and Medicine,* by Bicknell and Prescott, appears an even stronger statement. In a number of human experiments, with 75 out of 100 patients rutin apparently protected the possibility of stroke *in spite of high blood pressure.*

Dr. Somerville-Large prescribes doses of 120 mg. of rutin three times daily, plus 200 mg. of vitamin C. He says, "I find that the larger doses give a more rapid . . . result. . . . I have never met a case in which the capillary fragility skin test has not been reduced with rutin to well within normal limits." (*Transactions of the Opthalmological Society of the United Kingdom,* Vol. 69; 1949-50.)

As for serious strokes, successful vitamin therapy used by Dr. Morrison and other physicians combines B complex, wheat germ oil in concentrated form (1 teaspoon equals 15 teaspoons of usual strength), bioflavonoids plus extra vitamin C, vitamin K, and vitamin E. To prove that stroke victims can be helped, Dr. Morrison cites one case among others, of a 65-year-old maiden lady who had had a stroke. Her vision was poor, she was partially paralyzed, and with only one friend in the world, was desperate and depressed. After several months of nutritional therapy, she recovered much of her muscular power, lost her paralysis, became radiantly cheerful and optimistic, and asked permission to go swimming.

ADDITIONAL FACTORS TO REMEMBER

There are a few other items to keep in mind in relation to heart disturbance:

Obesity should be avoided.

There is evidence that there is less heart disease among those who drink hard water than those who drink soft water. If you have hard water, it may be wise to have your softener attached only to the hot-water tap. Let the cold-water tap alone, from which drinking, coffee-making, and cooking water should be drawn. (*Consumers' Bulletin*, March, 1963.)

There is also evidence that chlorinated water, because chlorine destroys vitamin E, may be an incidence in heart disease. Dr. H. M. Sinclair says, "It is possible that one of the greatest public health measures ever introduced—the chlorination of public water supply could assist the disease." (*Journal of the American Medical Association*, July 28, 1951.) The way out of this dilemma is to have your own well, buy bottled water, or boil chlorinated water, which removes the chlorine.

There are false heart attacks. A catch in the chest, lasting for one-half to five minutes and followed by a dull ache is called a "precordial" catch and has no relationship to heart trouble at all. Taking a deep breath, even though painful, produces sudden and dramatic relief. (*Annals of Internal Medicine*, Vol. 51, p. 461.) Sometimes as you straighten up after bending over, you may encounter a cramp in your rib section. It may frighten the daylights out of you. It is not a heart attack, but a cramp, possibly arising from the same cause as leg cramps. (See ch. 41.) It is easily prevented.

SUMMARY

To prevent heart attacks:

    Get plenty of sleep.
    Get plenty of exercise.
    Stop trying to compete with other people or with living. Take things in your stride. If someone gets ahead of you, let him. It's his heart, not yours.
    Include in your all around nutritional program:
    Vitamin E.
    Vitamin C.
    Bioflavonoids with added rutin.
    Vitamin B complex (found in brewer's yeast and liver).
    Lecithin granules.
    Minerals: calcium, potassium, magnesium (see previous list of sources).
    Dairy products from *un*pasteurized, certified raw milk.
    Oils which are *un*refined and *cold* pressed.
    Don't be afraid of fat, as long as one-third of it is taken from cold pressed oils. It can be used in salad dressings, mayonnaise, or special margarines. Do not use hydrogenated fat.
    Avoid sugar.

Royal Lee, D.D.S., suggests a natural remedy for artery hardening: flaxseed tea, flaxseed added to breakfast cereals, or flaxseed oil taken in perles. Flaxseed contains all the protective substances usually removed by the oil-refining process. Dr. Lee warns against rancid oils, which seem to encourage cancer.

All these items are available at health food centers. And don't let it deter you if some of your friends call you a quack.

38   Indigestion—gallstones —kidney stones

WATCH THOSE ALKALIZERS

Most people are confused by the term "acid stomach." According to Boris Sokoloff, M.D., millions of people are taking enormous amounts of alkaline preparations for "acid stomach" without their doctor's recommendation. Actually, nature has purposely endowed man with acid to protect him from infection. Hostile germs thrive on alkalinity but cannot survive in acidity. Instead of taking alkalizers or antacids, Dr. Sokoloff advises cultured milks and B vitamins to correct indigestion, adding that if you maintain a balanced diet, with sufficient minerals and vitamins, nature will automatically regulate your acid-base balance.

Alkalizers destroy vitamins. Still worse, the Animal Nutrition Laboratory at Cornell University discovered that calculi, one form of kidney stones, were caused in animals given bicarbonate of soda and milk.

Excessive use of one very popular antacid may lead to calcium deposits in various parts of the body, according to Dr. Frank J. Talbot. (*Medical Annals*, April, 1964.) Dr. Talbot feels that warnings of maximum use should be included on the labels.

Consumers' Report (August, 1960) states, "There is a widespread misbelief, encouraged by the advertising of hundreds of patent medicines, that indigestion results from 'too much stomach acidity' and that an alkalizer or antacid drug can restore the digestive tract to normal. . . . In many such cases alkalizers or antacids will 'cure' the indigestion, lulling the victim into a belief that he is not ill.

"Indigestion is not a disease; it is a symptom—or rather a number of symptoms. The term is a catch-all having no precise medical meaning.

Modern living causes many people to gulp their food, due to stress and hurry. When food is swallowed in large chunks and not chewed, the stomach has to work harder and more hydrochloric acid is secreted. Up to three to four times as much acid is secreted when food is bolted than when it is properly chewed. Eating too fast also causes one to swallow air. These bad habits force some of the digestive fluid into the esophagus, resulting in burping, a stinging sensation, or a sour taste. This gives the illusion of "an acid stomach."

Sodium bicarbonate is no longer recommended by many doctors since it has been found to cause alkalosis, particularly in those with a kidney condition. Even antacids are falling into disrepute. One physician who does prescribe them for temporary relief will not allow a refill of the prescription. Dr. Frederick J. Cullen, a medical consultant, says, "We must realize that any drug that is sufficiently potent to be effective is sufficiently potent to be harmful if misused."

Yet millions of Americans doctor themselves with nonprescription antacids because radio, television, and newspaper commercials tell them to. It is true that some foods upset some people, but most physicians will agree that the usual cause of indigestion is cramming or bolting food without chewing; or eating too fast. After all, teeth were put there to use.

Many people need more, not less acid, as you will soon see.

If you are tired or already have indigestion, instead of taking an antacid, stop eating altogether for a few hours, then eat easily digested, simple food. If indigestion persists, check with your physician.

HEARTBURN

Drs. Henry J. Tumen and Edwin M. Cohn reported in the *Journal of the American Medical Association* that of 120 cases of complaints of heartburn, none could be traced to an organic disease. Occasionally, tension or personality problems needed to be overcome, but more often heartburn was due to the following causes and did *not* need to be relieved by drugs or bicarbonates.

Eating too fast.
Drinking large amounts of fluids with meals.
Indulging too frequently in carbonated beverages.
Developing the burping habit to relieve distress.
Swallowing air when eating, or in chewing gum.
Eating irregularly.
Crowding too much food in at one meal.

Consumers' Report adds, "The type of indigestion dear to the hearts of the patent medicine copy writers undoubtedly is 'hyperacidity' and its supposed corollary, heartburn.

"Formerly, it was an accepted theory that heartburn always was due to overproduction of acid in the stomach. . . . Later studies have shown that this symptom can occur with normal, low, or no acid at all. . . . Hyperacidity has little to do with heartburn."

"Unfortunately, some of the symptoms of acid deficiency are similar to those of hyperacidity, or an oversupply of acid," says Frank B. Hamilton, B.S., Ph.D., "and an antacid is often taken when it may be the worst thing that could be done.

"The saliva . . . is the normal trigger that starts the flow of hydrochloric acid in the stomach . . . [and] hydrochloric acid is the fuse that sets off the flow of pepsin. . . . Any absorption of protein depends on the hydrochloric acid and the pepsin."

Dr. Hamilton points out, "It is almost a foregone conclusion that every one over 65 is short of hydrochloric acid. Why? Older people often have trouble chewing their food properly, usually because of poor-fitting dentures. There is also the possibility that salivary glands were damaged when their teeth were extracted." (From "Hydrochloric Acid Is Vital to Digestion and Health," *Let's Live.*)

MORE, NOT LESS ACID

Dr. Sokoloff agrees, "About one half of the middle aged and elderly people are suffering from low or non-acid stomachs."

Other investigators believe that at least 50 per cent of the population lack hydrochloric acid.

Dr. E. Hugh Tuckey adds, "No matter how good your diet is, if you have an insufficiency of hydrochloric acid your food is not digested and your body is not properly nourished. Lack of it may cause gas, burping, regurgitating, as well as putrefaction of food, even 24 to 36 hours after eating. Lack of it almost always causes anemia, distention, bloating, and sometimes heart pressure—even attacks. Upset emotions before or after a meal can halt the manufacture of HCL even though you normally have a sufficient supply."

Dr. Michael J. Walsh, consulting nutritionist, adds, "In the aging process, everything conspires to slow down our degree of hydrochloric acid. And there is only one fool-proof way of getting adequate amounts of acid—that is in the form of hydrochloric acid.

"The doctor believes that a person can have all the protein in the world but if he doesn't have sufficient hydrochloric acid, the protein isn't going to do much good." This applies to assimilating calcium and iron too.

"What you need for digestion of proteins is lots of acid. . . . If you need supplemental hydrochloric acid, you should have it in a buffered state. If you take it straight, it may destroy your tooth enamel. A better way to take it is by drops in buttermilk or skim milk. This is called 'buffering.' Buffering will help digest food without a jarring effect. An easier way is to take glutamic-acid hydrochloride capsules or tablets, available at health or drug stores. The glutamic acid acts as a buffer for the hydrochloric acid."

Henry A. Monat, M.D., writes, "Of all the proteins stimulating the secretion of hydrochloric acid, beef and beef extract are the most potent; gelatin and milk the least potent." (*American Journal of Clinical Nutrition*, Vol. 14, 3: 40.)

WHAT CAUSES GAS?

Gas can be caused by an oversupply of hostile bacteria, correctable by cultured milks and B vitamins; by an allergy (see "Allergies," ch. 22); by a lack of hydrochloric acid; or by a shortage of bile.

Arnold and Brody showed that when people with a normal acid secretion were given a considerable amount of alkaline preparation, hostile bacteria began to appear. This produced gas.

If gas is a problem, Adelle Davis advises hydrochloric acid in later years as a supplement. She suggests one capsule, such as glutamic-acid hydrochloride after each meal, to be increased later if gas persists, or stopped as soon as digestion becomes normal. B vitamins often stimulate the natural flow of hydrochloric acid and after a month of a good nutritional program, improvement is often noted. However, some people because of a prolonged vitamin B starvation may need to continue HCL indefinitely.

Dr. Jarvis' vinegar-in-water sipped before or during meals may be of help to some.

If you are still unconvinced that more, not less, acid may be necessary, your doctor can determine your need for hydrochloric acid.

The newer test for HCL is much more pleasant than the old uncomfortable method of swallowing a stomach tube. The new test is accomplished by measurement of an enzyme in the urine.

If it has been definitely established that you really have too much acid, rather than not enough, then, according to Dr. Michael Walsh, protein will help reduce the acidity. He adds, "Such people would also benefit by taking more acid in the form of buttermilk, yogurt and sauerkraut."

MORE HELP FOR INDIGESTION

Dr. Monat has some further helps: "Solids when finely ground up (by chewing) and mixed with saliva, receive the best reception in the stomach. . . . Eating a large quantity of food at one sitting may distend the stomach."

For those who have difficulty in chewing, blending raw vegetables or fruits (liquified in a blender) or juices extracted from fresh raw vegetables by means of a juice extractor, can deliver good nutrition. Canned baby foods can also be used. Dr. Monat adds:

"No food can be well digested if the patient is not relaxed mentally and physically. Short exercises such as walking, golf, swimming and Swedish gymnastics help digestion. Overwork, too vigorous exercise such as tennis, handball, hockey and horseback riding interfere with digestion, if performed within two hours of utilization of foods.

"Tepid baths from 15 to 30 minutes before partaking of food will promote digestion. Hot or cold baths interfere with digestion. Extreme cold or hot foods also interfere. Warm foods have the optimum chance of being utilized. Hard fats are absorbed slowly and sometimes not at all, whereas soft fats are absorbed almost completely. Fat depresses the motility of the stomach and secretion of HCL. . . . Also an excess of fats produces a sense of fullness and nausea."

The macrobiotic diet recommends chewing each bite of food 30 or more times. This makes drinking liquids with meals (which can dilute digestive juices) less necessary. (See ch. 18.)

A Russian study found that parsley juice increased acid secretion in the stomach, and stimulated bile secretion by increasing liver function. Parsley was found as effective as cabbage juice in stimulating gastric activity, and less was needed. Papaya has also proved helpful.

H. E. Kirschner, M.D., reports that alfalfa, either in tablets or in tea, acts as a good digestant.

IS YOUR GALL BLADDER RESPONSIBLE?

I remember an elderly woman, who at 70 complained bitterly of gas. She was positive it was caused one day by cucumbers, another day by radishes, another day by something else. Her physician suggested that she have her gall bladder removed. After a few weeks of relief following the operation, her original symptoms returned. Finally, a clinic discovered that she was secreting no hydrochloric acid. This meant that she had not been properly digesting protein, such as meat, fish, eggs, milk—even brewer's yeast, which is largely protein. Since symptoms are sometimes similar, lack of HCL had been confused with gall bladder disturbance in this patient.

Bile salts help people with a problem of fat digestion. (*American Journal of Clinical Nutrition*, March, 1963.) For disturbed gall bladders, physicians formerly recommended fat-free diets but this is now falling into disrepute. The gall bladder needs some fat in order to manufacture bile and assimilate the fat-soluble vitamins A, E, and K. Otherwise, it atrophies and causes even greater trouble.

Dr. Walter C. Alvarez admits that one of the main causes of indigestion is emotion. One patient suffering from an undiagnosable case of indigestion had a spontaneous recovery when her mortgage was paid! Another girl, in love, suffered from intestinal disturbance whenever she had a fit of jealousy.

The gall bladder, particularly, reacts to emotion and tension. Leland Kordel tells of a man who suffered from gall bladder trouble while working at his job in the city. When he took a leave of absence and moved to the country, his gall bladder trouble ceased. But when he returned to his tense city job again, his gall bladder problem returned, too.

GALLSTONES AND WHAT TO DO ABOUT THEM

Pauline Beregoff-Gillow, M.D., of Montreal and an internationally known physician who has practiced preventive medicine for 30 years, says, "The general practitioner frequently is visited by patients who report gallstones and ask if the gall bladder must be removed. Often these patients say that they have bilious attacks when eating too much fat, but never have pain.

"Gallstones are not due to defective gall bladders. When stones are large they cause no pain. When the stones are small and attempt to pass through a duct, then severe pain is felt. Even in the latter situation a mild sedative will bring relief.

"*Stones are due to dietary indiscretions.* The bile that forms in the liver cells, normally clear and thin, thickens when the diet is of fatty and undigestible foodstuff. Normally, bile flows rapidly through the ducts of the gall bladder and from the bladder empties periodically. *When the bile is thickened,* the flow is slow and the gall bladder does not fully empty. The remaining thickened bile precipitates and thus stones are formed.

"Removing the gall bladder does not cure the condition. *Remove the cause.* Correct your unbalanced diet (cut down on fats, rich food, and alcoholic beverages). Partake of fresh vegetables, salads, and fruit. Such a diet will help proper elimination, prevent stone formation.

"Stones may diminish in size and sometimes even dissolve, by a complete change in diet. You may live to be a hundred with your gall bladder and the stones. Have your doctor give you a thorough check-up and recommend a proper diet, according to your constitution." (*Herald of Health,* December, 1961.)

In 1962, the Department of Biochemistry and Nutrition, Polytechnic Institute of Copenhagen, conducted a study with hamsters to find out exactly what produced gallstones. First, the researchers found two types of stones: amorphous (which were formless), noncrystalline; and those composed of cholesterol.

In this study, a fat-free diet *favored* formation of cholesterol stones, whereas *unsaturated* fats tended to favor the amorphous stones (less troublesome). Bile salts appeared to give protection against cholesterol stones. Many people respond to bile salts. Ask your doctor.

Even if cholesterol foods are avoided, the body still manufactures its own cholesterol. Dr. Hulda Magalhaes of Bucknell University reported that a diet free of cholesterol leads to formation of gallstones in experimental animals, and that a fat-free diet also produces them.

Other studies with hamsters confirm that a nonfat or low-fat diet produces gallstones. The explanation is that "the diet being low in fat may be responsible for a decreased contraction of the gall bladder (which needs fat to perform smoothly) and this in turn may be an important factor in the stone formation." (*Nutrition Reviews,* September, 1960.)

Diet can definitely help. Carlton Fredericks reported a study with 702 people, all gall bladder victims. They were given multiple vitamins and minerals, B complex, vitamin E, a diet high in protein, low in carbohydrates. Sugar, fried and greasy foods, gravy, chocolate, and mayonnaise were forbidden; 700 recovered.

Imbalance in diet or vitamin intake is not wise. The *Journal of the American Medical Association* (June, 1943) states that vitamin B-1 (thiamin) used alone can cause gallstones. Any B factor should be accompanied by the rest of the B complex.

Here are various home remedies for naturally removing gallstones which I shall pass on for you to discuss with your doctor:

Two physicians have told me about an old folk remedy they have used for sluggish gall bladders. It consists of one-half cup of olive oil plus one-half cup of grapefruit juice stirred thoroughly and drunk at bedtime, followed next morning with a glass of hot water or coffee. The oil and juice may cause slight nausea, hence the reason for taking it at bedtime. One of the physicians says he tries this several times before recommending surgery. If, however, an X ray has revealed a large stone, doctors feel this method is not wise since it may tend to force the stone through the duct.

John E. Eichenlaub, M.D., gives his home cure for indigestion arising from a lazy gall bladder. He says, "When a person who has a high gall bladder index and who gets very little exercise complains of belching, uncomfortable fullness in the upper abdomen, and bloating after meals, lazy gall bladder is usually at fault. So long as no attacks of colic have occurred, a trial of home treatment is usually worthwhile.

"You can usually get a lazy gall bladder into action by taking one or two tablespoons of olive oil before each meal. This starts the flow of bile before the rest of the food enters your stomach. Although you may get a bit more indigestion from the oil for the first few days, you should see marked improvement inside of two weeks."

Italians use olive oil abundantly and are said to be quite free of gall bladder trouble. But most Italians I know insist on taking, not the super deluxe purified olive oil, but the virgin quality, which is the more natural and less refined of the two products. Some people find it helpful to start oil gradually and increase the amount as soon as it can be tolerated. If nausea occurs, apparently you have taken too much too soon.

Russian black radish (available in tablet form at health food stores) has been found helpful for gall bladder and related indigestion problems.

CAN GALLSTONES BE DISSOLVED?

A folk remedy suggests grape juice for dissolving gallstones, if catarrh has been involved.

Another old-time remedy, supposed to break up gallstones, prescribes two tall glasses of apple juice (fresh if possible) every two hours for two days; follow with 4 ounces undiluted olive oil.

Still another folk remedy: A generous pinch of cream of tartar (derived from grapes) in a glass of water sweetened with sugar, daily, one hour before breakfast.

Claudia James writes, "Nechessor, the Egyptian, dedicated chamomile to the Sun in recognition of its curative power. 'It most wonderfully breaketh the stone,' noted Culpepper a thousand years later. I worked out a little experiment of this myself. A man who had just paid $300.00 to have 64 gallstones removed gave me a few of them. 'You can't dissolve these with chamomile flowers,' he said. 'My wife and I have been pounding them with a big hammer and we can't break them.'

" 'Wait and see,' " was my reply. . . . So I made a solution of 14 [chamomile] flowers in a tablespoon of boiling water, poured it into a small glass and dropped two gallstones into it. The next day they were in four pieces. In five days they were like grit, and in ten days they had disappeared altogether." (See Bibliography.) Some people report that chamomile tea produces good results.

Beet greens have been found to contain a gallstone-dissolving ingredient. For those who hesitate to eat them regularly, a preparation called "Betaris" is available through your doctor who can order it from Vitamin Products, Milwaukee 1, Wisconsin.

R. Swinburne Clymer, M.D., lists two herbal remedies. He says, "In many instances it is possible to dissolve formed gall stones, or prevent their formation by proper medication." His formulas which have proved effective are:

Tincture of Tetterwort (*Sanguinaria canadensis*)	5 to 10 drops
Tincture of Barberry (*Berberis vulgaris*)	3 to 5 drops
Tincture of Fringe Tree (*Chiolanthus virginica*)	3 to 5 drops
Tincture of Bitter Root (*Apocynum androsaemifolium*)	1 to 2 drops

In water three times a day, best one-half hour after meals.

-or-

Tincture of Wormseed	8 to 10 drops
Tincture of Rheumatism Root (*Discores villosa*)	1 to 5 drops
Tincture of Mandrake (*Podophyllum peltatum*)	1 to 3 drops
Tincture of Fringe Tree (*Chiolanthus virginica*)	3 to 5 drops

In water three to four times a day.

WHY KIDNEY STONES?

Kidney stones have been found to result from a lack of Vitamin B-6. In 18 adults, vitamin B-6 was followed by excretion of urinary oxalate (oxalic acid), the major ingredient of many kidney stones. (*American Journal of Clinical Nutrition*, November-December, 1960.)

In 256 cases with kidney stones, calcium oxalate was present in 27 stones and calcium phosphate in 26. Intakes of vitamin A, vitamin C and fat were low in the people who were affected with stones. (*British Journal Urology* [1962], 34, 160-177.)

One form of kidney stone was caused in animals by milk and bicarbonate. (*American Journal of Clinical Nutrition*, Vol. 6, March-April, No. 2.)

W. J. McCormick, M.D., finds that a deficiency of vitamin C can result in kidney stones. (*Medical Record*, Vol. 159, No. 7; July, 1946.)

Dr. J. W. Joly, in his book *Stones and Calculus Disease*, writes, "I believe that the hypothesis that stone is a deficiency disease is the most probable and plausible that has yet been advanced."

WHAT NATURAL REMEDIES MAY DISSOLVE KIDNEY STONES?

Dr. McCormick states, "In my own clinical experience, I believe I have discovered the secret of the beneficent effect of apple cider in

the dissolution and prevention of renal calculi (kidney stones)—its content of vitamin C (ascorbic acid). . . . I have found that the change (from a cloudy urine) can usually be brought about in a matter of hours by large doses of the vitamin, 500 to 2,000 mg. oral or parental. Subsequently, daily maintenance doses of 100 to 300 mg. are usually sufficient to keep the urine free from these deposits."

Lemon juice has been used successfully in some cases. Dr. Bertrand Bibus, chief urologist, Kaiser Franz Josef Hospital, Vienna, has stated that large urate stones have been dissolved by prescribing the juice of one or two lemons daily.

"As far back as 1879, Russian doctors had tested a very old 'folk medicine' remedy for kidney ailments. Remedy: an 'infusion' of ordinary corn tassels! About 10 years ago Soviet Dr. E. K. Goldberg confirmed that a simple water extract of corn tassels had pronounced therapeutic effects on some patients with kidney, liver and gall bladder disorders. Dr. Dzhamaleva claims that some kidney stones gradually broke into fine grains; this action she demonstrated on all kidney stones except the 'oxalate' variety. Treatment was extremely simple: a weak infusion of corn tassels in water, one tablespoon taken by mouth, three to four times per day. Often pain, nausea and other typical symptoms lessened quickly." (*Northern Neighbors*, December, 1963).

The newest and most dramatic method for obtaining freedom from kidney stones, is magnesium. For method see p. 120.

SOME FOLK REMEDIES FOR WEAK KIDNEYS

1 glass a day of cooled parsley tea made from one store-size bunch of parsley to 2 pints of water, boiled 15 minutes.

Asparagus water.

At least 6 cups daily of tea made from red clover blossoms.

Alternate eating pumpkin seeds with watermelon seeds for 7 days.

Flaxseed tea, or Fenugreek tea (an aid to dissolving mucus) have helped some people to stop getting up so much at night.

39 Infections

One of the most exciting nutritional discoveries is that of using massive doses of vitamin C as a natural antibiotic. Everyone who tries this almost magical formula becomes so enthusiastic that he rushes around telling everyone else. I am not sure who discovered the therapy first, W. J. McCormick, M.D., of Toronto, Canada, or F. R. Klenner, M.D., of Reidsville, North Carolina; but no matter. They both deserve credit for acquainting us with a natural antibiotic which neutralizes toxins and eliminates infections without the unpleasant or dangerous side effects of some antibiotic drugs.*

Not long ago a friend of ours canceled an appointment because he was coming down with a virus. He ached all over, had a sore throat, was feverish, and felt miserable. My husband mentioned the McCormick-Klenner formula to him. It is, in general for an infection, 1,000 mg. of vitamin C (ascorbic acid) plus 1 calcium tablet (lactate, gluconate, or bone meal) at least every hour until the infection disappears. These doctors who discovered its value consider it harmless (as a vitamin, not a drug) since any excess unused by the body will be excreted through the urine. Ascorbic acid is available at drugstores in 250 or 500 mg. tablets, so that four of the 250 mg. or two of the 500 mg. make the necessary dose.

"Sounds like a lot," our friend remarked dubiously. "That's just the point," my husband answered. "The physicians say the purpose is to raise the vitamin C level in the blood. In case of death from infections, autopsy has shown that not a single drop of vitamin C could be found in the blood. So when infection does strike, the vitamin C level needs to be raised to normal as rapidly as possi-

* See Bibliography.

ble. And when that point occurs, and not a minute sooner, will the infection disappear."

"Well," said our doubting friend, "if the doctors say it's safe, maybe it's worth a try."

Next day he called in great excitement. "It worked!" he shouted. "I never saw anything like it. And I don't feel all washed out as I do when taking a regular antibiotic. Will it cure a cold too?"

"It has for me," said my husband. "I start the minute I feel the first cold symptom and I keep it up till I am sure I've licked it. The doctors say you will know when you have had enough, by a slight burning of the urine (which almost never happens). I have also found that the formula can be used for diarrhea, sore throat, upset stomach and all manners of infections, with tremendous success." (My husband, a Ph.D., is nutritionally oriented.)

The next time we saw our friend he told us he felt like standing on the streetcorner and shouting the good news about vitamin C as an antibiotic. He said he was advocating it for everyone he saw coming down with a cold.

The first time I tried it was when I woke one morning with a temperature of 104, and faithfully began the four 250 mg. vitamin C plus 1 calcium tablet routine—although I took it every two hours. By noon there was no improvement. By the middle of the afternoon, although my temperature was still high, I noticed a surge of energy after each dose. But then I would backslide until the next dose. I was about to decide the whole thing didn't work, when about 10 P.M. my temperature suddenly left as if it had been cut off with a knife. I felt wonderful—no weakness, no signs of illness. Had I stopped earlier, even one or two doses short of recovery, I would not have had success. Later I learned that not until the vitamin C level in the blood has been restored will the infection disappear. Those who don't get results have stopped too soon.

During this treatment, don't be surprised if your kidneys are temporarily active, since large amounts of vitamin C act as a diuretic and rid the body of water. For this reason vitamin C has been successfully used as a diuretic for swelling ankles in cases of heart congestion.

Other cures by this method sound almost fantastic. Dr. McCormick reports he has had spectacular results in the treatment of serious cases of tuberculosis, meningitis, scarlet fever, pelvic infections, and septicemia. Dr. Klenner has reported dramatic results with the same method in the treatment of virus diseases, polio, encephalitis, measles, herpes zoster, and virus pneumonia.

For the serious diseases, these doctors give the large doses by injection. For less serious infections, they advocate the vitamin by mouth. In some cases they recommend 1,000 mg. every hour; in others, 1,500 every two hours. Dr. Klenner says, "The amount of vitamin C for optimal effect will vary greatly with the individual. The type of disease and the degree of toxemia are important guides in determining the dosage. Although the usual dose of vitamin C is calculated on the basis of 65 mg. per kg. of body weight, and given two to four hours by needle, under certain conditions larger single injections can be used to good advantage. Vitamin C given to a child with measles, mumps, or chickenpox will abort or modify the attack, depending upon the intensity of the treatment. If the activity of the pathogen is stopped, the development of active immunity will be interrupted. . . . The itch of the measles and of chickenpox, the occasional vomiting accompanying these illnesses, and the pain of mumps were fully controlled within one hour when 250 mg. per kg. body weight was used."

Adelle Davis says she cured her son of mumps with vitamin C in one day. For chickenpox she dissolves fifty 500-mg. tablets or one hundred 250-mg. vitamin C tablets to 1 cup of boiling water, then refrigerates the mixture in a jar. One teaspoon of this liquid equals 500 mg. of vitamin C and can be added to fruit juice. Beginning at 7 A.M., she gave her son 1,000 mg. of vitamin C plus a little calcium powder in fruit juice every hour. By evening all swelling and illness were gone.

Dr. Klenner says, "Calcium in vivo, duplicates the chemical behavior of vitamin C in many respects. Calcium gluconate and calcium levulinate were used in conjunction with vitamin C therapy in a small series of pulmonary virus infections and in mild cases of influenza. There was definite synergistic response. Patients with colds derived most benefit from the combined treatment."

Dr. Klenner tells of case after case of polio which obtained complete recovery by this method. Allergies, asthma, lead poisoning, and hay fever (C in high doses becomes an antihistamine) are other disturbances which yield to this therapy. Physicians who examine the literature and employ the technique will chalk up additional successes.

WE ARE ALL VITAMIN C SPENDTHRIFTS

Apparently, we are constantly besieged with vitamin C destroyers. Even inhaling the fumes from a passing car uses up some of the vitamin. Dr. McCormick says every cigarette you smoke and every aspirin you take uses the amount of vitamin C found in a medium-sized orange. In normal health the body's supply is used up in 4 or 5 hours. But under sudden stress such as shock, an infection, an operation, or even an argument with your mate, the vitamin C supply stored in the adrenal glands is used up immediately. Dr. Klenner adds that one severe fit of anger burns up between 3,000 to 4,000 mg. of C in minutes!

Perhaps you have noticed, or maybe you didn't connect the fact, that a cold or other infection sometimes comes on the heels of a siege of emotional tension. So following any emotional upset, it is wise to raise your intake of vitamin C for a few days. Often, for no reason I can recall, I have felt low, draggy, or even depressed. After taking 1,000 mg. of C plus the calcium tablet, my energy returns, I experience a lift and soon feel normal.

Animal studies reveal there is a direct relationship between the amount of vitamin C in the diet and success in healing wounds. The studies found a higher concentration of vitamin C in wound and scar tissue than in other muscle tissues.

According to a study at Long Island Jewish Hospital and Yeshiva University College of Medicine, a substance called collagen (a gluelike substance) holds the body's joints together and its organs in place. In vitamin C deficiency, this gluelike substance becomes water, and infection can travel through the body more quickly via this watery network. A tightly knit collagen keeps the tissues firm and well "glued" together. Doctors can diagnose the watery condition of vitamin C deficiency by viewing the tissues under black light. You can observe your own vitamin C deficiency if you are subject to black-and-blue marks, bruise easily, have pink toothbrush, or in case of a cut or wound, heal slowly.

WHAT TYPE OF VITAMIN C IS BEST?

For massive doses, ascorbic acid seems to do the job for most people. Ascorbic acid is the one synthetic vitamin which is considered useful for such purposes. However, for day-in, day-out vitamin C maintenance, the bioflavonoids from natural sources are probably best because of the added factors present. The bioflavonoids are the entire C family or complex, including rutin (a capillary strengthening vitamin) hesperidin, ascorbic acid, and other factors. Bioflavonoids have been used—and good results claimed—for colds, retinal hemorrhages, pink toothbrush, and in RH-negative pregnancies and other cases. Bioflavonoids are found in the pulp, rather than the juice, of citrus fruits. If you drink a glass of strained orange juice, you are getting only 100 mg. of citrus bioflavonoids, whereas if you eat one orange, thinly peeled, leaving on as much white skin as possible, you will be getting 1,000 mg.

One man who told me he had not had a cold for 16 years, said he eats daily one-half lemon, skin and all. (Liquefied in a blender with water and honey, it is delicious.) Make sure there is no pesticide residue on the skin.

The citrus bioflavonoid tablets come under different trade names. They usually combine 100 mg. of vitamin C with 100 mg. of the flavonoids. Some doctors have been disappointed in claims made for bioflavonoids. Dr. Boris Sokoloff feels this is due to inadequate dosage and inactive brands of bioflavonoids. This parallels the reaction of American physicians to the use of vitamin E in this country where the cause was traced to inadequate dosage and synthetic rather than natural sources of vitamin E. Most nutritionists consider one or two tablets of bioflavonoids daily sufficient if your tissues are already saturated and you have not recently suffered from infection or emotional stress.

In addition to citrus fruits, other natural sources of vitamin C are rose hips and acerola berries. The acerola berry is many times higher in C than rose hips. The newest and most potent source is derived from bilberries.

In the massive doses of synthetic C, Dr. Klenner reports a few cases of rash, which soon disappears. I have known two people among hundreds who developed a rash from the synthetic vitamin, which disappeared on taking rose-hip C. Reports of animals and people given natural versus synthetic C are conflicting, so apparently it is an individual matter. In my own case, I use the synthetic C for massive-dose treatment of infections, and for daily use I take the natural bioflavonoids-plus-C (available at health food stores).

WHAT ABOUT COLDS?

I have learned, as a result of watching myself and my family, that a cold can be prevented more easily than it can be cured. The secret is to catch it early! At the first indication of a cold—a sniffle, scratchy or sore throat, *immediate* action is necessary. I use the massive dose of ascorbic acid—1,000 mg. per hour plus 1 calcium tablet. Usually this aborts the cold within hours, though I have known it to take a day or more. My husband, on the other hand, uses ascorbic acid-plus-bioflavonoids. Even if he starts too late to stop the cold, he brings it to a halt within a day's time by using the hourly dose. I have never been this lucky. If a cold develops for me, although I use the massive dosage of vitamin C, it runs its course, although in a lighter and shorter form.

A doctor who is exposed to colds from his patients, told me that he takes six bioflavonoids daily during the winter and never catches his patients' colds. A health food store owner uses another method. The minute a customer with a cold leaves the store, she takes a large dose of vitamin C and vitamin A. She keeps herself well vitaminized and she testifies that the C plus A has never let her down.

Occasionally, in treating a cold, vitamin A works better for some people. Of my own two sons-in-law, at the first cold symptom, one rushes for the vitamin C bottle. The other seizes the 25,000-unit vitamin A capsules and follows Carlton Fredericks' formula of 250,000 units daily for three days. In both cases, they are freed of cold symptoms within a day. Then they use *one* maintenance dose daily for a few days for added insurance.

Dr. W. Coda Martin and Dr. Morton S. Biskind report success with bioflavonoids in treating colds. In deciding whether to use the massive doses of A or C for a cold, if one does not work, next time try the other until you determine which is better for you.

An effective folk remedy for treating virus or other infections is six cloves of garlic. These can be chopped and added to green salad, or crushed and blended with butter and spread on bread which can then be toasted or just warmed in the oven. With the six cloves of garlic, drink a glassful of hot water in which has been stirred four tablespoons of cider vinegar and two tablespoons honey.

Verification of the therapeutic effects of garlic comes from a German magazine, *Medical Monthly* (March, 1950), in which Dr. J. Klosa administered 10 to 25 drops of oil of garlic every four hours for various respiratory infections. The results were enhanced if fresh onion juice extract was added.

If you do not find garlic palatable, several manufacturers make garlic perles which contain garlic oil.

One variety, supposedly odor-free, is known as "Social Garlic". Chewing a bit of parsley is a time-honored method of chasing garlic and onion breath odor. Still another suggestion is to put chopped garlic far back on the tongue and swallow without chewing—followed by water.

In any case, do not underestimate the therapeutic effects of garlic or that magical vitamin C! Both are natural antibiotics, and safe.

40 Insomnia

For many years most doctors and scientists believed that sleep requirements varied with each person and that no two individuals responded alike. Today, there is a bit of an about-face. Our world is changing. It is more hectic. Nearly everyone is experiencing more stress than ever before, and one protection against this stress is sleep. Dr. George S. Stevenson of the National Association for Mental Health says, "I believe it can safely be said that *all* human beings need a minimum of six hours' sleep to be mentally healthy. Most people need more. Those who think they can get along on less are fooling themselves."

According to Robert O'Brien, in an article "Maybe You Need More Sleep": "Lack of sleep is frequently the real trouble with the husband who loses his temper at breakfast, the mother who flares up at her children, or the man who flies off the handle at the office. Lack of sleep can make normally cheerful people feel moody and depressed. . . . And sleep loss is a subtle poison; its victims are usually the last to realize what's wrong.

"It is now evident that disturbances in behavior from lack of sleep closely resemble the disorders produced by certain narcotics, alcohol, and oxygen starvation. Perceptions grow fuzzy. Our sense of timing is off. Our reflexes are a little late. Values slip out of focus. We are literally not 'ourselves.' . . . And it can happen to you, as many who have fallen asleep at the wheel of a car can testify."

Twenty-five members of a British North Greenland Expedition who spent from one to two years at a base near the North Pole were permitted to sleep any time they wished during the 24-hour nights. This demand-feeding of sleep, similar to the demand-feeding of babies who are given a bottle whenever they are hungry, was watched with interest. When the sleep was totaled for a month each member had averaged 7.9 hours a day. The result of the study was summed up: "The traditional eight hours' sleep seems to be what the body needs."

But inability to sleep eight hours apparently worries many people. A director of a home for the aged said the two problems which worried oldsters most were "their bowels and their sleep."

J. D. Ratcliff, reporting on sleep (*Family Weekly*, June 13, 1965) says that researchers find that sleep needs vary with individuals. Dr. Alton Ochsner, of New Orleans' Ochsner Clinic, feels that four hours are sufficient for his own needs. If he feels fatigued during the day, he is refreshed by a five minute catnap—he needs only a few seconds to fall into a sound refreshing sleep. Other people, who do not find daytime catnapping easy may probably need more hours of sleep at night.

Dr. Philip M. Tiller, Jr. of Louisiana School of Medicine has found a high correlation between various symptoms of poor health and inadequate sleep (seven or less hours a night). Dr. Tiller prescribed 10 hours of bed rest at night and an hour's nap in the afternoon for many aging people who were suffering from various minor complaints. If sleep did not come easily, Dr. Tiller asked that radio and TV be turned off and eyes be kept closed.

Surprisingly, Dr. Tiller found that his test subjects began to sleep more naturally; that the afternoon nap improved night sleeping; and most important of all, complaints which had brought many patients to a doctor's office disappeared.

William Kitay has recommended a sleep-break in the office for tired businessmen. It is a boon to tired executives. He says, "A bit of sleep to the tired businessman is as welcome to his nervous system as a snack to his hungry stomach."

Dr. Tiller agrees, and adds, "As the work load increases, so does the need for sleep. Yet the exact opposite course is usually followed—the busier the person, the less he sleeps."

Dr. Ochsner concludes, "The siesta habit is a good one. It is difficult for many people to store up a day's energy needs with a single stretch of night sleep."

It is a wise businessman who will take a few minutes at lunch or coffee break time to put his feet up on the desk and catch a few minutes snooze. This is far better than "whipping the tired horse" during the day and resorting to sleeping pills at night because of the effects of overstimulation of his nervous system.

In *Lancet* (February 8, 1958) a doctor writes, "I have been waging war on sleeping tablets. Every person who asks for them, or who obviously hopes for them, is submitted to a series of questions. The results of my investigations are startling. In my series of about fifty patients with insomnia:

"Only three patients went to their beds later than 10:30 P.M. Most went to bed at 9:30 or earlier. One went to bed at 5 P.M." These people were determined to sleep but tried too hard and overworried about not sleeping.

Sleep produced by sleeping pills is not as beneficial as you might think, according to Dr. Billy S. Taylor. He writes in *Western Medicine*, "The sleep induced by sedatives may not restore normal vigor."

Dr. Henry Beecher, of Massachusetts General Hospital, agrees. He believes that sleeping pills reduce a person's efficiency the next day.

WHAT IS A "SLEEP-CHEAT"?

A "sleep-cheat" is not to be confused with an insomniac. He *can* go to bed but he won't. He won't miss the late television show; he can't break loose from that poker game; he won't stop talking. These are the people who may be heading for health impairment by burning the candle at both ends.

Robert O'Brien comments, "Millions of people stay up too late out of habit. Many feel that the late evening hours are the only ones they can call their own. Tired housewives, for example, who have put their children to bed feel that now, at last, they are entitled to a little time to themselves. They guard these moments jealously, against all pleas that they get to bed. But the price of that extra hour is stiff.

"Many late stayer-uppers hang on simply because they are dissatisfied with how little they have accomplished during the day. The irony is that if they got the sleep they needed, their days might be better balanced . . . with greater efficiency. . . . For most of us, the price we pay for staying up later than we should is common irritability.

"The time spent in sleep is not lost. Adequate sleep is an essential ingredient in producing joy in life—that sudden rush of well-being that sometimes sweeps out of nowhere and makes us glad to be alive." (*Farm Journal*, 1960; reprinted in *Reader's Digest*, February, 1960.)

CAN YOU REPAY A SLEEP DEBT?

Yes. If it is a now-and-then loss of sleep. Sleeping late over the weekend will probably cancel the debt for an occasional late week night. A test showed that it took two good nights' sleep to help offset one night of only four hours' sleep.

WHEN DO YOU GET THE MOST RESTFUL SLEEP?

This appears to be an individual matter. Some people insist they get their best sleep before midnight. Others are late-morning sleepers and can't nap during the day. Everyone's sleep pattern differs.

William Gutman, M.D. (see Bibliography), says, "The amount of sleep one needs depends on its quality. As in the case of food, the quality of sleep is much more important than the quantity. A few hours' deep sleep with complete relaxation is far more refreshing than a long, superficial, restless sleep.

"Experiments have shown that the greatest depth of sleep is reached within the first two hours; then it decreases very quickly until after five or six hours it becomes rather superficial.

"There are two types of sleeper. The evening type feels drowsy in the evening, falls asleep and is at his best in the morning. The morning sleeper is more fully alive in the evening. He falls asleep comparatively late, often with difficulty, and sleeps well into the late morning hours. If awakened earlier, he feels bad and is more or less disinclined to work."

DO PEOPLE WAKE UP DIFFERENTLY?

Indeed they do. You can only wake up as fast as you warm up. Efficiency in the morning has a direct connection with the body temperature. Some people warm up faster—thus wake up much faster than others, according to Dr. Nathaniel Kleitman of the University of Chicago.

Nutritionists say that the slow wakers are possibly deficient in B vitamins and protein.

Your brain awakens you in reverse order to which it put you to sleep—in a gradual progression. First to wake up are your large muscles—legs, arms, back and neck. Then come the senses. The first to awake is touch, then hearing, vision, and lastly smell.

If you can arrange it, take plenty of time to wake up and thus avoid nervous irritations during the rest of the day.

DOES COFFEE KEEP YOU AWAKE?

Perhaps. If you think it does, it probably does. The reverse is also true. In one study, caffeine was removed from coffee and put into hot milk. All those patients receiving the caffeine in hot milk (unknown to them) slept like babies. The others who drank decaffeinated coffee without knowing it, couldn't sleep a wink!

WHAT TRICKS ARE HELPFUL?

In *Confessions of an Insomniac*, Dora Pantell lists six rules she learned from research and personal experience:

1. "Get rid of your conditioning. You probably don't need the eight to nine hours sleep you think you need. You may get along just fine on seven, or even five to six plus a few catnaps during the day.

2. "Put away that clock. Having it around will only worry you unnecessarily.

3. "Do what you feel like doing when you can't sleep.

4. "If you feel like worrying a problem through at night, go right ahead. Making a concrete plan—even if you revise it first thing in the morning—at least it will give you some peace of mind.

5. "If you must probe your subconscious at night, do. . . . If you don't know what's worrying you, try to find out. You've got to face it some time. The sooner the better!

6. "If you haven't a thing to worry about and still can't sleep, find something to think about. . . . If you are busy doing something, your insomnia will go—quietly."

The trick which helps most is to conjure up the pleasantest picture possible—that lake where you vacationed last summer, or that room you want to redecorate. Sometimes I wander mentally through my small garden, planning it in the winter, examining each plant in the summer. I am usually asleep before I get to the end of the garden.

ARE SLEEPING PILLS HARMFUL?

Yes. Dr. Walter C. Alvarez formerly of Mayo Clinic reports that they may lower your I.Q. because they dull the brain.

George P. Larrick of the Food and Drug Administration warns: "Barbiturates produce more mental, emotional and neurological impairment than morphine.

"Like morphine, barbiturates produce physical dependence, but withdrawal of barbiturates is even more serious. In some cases patients even die during withdrawal."

The New York Health Department estimates that 20 per cent of all prescriptions filled by druggists contain barbiturates. William Percival, staff writer for the New York *World-Telegram and Sun*, says that Benny and Barby, better known as benzedrine and barbiturates, are encouraged by big-time racketeers. "They make a charming couple; they will lead you down the primrose path straight to the hospital. Next stop, the morgue."

ARE THERE ANY SLEEPING POTIONS WHICH ARE SAFE?

Eating the day's largest meal before going to bed keeps many people awake or promotes restless sleep. Try a light meal and see if it doesn't help. There are calming food nutrients to take at bedtime for those who feel they can't sleep on a completely empty stomach: vitamin-B-rich brewer's yeast stirred into juice or water; vitamin E in capsule form or wheat germ; lecithin granules; and old-fashioned licorice.

Adelle Davis says, "A calcium deficiency shows itself by insomnia, another form of inability to relax. . . . For persons whose tissues are starved for calcium, however, the amount in a milk drink is a mere drop in the bucket. I usually tell persons whose insomnia is severe to take temporarily two or three calcium tablets before retiring and to keep both milk and the tablets on the bedside table and take more every hour if wakefulness persists."

Leland Kordel tells us that it is practically impossible to find a farmer or a lumberjack who can't sleep. It isn't only the fresh air, he says. Exercise releases calcium and lactic acid into the muscles. His advice then is, a walk during the day—the closer to bedtime the better. Or take calcium tablets plus lactic acid milk such as buttermilk or yogurt. Buttermilk is especially good for inducing sleep because it contains lecithin as well as calcium—both calming agents.

Avoid taking vitamin A at night. It is a stimulating vitamin and may keep you awake.

HOW TO GET TO SLEEP NATURALLY

Charles P. Kelly has written a book called *That Natural Way to Healthful Sleep* which, according to the publishers, is guaranteed to put you to sleep. He says, "The body produces its own sleep-inducing chemical, an internal tranquilizer, and by following a few simple directions, you can help the body put you to sleep, naturally."

It has been known for more than a hundred years that carbon

dioxide will produce anesthesia. Compared to drugs, the effect of carbon dioxide is completely natural. It already occurs in our own bodies in tissues and fluids and is in the air we breathe.

Mr. Kelly writes, "When very slightly increased, carbon dioxide acts as a sedative, quieting activity or excitement in the nervous system. . . . It tends to bring on drowsiness, which under favorable conditions may lead to sleep. This sleep-producing effect . . . can be easily brought about by merely reducing the volume of breathing.

"The anesthetic effect of carbon dioxide cannot be produced by controlling breathing, because when consciousness is lost, control is also lost, and breathing goes back to normal. . . . No overdosage is possible, either by accident or by deliberate intention. . . . Sleep induced by carbon dioxide is natural sleep.

"For the past seventeen years," he says, "I have been using controlled breathing as a sleep inducer whenever sleep did not come promptly. . . . I have never been able to detect even the slightest undesirable or unpleasant effect. Now at the age of eighty-six, I am in good health, with near perfect digestion and few aches or pains . . . and my mental alertness seemingly unimpaired. This prolonged vigor I attribute largely to the adequate sleep which I have always managed to get and which I am now continuing to ensure by the use of controlled breathing."

Here is Mr. Kelly's formula: Lying on your side in bed, take three *deep* breaths expanding the abdomen completely. Then hold your breath until you can no longer resist breathing again. Then take three more deep breaths followed by more breath-holding. You may need to do this several times. Don't worry while you're holding your breath. It won't hurt you. Mr Kelly suggests diverting your attention by mentally reciting "Twinkle, Twinkle Little Star" or some other nursery rhyme. While the breath-holding continues, the "accumulation of carbon dioxide in the body is carried much further," he explains.

After you have completed several rounds of deep breaths followed by breath-holding, Mr. Kelly then advises minimum breathing—shallow, short breaths which are so slight that movement of air in through the nose is barely discernible. When you feel you *must* breathe deeply again, by all means do so. However, as you now concentrate on minimum breathing, you will no doubt fall asleep. If for some reason you are the exception to the rule and the system doesn't work, read Mr. Kelley's book to get the complete story plus other helpful hints to make good that guarantee! But to summarize his system: Three deep breaths, hold breath. Repeat several times. Follow with regular minimum (shallow) breathing. Then, sleep!

Chuck Coker, football coach, suggests, "If you want to go into a deep sleep when you go to bed, lie flat on your back. Contract the muscles in your toes, your knees, your abdomen, your back and your neck—then relax. If necessary, repeat. Think about pleasant things. (*Let's Live*, May, 1962.)

Johnnie Lee MacFadden advises lying on your back, relaxing, and then giving yourself autosuggestion. Say to yourself, "I am completely relaxed. I'm tranquil. I'm at ease and allow no person, situation, or thing to take away my inner tranquility. My peace of mind, my joy, my enthusiasm, my happiness. I allow people, situations, and things to bring me happiness, but I absolutely refuse to give them the power over me to take away my peace of mind. I am falling asleep now, in a deep, peaceful, restful . . . sleep." (See Bibliography.)

John E. Eichenlaub, M.D., recommends tranquilizing tubs. He suggests putting a pillow or a rolled towel behind your neck, keeping a candy thermomenter in the tub and the water running gently so that the temperature stays around 100 degrees while you remain in the tub at least a half hour. You can stay there two or three hours, he says, if you need extra tranquilizing. (See Bibliography.)

And here is a delightful collection of old-time remedies for insomnia:

Place your bed in a north-south direction—head toward the north, feet pointing south. (It's worth a try.)

Brush your hair before retiring and after a warm foot bath, rub your feet gently.

Drink hot lemon tea or hot grapefruit juice.

Eat a slice of onion on toast just before bedtime.

Use 1 teaspoon of apple cider vinegar and a little honey in 1 cup of water before meals, three times daily.

Wash celery and put it with a few leaves through the juicer. (Good for nerves, too.)

Make a tea from a heaping tablespoon of thyme and boiling water. (Also good for nerves.)

Take six deep, deep breaths. You should fall asleep.

Drink a glass of warm milk with a teaspoon of honey added.

One of the sleep tips included in this section is bound to work. If it doesn't, the best tip I can pass on to you is—if you can't go to sleep, try staying awake!

41 Leg cramps

Many a person has been awakened in the middle of the night with a clutching, tearing cramp in a foot or leg accompanied by terrific pain. Though it *may* come from more serious disturbances, the usual, simple cause is a lack of calcium.

My Harrow and Mazur textbook of biochemistry (see Bibliography) explains, "A concentration of calcium below the normal amount, brought about by a deficiency of the parathyroid hormone, affects the central nervous system and produces an increased irritability of the peripheral nerves. At a later stage, muscle spasms (affecting the face, hands and feet) . . . make their appearance."

It is possible that, though a person takes adequate calcium, he is not absorbing it properly, in which case the lack of vitamin D, a calcium co-worker, may cause the cramp. The biochemical textbook says, "Vitamin D, possibly by regulating the utilization of calcium from the intestine, influences the extent to which the body uses the element."

Don't be too sure that you are not calcium deficient. At Bellevue Hospital in New York City, 4,200 people ranging in age from 2 to 72 years old, were tested. Only *two* were *not* calcium deficient!

Albert E. Holand, Jr., consulting nutritionist, says, "I dare say that scarcely a medical doctor exists who has not given a calcium shot to quiet a jittery patient, or relax a 'charley-horsed' muscle. These physicians can testify to the often dramatic results when calcium lactate or calcium gluconate is injected directly into the blood stream." (These calcium compounds can also be taken by mouth.)

The thyroid and parathyroid glands can control the assimilation of calcium, providing they are given the proper raw material. A calcium deficiency is aggravated when the body's metabolic rate is lowered during sleep and rest. This explains why foot and leg cramps usually take place at night.

There are other co-workers, though, that calcium must have to be properly used by the body. Albert Holand adds, "For example, it is well known that calcium is best prepared for absorption in an acid medium. Therefore a deficiency of stomach acids (hydrochloric acid in the main) could very well inhibit calcium absorption. Phosphorus and potassium, iodine and protein are interrelated in helping the thyroid and parathyroid glands do their duty. Mr. Holand concludes, "Following this line of reasoning, it would seem logical to supply with calcium the mineral co-partners that help. I know of no mineral source which supplies these factors better than sea kelp—a rich source of potassium, iodine and a host of nutrients which could well assist in the assimilation of calcium." (*Let's Live*, June, 1963.) Magnesium has also proved helpful.

In a prenatal clinic in Brazil, one-third of 980 pregnant women complained of leg cramps, particularly toward the last three months. Sixty, in whom the cramps were frequent and severe, were treated with minerals, vitamins and six daily intravenous injections of one gram of calcium gluconate, followed by oral doses of 3 to 5 grams of calcium gluconate three times daily for three weeks. Thirty-six were cured and 19 improved.

Royal Lee, D.D.S., suggests riboflavin, a B vitamin, for leg cramps. He makes an impressive statement about the type of calcium which can be used: "Calcium lactate is the most soluble and most easily absorbed of the calcium group and the most desirable from a nutritional standpoint. Bone meal—the calcium derived from *cooked* bone meal is almost completely insoluble and therefore of little use to the body. If the bone meal is uncooked, there is a certain amount of soluble calcium, although this product is especially valuable because of its amino acid and protein content." (*Let's Live*, October, 1963.)

A late issue of *Organic Consumer Report* (September 1, 1964) says, "Muscular cramps, most often troublesome at night, can be relieved in 15 or 20 minutes through the use of a tablespoon of calcium lactate, taken with one teaspoon each of cider vinegar and honey, in hot water."

Dr. D. C. Jarvis writes, "When calcium is precipitated in the body we notice the appearance of muscle cramps. These are painful, commonly occurring in the legs during the night. They may also appear in the stomach, the intestines and the heart. The taking of two teaspoonsful of apple cider vinegar and two of honey in a glass of water with each meal allows the precipitated calcium to enter solution, and the muscle cramps disappear."

Adelle Davis (see Bibliography) reports that people who live on a fat-free diet absorb little or no calcium from their food. The addition of oil may bring relief. Vitamin C, too, has been helpful, she says, to soldiers who tramped many miles and suffered no leg cramps as compared with untreated soldiers who did suffer and did not recover for days.

One woman wrote to *Organic Consumer Report* (April 2, 1963): "After suffering painful muscular cramps in the legs and feet and trying almost everything . . . my nutritionist suggested calcium lactate, a food supplement available without prescription at drug or health stores at a nominal cost. I took four tablets each morning along with vitamin F (unsaturated fatty acids) and in a short time my problems had been solved." (Calcium is also recommended in *Annals of Surgery*, Vol. 131 [1950], p. 652.)

Buttermilk may help because it contains vitamin F, calcium and acids. (Peters and Van Slyke, *Quantitative Chemistry*, Vol. 1, p. 828.) Leg cramps and pain may also be due to:

ATHEROSCLEROSIS, or cholesterol deposits in the arteries, resulting in decreased circulation. Adelle Davis, in her article "Keep Your Heart Young" (*Modern Nutrition*, March, 1959), writes: "Witness the postman who was carried in to see me with such painful atherosclerosis in his legs that walking was impossible. Three physicians had suggested amputation. I gave him lecithin and choline and yeast and unsaturated fatty acids and so on. Now he can walk several miles with no trouble at all. And another man who had always been weak and sickly and who developed cramps in his legs from high blood cholesterol started to take nutrition seriously. Last summer he climbed Mt. Rainier."

PHLEBITIS. Catharyn Elwood (see Bibliography) writes, "Vitamin E has been used for phlebitis. This nasty inflammation of the veins of the leg kept one woman from working for five years. In six days the pain was gone; in 10 days . . . the swelling had completely disappeared."

Drs. Evan and Wilfred Shute of Canada. (See Bibliography.) "Clots in the veins . . . are all too common. . . . These are not only temporarily disabling, but they tend to promote chronic disability, with swollen, tender, painful legs hindering locomotion for years. . . .

"The popular agents used by the medical men to date have been the so-called anticoagulants, drugs, which hinder further blood clotting but do little or nothing to dissolve existing clots or provide detours around the plugged veins. They are dangerous, too—so dangerous that it is questionable if they have any place at all in medical treatment. Indeed there is a good deal of medical debate on this issue at the moment.

"Alpha tocopherol (a form of vitamin E) is a happier answer and a *safe* one. In large doses, it not only prevents clots from spreading, but it often melts them away rapidly, provides collateral circulation around the obstructed vein, and seems to prevent clots breaking loose as emboli. Its effect on a fresh thrombosis is truly amazing. Even the chronic case is occasionally helped, something that no other agent can achieve. . . . Moreover, alpha tocopherol can prevent a recurrence. . . . Some hospitals around the world have already begun to use it as a routine post-operative measure.

"We suspect that the patient who has had one or more attacks of thrombosis should always take some alpha tocopherol thereafter. . . .

A chance blow, a kick by a child, bumping a chair, even influenza can flare a phlebitis even 7 to 20 years after the initial attack. . . . If such a recurrence does appear in a patient already taking a small prophylactic dose of alpha tocopherol, all she has to do is increase the dosage . . . at once, and the recurrence will be headed off."

Lancet (Vol. 2, 1949) states that vitamin E helps cramps in calves of the leg.

The biochemistry textbook gives still another reason for leg cramps: "Extreme sweating due to high temperature or much exertion may cause so much loss of sodium chloride from the body as to develop leg and abdominal cramps."

Nevin S. Scrimshaw, M.D., reporting in the *American Journal of Clinical Nutrition* (February, 1964), says, "Excessive sodium chloride losses in sweat must be replaced or muscle cramps will develop."

A final suggestion: *New England Medical Journal* (January 28, 1954) advises exercise to help leg circulation. Move the toes, legs, and feet after prolonged sitting, television, viewing, air flights, and automobile trips. Get up and move around at every opportunity.

42 Overweight and fasting

Most of us overeat. Mildred McKie, M.D., says, "So strong is the habit of eating that most people feel they will starve to death if they miss a meal. Many feel they must eat to keep up their strength."

Hereward Carrington reports, "Louis Cornaro [briefly mentioned in Chapter 21] lived a reckless and dissipated life, the result being that he completely broke down at the age of forty, and was given up by his physician to die. He was indeed a physical wreck!

"Taking matters into his own hands, however, Cornaro decided to reform his life, and see what the results would be. He simplified his diet and cut down on the quantity of food to the barest minimum. Within a few days he began to see the difference, and at the end of the year found himself completely restored to health. Seeing this, he continued this simple and abstemious life for the rest of his life. He limited himself to twelve ounces of solid food daily—and fourteen ounces of wine."

Food in those days (1467-1566) was not refined as it is today. Modern studies have shown, in agreement, that less food, high in vitamins and minerals, can produce a longer life. The 14-ounce daily ration of wine in Cornaro's diet was "new wine" which is also reputedly richer in vitamins and minerals. His diet included bread made from wheat meal, egg yolk, poultry, fish, soups, meat, milk (raw, presumably), and vegetables. As you may suspect, Cornaro was not overweight!

It is becoming more and more a belief that frequent, smaller feedings are more beneficial than fewer, voluminous meals. In Bali, fat women are almost unknown. Yet Balinese women seem to be nibbling all day long. (Nibbling may be a reversion to the eating habits of primitive people who obtained much of their food by foraging.) Dr. Clarence Cohn warns that nibbling isn't just a free ticket to eat all you want all of the time. You must choose intelligently the amount of calories best for your need and then distribute them throughout the day in frequent feedings. This is scientific nibbling. (*American Journal of Clinical Nutrition*, November, 1962.)

Just because your foods are natural is no excuse for overeating, either. Ruth Rosevear, a nutrition counselor, says, "A few people read all about the good things in natural foods (eat them) and gain tremendously. Think of this: You don't need everything every day. We do not store protein or vitamin C, so they are essential, but the extra things like nuts or dried fruit can be spaced out. Tell yourself, 'Come Tuesday, I will have nuts.' Or, knowing a fancy dinner is coming, save calories ahead for it. [For weight control] it is better to have ⅓ of the daily calories at each meal, so as to 'work them off' rather than have them 'pile on' after a heavy dinner." (*Modern Nutrition*, July, 1962).

Charles De Coti Marsh advises eating a different meal on each of 28 days in order to ensure a well-rounded diet.

WHAT, BESIDES FOOD, CAUSES OVERWEIGHT?

Underactivity can cause weight gain. Lawrence Galton in an article, "Why We Are Overly Larded," reports, "Today's carpenter saws boards with a mechanized saw; teamsters now use mechanical lifts; Junior has a car instead of a bicycle. At home and on the farm, as well as in industry, labor-saving devices make life increasingly sedentary. So do today's recreational habits: TV occupies many of our free hours and spectator sports have largely superseded individual participation in athletics. (*New York Times Magazine*, January 15, 1962.)

"We just don't need as many calories as we did in years gone by," adds Dr. Herbert Pollack. We do need more exercise.

There are a relatively few cases of overweight which can be traced to biological causes, according to Irving B. Perlstein, M.D. (See Bibliography.) The psychological causes of overweight are by far the most important. Some people use narcotics to anesthetize their anxieties and conflicts. Others use alcohol. But the majority resort to food—a sedative that is cheaper, easier to get, and far more respectable.

Dr. Perlstein feels that in order to grow thinner, the emotional eater must grow up psychologically. He must stop trying to escape from his difficulties and learn to live with them or in spite of them.

Rebecca Beard, M.D., agrees. She adds, "We can learn to live without tension and strain. We can learn to live so that it doesn't make any difference whether things are upside down, right side out or hind side before."

Dr. Perlstein has found that once an overweight person makes such an adjustment, he has little or no trouble in sticking to a weight-reduction program. His excess pounds then permanently vanish. How do you make this all-important adjustment?

"You must recognize that you cannot isolate your weight problem from your other problems and solve it separately. In order permanently to change your weight, you will have to, in some manner, change yourself. . . . It is your moment of truth when you say, . . . 'I am not going to go on this way any longer; I am going to take action, meet this thing head on and do whatever is necessary to rid myself of this burden now and forever.'"

Dr. Perlstein's book, *Diet Is Not Enough*, gives further help with the method he uses to permanently and psychologically "cure" overeaters.

WHAT DIETS REALLY WORK?

Because so many people wail that they get so hungry they *can't* stay on a reducing diet, I am going to repeat the DuPont Diet previously mentioned in *Stay Young Longer*. This diet is an application of the one which Stefansson, the explorer, developed as a result of his arctic research. The diet appeared twice, many years ago, in *Holiday* magazine. It was tested in the DuPont Company under the supervision of Dr. George H. Gehrmann and an associate, Dr. A. W. Pennington. The original study called, "Obesity in Industry, the Problem and the Solution," appeared in *Industrial Medicine*, June, 1949. Of the 20 men and women taking part in the test, *all lost weight on a diet in which the total calorie intake was unrestricted*. In other words, the subjects could eat all they wanted. They ate, for the most part, about 3,000 calories a day but extra meat and fat were allowed those who were hungry and wanted to eat more. The dieters reported that they felt well, enjoyed their meals and were never hungry between meals. Many said they were more energetic than usual. Not one complained of fatigue. As their weight dropped, those with high blood pressure also reported a blood pressure drop. Weight losers lost from 9 to 54 pounds in from one and one-half to six months.

The DuPont diet is a high-fat, high-protein diet. It is not necessary to trim off all visible fat in this diet; in fact the diet advises *extra* fat along with the meat. The DuPont diet calls for three parts protein to one part fat. Sugar is omitted and starch is kept low.

The reason you don't get hungry on this diet, according to the doctors who supervised it, is that fat stays in the stomach for a longer time than most foods and gives a feeling of satisfaction.

The diet: First course: one-half pound or more of fresh meat with the fat at each meal. You can eat as much as you want. Second course: one helping (no seconds) of white potatoes fixed in any manner—boiled, baked, pan or french fried, or rice [natural brown], or fresh fruit. You must use little or no salt and no sugar or flour. You may have a cup of black coffee or clear tea with each meal. You may season the meat with pepper, paprika, celery seed, chopped parsley or other seasoning which does not contain salt. You need not count calories or stop eating while you are still hungry or take strenuous exercise. You should, of course, have a precheck with your doctor. The diet doesn't, because of the added fat, upset the gall bladder, according to supervising doctors. If it does, less fat can be used at first and later gradually increased, using nausea as the guide to stop for the time being.

Weight loss can and does occur on this low carbohydrate diet. Many people *live* on it and stay slim and well. Carlton Fredericks suggests dividing it into six small meals daily. You will not get hungry. The Drinking Man's Diet, or Air Force Diet, is merely another variation of the same, except that it allows alcohol. Be sure to read Chapter 21 (Alcohol) for the amount of alcohol that is safe to consume.

In case you get hungry between meals or during a reducing diet, eat a tablespoonful of natural, unhomogenized peanut butter. It will stay your hunger for hours.

WHAT ABOUT FASTING?

Fasting goes back to the Bible. There are people who still advocate it. In spite of its recommendation, however, something new has happened to our civilization which now makes it exceedingly dangerous.

It is important to clarify the definition of the word "fasting." To one person it means complete abstinence from food; to another it means limiting the amount of food eaten, or cutting out certain foods temporarily. Those who give up certain foods for Lent, for instance, may consider this a "fast."

A nutritionist in Australia reports two hazards of fasting today. She says, "The world is not what it once was; it is not what it was 15 years ago. We forget this and forget to adjust.

"The first hazard of fasting is the fact that nearly every individual in some degree is contaminated with DDT or a similar insecticide. It is in our food; it is in our soil. We cannot completely escape it. It is cumulative and is stored in fatty tissue in the body. When a person fasts, the insecticide is released into the blood stream and as the fat breaks up, it becomes a self-poisoner.

"Still more serious is the fact that fasting allows the strontium stored within the body to burrow deeper into the bones. Released from various storage depots in the body, it has no other place to go but toward the areas for which it has the greatest affinity—the bones.

"I have seen people who advocate fasting and who formerly thrived on it, now look emaciated, like walking skeletons, as a result of fasting. Our world, our lives have changed and so must we."

This principle has already been demonstrated in the case of wild life. Birds, prior to a long migratory trip, are known to eat heartily to build up a reservoir of fat, to use as needed, for energy. If this preparatory diet has been contaminated with insecticides, death may take place—not immediately, but later—as the poisons, together with the fat, are released into the blood stream.

In Louisiana, fishermen have reported hordes of dead geese, cranes, and small birds as well as large numbers of dead fish. The fishermen have noted that the deaths increase with the onset of cold weather. The U.S. Public Health Service scientists, after establishing the fact that the deaths were due to insecticides, endrin and dieldrin, explained that "the deaths took place in cold weather because that is when fat, in which the poisons accumulate, is released into the blood stream for metabolic sustenance." (*New York Times*, March 20, 1964.)

The nutritionist who considers fasting a dangerous procedure in this present age is referring, for the most part, to complete abstinence from food except for water. It is true, however, that even a drastic curtailment of food, causing sudden weight loss, has proved not only disturbing but dangerous.

Four physicians at the University of California Department of Medicine and School of Public Health (Los Angeles)studied 11 obese patients who maintained a prolonged fast on water and vitamin pills. Serious complications developed in every one of the cases, including temporary anemia, low blood pressure, and gout. The problems usually disappeared after the patients began to eat again. (*Journal of the American Medical Association* [1964], 187:90.) The conclusion of the study: Prolonged fasting is hazardous.

A dentist has told me that he has observed signs of damage in the mouth after only three days of total fasting.

I asked a nutritionally oriented physician, whose methods I respect, for his opinion of fasting. He said, "I wish you could see tests of the effects of some of the body organs of my patients as a result of fasting. They have deteriorated seriously."

The complete absence of food for a number of days produces fatty livers in a number of animal species. (*Nutrition Reviews*, August, 1963.)

Two wrestling competitors collapsed before they could take part in a tournament because they had been placed on starvation diets to reduce weight. (*Science News Letter*, March 30, 1963.)

One man I know says he cannot diet successfully without taking a full array of vitamins to maintain his energy level.

If you wish to rid your body of toxicity, according to one physician, you may—but only under a doctor's supervision—follow a partial fasting regime for 48 hours (once a week, if your doctor approves) of celery and raw grapefruit.

MODIFIED FASTING WITH JUICES

Many have reported a certain type of eating, which they call fasting, and which they feel has proved beneficial by allowing body process to rest now and then and body poisons to be eliminated instead of absorbed. This modified version of a "fast" includes fresh, raw vegetable juices one day per week, or substituting fresh raw fruits and vegetables for the regular diet for a week or more. (The fruits and vegetables should obviously be spray-free).

Organic Consumer Report (February 18, 1964) says, "Generous additions of more raw fruits and vegetables to the daily diet for a period of one week to one month will usually put new spring in the step, clear the mind, improve the memory, and sensitize the taste buds. . . . You'll feel as if you're walking on Cloud 7."

You might consider two other partial fasts mentioned elsewhere in this book—the grape juice diet (see "Cancer," p. 242) and Macrobiotics (see chap. 18).

HOW TO REDUCE AND STAY REDUCED

There may be days when you wake up with great will power and decide that you will start reducing immediately. Psychologically, this is the day to start! As everyone knows, the first day or so is the hardest. Whether you avail yourself of a raw-fruit, vegetable, or juice diet, or merely eat less at each meal, something happens: your stomach begins to shrink. Herein lies your key to successful reducing, usually overlooked.

As your stomach is first given less food, it complains and you are ravenously hungry (unless you take a bit of brewer's yeast stirred up in water with a tablespoonful of vegetable oil; this keeps hunger at bay for hours). After the initial shock, your stomach shrinks, demands less food, and the going is easier. You may even take off some of those unwanted pounds with ease. But what happens next, determines the future success or failure.

Once your stomach is shrunk, by all means keep it that way and your battle is largely won! If you decide, rather, to reward yourself and fill up with your former pattern of eating large or second helpings, you will have undone all the hard work. Your stomach will again expand, it will again demand large helpings, and again you will gain weight. It is this on-again, off-again dieting which leads nowhere but to continuous overweight.

So grit your teeth on the day you or your mirror decides the time is *now*. After you have once shrunk your stomach, don't ever again overfill it. The very *second* you begin to get that "full" feeling is the time to stop. Watch for, and follow the inner warning, regardless of how much is still left on your plate. Thus your food control—and weight control—will become self-regulatory and automatic.

A simple method of losing weight is the "eat just half" plan. Robert Peterson has reported this in his column, "Life Begins at Forty," and for one man it worked like a charm. If you have been accustomed to eating two sandwiches, eat just one. If you have always eaten two helpings, eat just half—or one helping. Whatever you have been eating or drinking, eat or drink just half. It should become a way of life, and if you stick to it, you should maintain your ideal weight without starvation, and with little effort.

There is an even simpler way to lose excess weight and maintain a normal weight as well as improved health for the rest of your life. Instead of bolting your food, if you chew each mouthful until it liquefies, until it "swallows itself," you will extract more enjoyment and flavor from your food; you will place less strain on your digestion; and you will need far less food to satisfy your appetite. This in turn should help your weight to remain normal without effort, since the greatest good is extracted from the least food.

This technique was originated by Horace Fletcher, in the early 1900's. His system was called Fletcherism and, of course, was considered a fad by the medical profession at that time. Nevertheless it was endorsed by such people as John D. Rockefeller, who tried it with success on himself. The results of this method of eating were also proved valid by tests at Yale University. Furthermore it was considered sufficiently important to be incorporated in the manual of the U.S. Army.

Horace Fletcher spent nearly a lifetime and over $100,000 perfecting and testing his technique, which included other precepts, in addition to thorough chewing. Fletcher found that one should never eat until he was extremely hungry, and that on should not eat under the pressure of tension, fatigue, or other disturbing conditions. In other words, Fletcherism encouraged maximum digestion of a minimum amount of food in every way possible. As a result of trying this new way of eating on himself, he lost 60 pounds in five months, and reported that his head felt lighter, his vitality increased, and his chronic fatigue of many years disappeared. Twenty years after he began to "Fletcherize," he broke a world record of muscular endurance as proved by Yale tests.

WHAT ABOUT WATER STORED IN TISSUES?

For those who are fat because they store water, there are other courses of action. Cut down on salt, and increase vitamin C and vegetable oils. Adelle Davis cites instances in which people who were unable to reduce by any other method, did so by taking at least two tablespoons of vegetable oil daily. Magnesium also helps.

Scientists at the University of California found that rats deprived of water with their meals ate less. Apparently, they regulated their food to maintain the proper food-water ration. Withholding water did not interfere with their digestion.

One physician told me that in order to cut down on water retention he first checks the condition of his patient's thyroid, pituitary, adrenals, sex organs. He then prescribes natural oils because they contain hormone factors, he says. And he prescribes 1,000 to 2,000 mg. of natural C complex daily as a diuretic until excess water is eliminated.

Remember, "It takes more energy to carry 50 pounds of excess fat than to carry 50 pounds of lead." (*Science News Letter*, October 29, 1960.)

Dr. Clive McCay has a set of rules for reducing:

Spend about $6.00 for a bathroom scale.
Weigh yourself at the same time in the same clothing at the same hour, once a week.
Buy a table of food values for about five cents.
Cut your diet approximately in half, or eat 1,100 calories a day.
Keep your dieting secret.
(*Natural Food and Farming*, February, 1960.)

43 Ulcers

WHAT IS AN ULCER?

An ulcer is an open sore on an external or internal body surface. Duodenal ulcers are three to four times more common than stomach ulcers. The assumption is that in a duodenal ulcer, the digestive acid glands are chronically overactive, producing too much acid, too much of the time. In a stomach ulcer, there is a normal amount of acid but the tissue has low resistance to even the normal amount of acid. A newer theory, however, is that the ulcer patient fails to secrete enough mucous to protect the stomach walls from acid invasion.

WHAT ARE THE SYMPTOMS?

Pain, usually described as a gnawing, burning sensation or pressure in the upper abdomen, or just below the breast bone. It often appears a few hours after meals or an hour or so after bedtime because there is little food in the stomach at that time to buffer or cushion the effect of the hydrochloric acid.

WHAT CAUSES ULCERS?

Careless eating, highly spiced foods, coffee, cigarettes, alcohol, even too much sugar have been blamed. But nervous tension is considered the most important cause, since tension works on a nonstop, full-time basis, constantly goading acid glands into production. An ulcer, once healed, has been known to flare again during a psychological crisis. The relaxed, easygoing person is seldom afflicted.

Ulcers may run in families and men seem to be more susceptible than women. Cold weather may make them worse since cold causes constriction of blood vessels. The Mayo Clinic has found that those who take aspirin regularly have four times as many ulcers as those who don't.

"Gastric ulcers occur in anywhere from 11 to 31 per cent of arthritic patients who are given cortisone—three times the usual rate for such patients," reports Morton M. Hunt in an article, "Side Effects: A New Worry for Doctors." (*Look* December 31, 1963.)

However, Dr. T. L. Cleave in a new book, *Peptic Ulcer, Causation, Prevention and Arrest* (Baltimore, Maryland: Williams and Wilkins Co., 1963) presents an entirely new theory about ulcers. It is his contention that people do not eat enough protein and that the idle gastric juices work on the stomach lining instead. He contends that the main reason for inadequate protein is that our natural foods have been processed to the point where whatever protein did exist is now removed.

He also considers ulcers a deficiency disease due to a prolonged poverty of vitamins and minerals in the diet. D. T. Quigley, M.D., is in complete accord with this theory. He says, "A healthy mucous membrane in a well-fed person will stand a good deal of stimulation from roughage with not only no ill effect but with good effect. This is natural and normal. . . .

"The so-called enriched flour is still lacking in many vital elements, and so is a menace to these patients. It should be forbidden the ulcer patient for life. Sugar furnishes calories without vitamins or minerals. It is a slow poison for the ulcer patient. . . . Honey contains all necessary minerals . . . and this can be used freely for sweetening. Other forbidden foods are canned and packaged foods. These have been robbed of their value by the application of high heat and long storage. They are stale and worthless and crowd out good foods. Exceptions: sea foods, canned acid fruits and vegetables."

After healing takes place, Dr. Quigley recommends:

Whole grain flour and cereals.
One pound to one and one-half pounds of fresh raw vegetables and
   fruit daily.
Fresh meat, rare.
Natural foods and natural vitamin supplements.

Both Drs. Quigley and Cleave warn against the following foods:

Sugar.
White flour.
Processed cereals and polished rice.
Pastry, cakes, cookies made from white flour.
Sugary foods; including chocolate, candies, ice cream, and other con-
   fections.
Alcohol. It should be regarded as a carbohydrate. According to Dr.
   Quigley, one-third of a pound of sugar daily (the average American
   intake) is equal to a pint of whiskey.

Both Dr. Cleave and Dr. Quigley deny that stress is a cause of
ulcers. Dr. Quigley explains why: "These persons [with ulcers]
are irritable and unstable. They are starved generally and specifically. In many cases the nervous symptoms overshadow the ulcer
symptoms. The reason is that the nerve disease and the ulcer both
go back to a common cause; an oversupply of refined carbohydrates which causes a dangerous reduction of the vitamin and mineral concentration in the blood stream. Peptic ulcer is never *caused*
by nervousness. It is *associated* with it."

In final analysis, the cause of ulcers still is something of a mystery, according to many experts.

WHAT ABOUT TREATMENT?

Doctors in India state that of 50 cases of peptic ulcer, *all* were cured
by a low salt diet. More than one gram of salt daily was found to
overstimulate hydrochloric acid. Dr. Quigley suggests other helps:
"In addition to natural foods, for the reason that deficiency-
diseased persons have an increased requirement for vitamins and

minerals depending on the time of such starvation and degree, we must resort to concentrates.

"Calcium may be supplied in milk, iron in meat, iron in seafood (in addition to iron and iodine supplements). All fat-soluble vitamins (A,D,E,K) must be used to make up for past dietary sins. Wheat-germ oil and ascorbic acid can be added to cod-liver oil.

"To summarize: Peptic ulcer is a deficiency disease reflecting a relatively high intake of refined carbohydrates and an inadequate amount of all vitamins and food minerals. A high vitamin and mineral diet should be prescribed with cod-liver oil concentrates and all water-soluble vitamins, the concentrates to be used in large doses for a limited time, the high vitamin-high mineral diet to be kept up for life." (*Nebraska State Medical Journal* [April, 1945], Vol. 30, No. 4. Also available in Reprint No. 17, Lee Foundation for Nutritional Research, Milwaukee 3, Wisconsin.)

WHAT REMEDIES PROVIDE RELIEF AND HASTEN HEALING?

H. E. Kirschner, M.D., recommends the use of fresh comfrey leaves blended in his "green drink." * Comfrey leaves are slightly mucilaginous.

Dr. John C. Houck recommends kelp, and dulse, as a source of iodine. Japanese "Nori" is another.

Dr. Arthur H. Bryan reports that ulcers respond to cultured milks (buttermilk and yogurt).

One study (*American Journal of Gastroenterology*, July, 1958) tells of the success of the Drs. Samuel, Jerome, and Bernard Weiss in their use of bioflavonoids (vitamin C complex) in the treatment of 36 cases of bleeding ulcers. The doctors used no other medication. Three to nine bioflavonoid capsules were given orally each day in addition to an orange juice-milk-gelatin mixture, plus the usual bland ulcer diet. Bleeding was arrested, usually on the fourth day, and complete healing, ascertained by X rays, took place in 12 to 22 days. Twenty-three of the 36 patients had no recurrence of bleeding in two years, 12 cases remained ulcer-

* For comfrey sources, see Bibliography for Cancer.

free for one year, and the remaining case was ulcer-free for four months at the time the study was reported. The bioflavonoid treatment seemed to provide lasting relief. Smoking, because it uses vitamin C in the body, has been found to slow the healing of ulcers.

In Moscow, pantothenic acid, a B vitamin, was used with excellent success. Of 30 ulcer patients, 24 had duodenal ulcers and 15 patients had had ulcers for more than three years. In treating them, .05 grams of pantothenic acid was given each patient daily (it was doubled for two severe cases). Most patients began to improve after two to five days' treatment. A few more began to respond after six to eight days. Pain was reduced in 12 out of 24 patients who had night pain and in 12 who had hunger pain. Disappearance of night pain led to better sleep and appetite improvement in 25 patients, and symptoms of dyspepsia disappeared.

Vitamin E (alpha tocopherol) fed daily to rats gave them complete protection against ulcers. (*Proceedings of the Society for Experimental Biology and Medicine*, March, 1947.)

Olive oil, vitamin B complex, and, of course, the well-known daily glassful of fresh raw cabbage juice, have all proved helpful.

Russians have used honey for healing of ulcers for many years. Home remedies include:

Raw potato juice.
Fenugreek tea.
Garlic.
Raw flaxseeds. Chew one-quarter teaspoon midway between meals and at bed time.
One-half milk plus one-half pure fresh orange juice for one week. (The mixture should curdle.) Nothing else. Next week add a raw egg yolk. The drink may be taken as often as desired. (Dr. Eleanor E. Amend; see Bibliography.)

A simple remedy, according to Captain Frank Roberts (see Bibliography) has affected thousands of X-ray proved cures in three to four months. It is:

THE HERBAL CURE OF DUODENAL ULCERS

3½ oz. Tincture of Echinacea
3½ oz. Poke Root
3½ oz. Marshmallow Rind
3½ oz. Goldenseal Root
3½ oz. Cranesbill Root

Captain Roberts says, "For dosage: 30 drops in a wineglass of water, three times daily between meals. Shake the mixture thoroughly before measuring out each dose or you will get a wrong proportion of the five remedies."

44 Miscellaneous natural remedies

Many folk remedies date back to pre-biblical times, or even to the beginning of civilization itself. Unfortunately they are being gradually lost, forgotten or suppressed.

Write down, in the space provided at the end of this section, any natural remedy you may learn, either from those of the older generation, while they still recall them, or from people from foreign countries where home remedies are still often used.

Help preserve this precious heritage in our own country before it is too late.

To start your collection, here are a few miscellaneous natural or folk remedies:

ATHLETE'S FOOT

Rub with apple cider vinegar, either plain or diluted.

BOILS OR ABSCESSES

Make a poultice of white, fluffy bread. Place two or three slices in a white cloth napkin. Fold napkin lengthwise. Using the ends, dip the napkin in boiling water and then twist ends to squeeze excess water. Apply poultice to abscess or boil. Cover with a towel so that body heat maintains the warmth. Leave on overnight or until boil opens naturally.

Or use a potato poultice by applying directly to the skin a scraped or grated potato. Cover with a cloth. Dr. Eleanor Amend explains the value of the potato poultice, "It has a cooling, soothing effect and will help draw to a head." She also suggests a slice of lemon or garlic tied on overnight. She adds, "Both are antiseptic and healing." Add ground linseeds (flaxseeds) or fenugreek seeds to water and cook to a porridge-like consistency; or use boiled, mashed potatoes. Apply as a poultice, hot as can be tolerated. (Dr. H. C. Vogel: *The Nature Doctor*).

BURNS

Gertrude Foster, writing in July, 1963 issue of *House Beautiful*, tells of the miraculous effect of the plant *Aloe vera*, used for burns. A guest at a party carelessly folded back a pack of paper matches to light one match. The whole packet exploded and burned the guest's fingers painfully. The hostess reached for the cactus-like flower on her kitchen window sill, cut off a piece of the leaf and rubbed it over the burned areas. A transparent glue formed over the burn and brought instant relief from pain. The next day there was no redness and the fingers were still free from pain. Others report similar experiences.

If your nurseryman cannot supply you with this plant, a succulent, write for sources of supply to *House Beautiful*, 572 Madison Ave., New York City 22, and mention the July 1963 issue. If you burn yourself before your plant arrives, the American Dermatological Association suggests plunging the burned area in ice water. For major or large area burns, see your doctor.

CATARRH (MUCOUS)

Albert Holand, Jr., consulting nutritionist, suggests fenugreek seed. It can be made either into a tea (a teaspoon of seeds to a cup of boiling water) or a teaspoonful of powdered seeds (ground in a blender or small electric nut mill) added to salads, cereals or other foods. Ten tablets daily can be used instead. Mr. Holand, who explains the use of fenugreek in his article, "Grandma's Favorite Remedy for Mucous," (*Let's Live* magazine) adds, "As a general rule, the beneficial results to be observed are clearing of post nasal drip (catarrh), diminished sinus congestion, improved kidney action, relief from uncomplicated sore mouth and irritated mucous membranes, as well as less coughing up of phlegm and diminution of other mucous secretions."

Mr. Holand points out that fenugreek has long been used by veterinarians as an animal conditioner. In India, it is used to improve the feminine figure! It is also an ingredient of curry powder.

CORNS

Soak feet in hot water. Apply lemon juice or kerosene oil nightly.
Cut a slice of onion through the center. Soak in vinegar 24 hours. Bandage onion slice on corn so it will remain through the night. Repeat every night for a week.
Place the end slice of lemon on corn and bind overnight. Repeat each night as needed.
Keep the corn moistened with castor oil until it disappears.

CUTS

Apply fresh lemon juice or slice of lemon.
Make a "band-aid" of a piece of fresh comfrey leaf.

EARACHE

Put a small slice of garlic button loosely in the ear, or put garlic powder on a piece of cotton and insert in ear. Cover with a heated wet towel.

HANDS

Chapped:
Rub with the yellow side of a lemon peel several times daily. Wash off with water.
Rub on apple cider vinegar, plain or diluted.
Rub on sesame oil (available in health food stores).

Brown spots (and moles):
Crush a clove of garlic. Rub on and leave for a short while. Repeat daily if necessary.
Rub in castor oil *daily*. Dr. D. C. Jarvis reports success with castor oil for brown spots on the hands. I have known two cases in which this treatment caused large moles on the face to disappear within a month or so. If the mole appears irritated in any way, before using castor oil application, see your doctor.

INSECT STINGS

Bee or wasp venom is highly toxic to a few people. A doctor can test you ahead of time to determine if you have a special allergy to the venom. If you are stung around the face, eyes or nose and exhibit any unusual symptoms such as chills, dizziness, fever, heavy perspiration, headache, nausea or vomiting, diarrhea, great thirst, throat or chest constriction, extreme weakness, rapid pulse or unconsciousness, take no chance! Call a doctor *immediately*.

For minor insect stings from an ant, bee, or wasp, try any of the following:

Rub with freshly cut onion or garlic.

Apply fresh lemon juice.

Touch the sting with chlorox, peroxide, liquid bluing from the laundry, alcohol or household ammonia. If you use ammonia, saturate a piece of cotton with water and ammonia and keep it on the sting for a short while to help neutralize the poison.

Apply garlic juice.

Use honey. Kathleen Hunter, who keeps bees and is stung constantly, says she touches the spot with honey and forgets about it. If you are in the garden, pick up a handful of damp earth or mud and apply.

POISON IVY OR POISON OAK

Equal parts of apple cider vinegar and water applied often.

Make a poultice of crushed garlic. Put several crushed cloves of garlic between layers of gauze and apply to the affected area for one-half hour.

Grind up any green leaves available. The best are leaves of the green bean vine. Plantain, dandelion, or plain grass or tree leaves will do. (Green plants contain healing chlorophyl). Apply

One physical therapist reports the case of a young boy who was hospitalized and covered with rash and blisters from head to toe. Doctors had about given up but gave permission for the green leaf therapy. The therapist used the quickest thing at hand—green spinach leaves. Liquefying the leaves, he applied the mixture as an ointment. Relief appeared in one afternoon; the boy was released from the hospital the next day, much to the amazement of the hospital staff. (*Journal of Natural Living*, Vol. 3, No. 6)

A well-known American Indian remedy, which is said to work very well, is the common jewel-weed (*Impatiens pallida*). Bruise the leaves and stems and rub in the juice.

ANTIDOTE FOR POISONS

Two doctors, Jay M. Arena and Grant Taylor, of Duke University School of Medicine, offer an antidote for poisoning when the cause is unknown. The ingredients: burned toast, strong tea and milk of magnesia. The burned toast contains pulverized charcoal to help absorb poisonous materials in the stomach; the tea contains tannic acid to offset an alkaline poison; and the milk of magnesia is to help counteract an acid poison. Used together, these doctors state, the ingredients provide over-all protection.

SEA OR AIR SICKNESS

Dr. H. C. A. Vogel writes, "Vitamin B-6 (pyridoxine) has proved itself an exceptionally efficacious remedy against seasickness and even air sickness. Begin taking these vitamins two to three days before setting out on a journey . . . eat naturally and don't make any excessive demands on the body merely because the airline, ship or the railways offer extensive menus."

SORE THROAT

Dr. Eleanor Amend suggests two tablespoons of fenugreek seeds simmered in a quart of cold water for an hour. Use as a gargle and drink three cups daily.
Gargle with salt and vinegar, diluted with water.

SPRAINS

Alternate hot and cold water applications.
Make a paste of iodized salt and apple cider vinegar. Massage gently into sprained area. (Dr. Amend)

SUNBURN

Aloe vera (see Burns).
Weak solution of vinegar.
Rub on ordinary tea (contains tannic acid).

TARTER ON TEETH

Dr. D. C. Jarvis suggests one teaspoon apple cider vinegar to a glass of water and sipped at meal time. Dentists corroborate the effect of this treatment, according to Dr. Jarvis. After several months, patients have reported less tooth decay, stronger fingernails, and hair falling stopped. He also considers this mixture a good "settler" for upset stomach.

TOOTHACHE

Place a hot water bottle on your feet.

WARTS

For plantar warts (those on the bottom of the feet) complete cures have been noted in 208 out of 238 cases as a result of the use of a water-soluble vitamin A, given orally. Only in one case did the warts reappear. Vitamin A injections were also helpful, or keep bandaged with cotton soaked in castor oil. (*Clinical Medicine,* July 1959)
For ordinary warts, Dr. Amend suggests the following:
Keep moist with castor oil till removed.
Rub with a piece of garlic nightly.
    According to Irwin I. Lubowe, M.D. in his book, *New Hope for Your Skin*, (New York, 1963, E. P. Dutton and Co.,) warts are caused by a specific wart virus. They can be spread by rubbing the wart on the side of one finger against other fingers or skin

areas, possibly starting a whole new colony of warts. Neither should they be gnawed with the teeth or picked at by the fingernails.

Some warts go away spontaneously, perhaps due to a strengthening of the body defenses. Dr. John Locricchio, Jr., and John R. Haserick of the Cleveland Clinic found that immersion of warm water (between 113 and 119 degrees) for thirty to ninety minutes once or twice weekly had good results. Nine out of fifteen patients lost their warts completely and another four were greatly improved. Dr. Lubowe warns that a hair growing from a wart or mole should not be plucked. It should be clipped only. Medical consultation is advisable, he says.

Bibliography

Most of the following books are available either through your local bookstore, health food store, public library, or from Mildred Hatch Library, St. Johnsbury, Vermont. In a few cases special sources will be given for hard-to-find items.

PART I
Some Unusual Treatments
CHAPTER 1
Believe It or Not

D. T. Atkinson, M.D. *Magic, Myth and Medicine*. New York, Premier Books, 1956.
Gilbert E. Brooke, "Handbook, Tropical Medicine", *Hygiene and Parasitology*, 1908.
Elizabeth Terry, "Quacks", *National Health Federation Bulletin*, April 1963.

CHAPTER 2
How to Be Healthy

R. Swinburne Clymer, M.D., *The Medicines of Nature—The Thomsonian System*. Quakertown, Pa. P.O. Box 77, The Humanitarian Society, 1960.
Harvey Graham, *The Story of Surgery*. New York, Doran and Co., 1939.
William Gutman, M.D., *Prolongation of Life*. Rustington, Sussex, England. Health Science Press, 1961. (Available Harmony Bookshop, New Castle, Pa.)
Earl L. Shaub, *Creative Power*. New York, G. S. Rand, 1958.

CHAPTER 6
Who Can Help You?

Carter Harrison Downing, M.D., D.O., *Osteopathic Principles in Disease*, San Francisco, Ricardo J. Orozco, 1935.
Pyramid Books, 1962.

George A. Wilson, D.C., *Second Factor in Chiropractic*, Long Beach, California, Standard Research Laboratories, 6455 Don Julio St., 1959.

CHAPTER 7
Homeopathy

J. Ellis Barker, *Miracles of Healing, A New Path To Health*, London, Maxwell Love and Co., Ltd. (Available from Harmony Book Shop, New Castle, Pa.)

Alonzo J. Shadman, M.D. *Who Is Your Doctor and Why?* Boston, 1958; Available from Lee Foundation for Nutritional Research, Milwaukee 1, Wisc. or Harmony Book Shop, New Castle, Pa.

A directory of Homeopathic Physicians is available for $2.50 from American Institute of Homeopathy, 1011 Arch Street, Philadelphia 7, Pa.

Homeopathic Pharmacies: where remedies may be ordered (write for prices):
Boericke & Tafel, 1011 Arch St., Philadelphia 7, Pa.
Erhart & Karl, Inc., 17 N. Wabash, Chicago 2, Ill.
Hahn & Hahn, 324 Saratoga St., Baltimore 1, Md.
Luyties Pharmaceutical Co., 4200 Laclede Ave., St. Louis 8, Mo.
Standard Homeopathic Pharmacy, 204 W. 8th St. Los Angeles 14, Calif.
Mylans Pharmacy, 220 O'Farrell, San Francisco 2, Calif.
Homeopathic Pharmacy, 844 Yonge St., Toronto, Ontario, Canada.

CHAPTER 8
The Biochemical Cell-Salts

Edward Bach, M.D., *The Twelve Healers and Other Remedies*. Ashington, Rockford, Essex, England. C. W. Daniel Co., Ltd., 1960. (Available Harmony Book Shop, New Castle, Pa.)

J. B. Chapman, M.D., *Dr. Schuessler's Biochemistry*, Mokelumne Hill, Calif., reprinted 1963.

Mira Louise, *More About Biochemistry*. Adelaide, South Australia. Sharples, Printers Ltd. 1959. Also, *What To Do About Functional Disorders*. (Available Harmony Book Shop, New Castle, Pa.)

Schuessler Remedies available from Homeopathic Pharmacies (See list above.).

Dr. Marcus Bach, "Let the Flowers Heal You." *Fate*, July, 1963 also

Bach Remedies available from Keene and Ashwell, Ltd. 226 Venner Rd., Sydenham, London, S.E.26., England. $8.00 surface mail; $9.50 air mail.

Aubrey Westlake, *The Pattern of Health*. New York, Devin-Adair, 1963.

CHAPTER 9
Do Herbs Help?

Kathleen Hunter, *Health Foods and Herbs*. New York, Arc Books, Inc. 1963.

F. Ellingwood, M.D., *Materia Medica and Therapeutics*. Chicago, Ill. Medical Press, 1898 p. 264.

Claude V. James, *Herbs and the Fountain of Youth*. Edmonton, Alberta, Canada, Amrita Books, 12114 93rd St. 8th Printing, 1957.

W. N. McCartney, M.D. *Fifty Years a Country Doctor*. New York, E. P. Dutton, 1938.

Dr. Nehru's reference to onions: *Electronic Medical Digest*, Special Ed., 1960,

Available from Lee Foundation for Nutritional Research, 612 N. Vermont Ave., Los Angeles 5, Calif.

Ebba Waerland, *Rebuilding Health*. New York, Arc Books, Inc. 1968.

CHAPTER 10
Pressure Therapy—Acupuncture

William H. Fitzgerald, M.D. and Edwin F. Bowers, M.D. and George Starr White, M.D., *Zone Therapy, or Relieving Pain at Home and Zone Therapy* (Combined editions). Mokelumne Hill, Calif. Health Research, 1952

F. M. Houston, D.C.Ph. C., *Contact Healing*. Long Beach 3, Calif. 5600 E. 2nd St. Order direct from Dr. Houston.

Leslie O. Korth, D.O.M.R.O., *Some Unusual Healing Methods*, Wayside, Grayshott, Hindhede, Surrey, England, Health Science Press, 1960.

D. and J. Lawson-Wood, *First Aid At Your Finger Tips*. Health Science Press, Sussex, England.

Felix Mann, M.B., *Acupuncture*. New York, Random House, 1963.

George A. Wilson, D.C., Chief Emeritus of Research, Spears Chiropractic Hospital and Research Director of the International Chiropractic Biophysical Research Society, *Emotions In Sickness*. 6455 Don Julio Street, Long Beach, Calif. 1963.

CHAPTER 12
Human Electronics-Radieathesia

Thomas Colson, D.O., B.S. L.L.B., *The Electron Theory in Medicine*. Compiled and edited by Fred J. Hart, San Francisco, Calif. Electronic Medicine Foundation, 1953. (Available Lee Foundation for Nutritional Research, 612 Vermont Ave., Los Angeles 5, Calif.)

Langston Day, with George De La Warr, *New Worlds Beyond the Atom*. New York, Devin-Adair, 1963.

Ruth B. Drown, *The Theory and Technique of the Drown Therapy and Radio Vision Instruments*. London, W. 1. England, Hatchard and Co. 1939.

Electronic Medical Digest. Special Edition, 1960, San Francisco; Electronic Medical Foundation. Available from Lee Foundation for Nutritional Research, 612 N. Vermont Ave., Los Angeles 5, Calif.

John H. Heller, *Mice Men and Molecules*. New York, Charles Scribner & Sons, 1960.

Abbe Mermet, *Principles and Practice of Radiesthesia*, New York, Thomas Nelson and Sons, 1959.

Aubrey Westlake, B.A.M.B., The Pattern of Health, New York, Devin-Adair, 1963.

CHAPTER 13
Do-It-Yourself Radiesthesia

Dr. Vernon Wethered, B.Sc., *An Introduction to Medical Radiesthesia*, Ashingdon, Rochford, Essex, England, C. W. Daniel Co. 1957.

James Crenshaw, "Science and Industry Look at Dowsing." *Fate*, Sept. 1965.

Hardwood, hand-turned, perfectly-balanced Pendulums available Harmony Book Shop, New Castle, Pa. $2.00.

PART II
Health Through Nutrition
CHAPTER 15
Our "Good" American Diet?

To learn more about the use and sources of where safe, natural foods may be purchased, subscribe to Natural Food Associates' magazine, *Natural Food and Farming*, membership fee of $5.00 includes magazine. Address: Natural Food Associates, Atlanta, Texas. (Joe D. Nichols, M.D., is president of this fine group, which has regional Associations throughout the United States.

Dr. Carlton Fredericks and Herbert Bailey, *Food Facts and Fallacies*. New York, Arc Books, Inc. 1968.

Agnes Toms, *Eat Drink and Be Healthy*, New York, Devin-Adair, 1963. (A complete natural foods cookbook).

Beatrice Trum Hunter, *The National Foods Cook Book*. New York, Simon & Schuster, 1961.

Adelle Davis, *Let's Cook It Right*. New York, Harcourt, Brace.

Sonya Richmond, *International Vegetarian Cookery*. New York, Arc Books, Inc. 1967.

Edward E. Marsh, *How to be Healthy with Natural Foods*. New York, Arc Books, Inc. 1968.

CHAPTER 18
Macrobiotics

George Ohsawa, *Zen Macrobiotics The Art of Longevity and Rejuvenation;* also *The Philosophy of Oriental Medicine*. Printed in Japan; available from Ohsawa Foundation, 61 W. 56th St., New York City, N.Y.

CHAPTER 20
The Star Exercise

The Star Exercise, contributed by Eugene Fersen (deceased). Further information available from The Lightbearers, 1409 E. Prospect, Seattle, Wash.

Spiritual Healing Books:

Rebecca Beard, M.D. *Everyman's Search*, New York, Harpers, 1950.

Dr. William R. Parker and Elaine St. Johns, *Prayer Can Change Your Life*. New York, Prentice Hall, 13th Printing, April 1962.

PART III
Treating Diseases Naturally
CHAPTER 21
Alcohol and Alcoholism

Charlotte Carter, R.N., and Dyson Carter, M.Sc., *Cancer, Smoking, Heart Disease, Drinking in Our Two World Systems Today*, Toronto, Ontario, Canada, Northern Book House, 1957.

Charles De Coti Marsh, *Rheumatism, Arthritis, The Conquest*, (1958), *Prescription For Energy*, (1959); both London, Eng., Thorson's Ltd. (Available from Harmony Book Shop, New Castle, Penna.).

Harold Sherman, *Anyone Can Stop Drinking*, New York, C. and R. Anthony, 1959.

Peter J. Steincrohn, M.D., *Your Life To Enjoy*, Englewood Cliffs, N.J. Prentice Hall, 1963.

Roger J. Williams, Ph.D., Alcoholism, *The Nutritional Approach*, Austin, Tex., University of Texas Press, 1951.

CHAPTER 22
Allergies

Arthur F. Coca, M.D., *The Pulse Test*, New York, University Books (Lyle Stuart), 225 Lafayette Street, New York City 12, 1956.

Adelle Davis, *Let's Eat Right To Keep Fit*, New York, Harcourt, Brace, 1954.

Catharyn Elwood, *Feel Like A Million*, New York, Devin-Adair, 1956.

Theron G. Randolph, M.D., *Human Ecology and Susceptibility to the Chemical Environment*, Springfield, Ill., Charles C. Thomas, 1962.

Herman Hirschfeld, M.D., *The Whole Truth About Allergy*. New York, Arc Books, Inc. 1963.

CHAPTER 24
Arthritis

Charles B. Ahlson, *Health From the Sea and Soil*, New York, Exposition-Banner, 1962, (available from Charles B. Ahlson, 211 Mariposa Ave., Watsonville, Cal., $4.00).

Dan Dale Alexander, *Arthritis and Common Sense*, Hartford, Conn., Witkower Press, 1956, rev. ed.

Rebecca Beard, M.D., *Everyman's Search*. New York, Harper & Bros., 1950.

Joseph Broadman, M.D., *Bee Venom, the Natural Curative for Arthritis and Rheumatism*. New York, G. P. Putnam and Sons, 1962.

D. C. Jarvis, M.D., *Arthritis and Folk Medicine*. New York, Holt, Rinehart and Winston, 1960.

Mildred W. McKie, M.D., *Natural Aids for Common Ills*. Northboro, Iowa.

John Ott, *My Ivory Cellar*. Chicago, Twentieth Century Press, 1958.

Melvin E. Page, D.D.S., and H. Leon Abrams Jr., *Health Versus Disease.* St. Petersburg, Fla., Page Foundation (2810 First St. North), 1960.

Max Warmbrand, N.D., D.O., *Encyclopedia of Natural Health.* New York, Julian Press, 1962, and *New Hope for Arthritis Sufferers.* New York, Whittier Books, 1959.

H. Curtis Wood Jr., M.D., *Overfed but Undernourished.* New York, Exposition-Banner Press, 1959.

Bernard Aschner, M.D., *Arthritis Can be Cured.* New York, Arc Books, Inc. 1968.

Sea Water available from the following sources. *Write for prices:* Delamer Solution (sea water plus calcium, iron, and iodine), Del Monte Laboratories, 908 W. 17th St., Costa Mesa, Calif.; Sea Val (sea water plus four vitamins), Sea Water Enterprises, P.O. Box 302, Watsonville, Calif. Mineralized Calodine, 3401 MacArthur Blvd., Oakland 2, Calif.

Desert Tea, available from Governor Herbs, Inc. P.O. Box 3095, Inglewood, Calif. 90304.

CHAPTER 25
Asthma

E. M. Abrahamson, M.D. and A. W. Pezet, *Body, Mind and Sugar.* New York, Henry Holt, 1951.

H. E. Kirschner, M.D. *Nature's Healing Grasses.* Yucaipa, Calif., H. C. White Co., 1960.

Eric F. W. Powell, *Health Secrets of All Ages.* Rustington, Essex, Eng. Health Science Press (Available from Harmony Book Store, New Castle, Penna.)

Herman Hirschfeld, M.D., *Your Allergic Child.* New York, Arc Books, Inc. 1965.

Russian Comfrey Plants: Shafers, 238 Sinclair, Glendale 6, Calif. No orders less than $3.00. For other sources, see ch. 28-29, Bibliography.

CHAPTER 26
Backache

Kenneth C. Hutchin, M.D., *Slipped Discs.* New York, Arc Books, Inc. 1964.

Harry Clements, D.O., *Banishing Backache and Disc Trouble.* London, Eng., Health for All Publishers, 1959.

CHAPTER 27
High Blood Pressure—Hypertension

E. M. Abrahamson, M.D. and A. W. Pezet, *Body, Mind and Sugar.* New York, Henry Holt, 1951.

Virginia Z. Barth, *There Is An Art to Breathing.* Los Angeles, Llewellyn Publications, 1960.

Kenneth C. Hutchin, M.D., *Heart Disease and High Blood Pressure.* New York, Arc Books, Inc. 1964.

R. Swinburne Clymer, M.D., *Nature's Healing Agents*. 1963, 4th ed. Phil. Dorrance & Co.

Arthur F. Coca, M.D., *The Pulse Test*. New York, University Books, 1956.

Catharyn Elwood, *Feel Like a Million*. New York, Devin-Adair, 1956.

Kathleen Hunter, *Health Foods and Herbs*. New York, Arc Books, 1965

Melvin E. Page and H. Leon Abrams Jr., *Health Versus Disease*. St. Petersburg, Fla., Page Foundation, Inc., 1960.

Herman Pomeranz, M.D., *Control High Blood Pressure*. London, Eng.; Health for All Publishers, 1959.

Eric F. W. Powell, *Health Secrets of All Ages*. Rustington, Essex, Eng. Health Science Press (Available from Harmony Book Shop, New Castle, Penna.)

Benjamin P. Sandler, M.D., *How to Prevent a Heart Attack*. Milwaukee, Wisc., Lee Foundation for Nutritional Research, 1958.

Evan Shute, *Your Heart and Vitamin E*. New York, Devin-Adair, 1956.

George A. Wilson, D.C., *A New Slant to Diet*. Long Beach, Calif., Standard Research Labs., 6455 Don Julio Street: 1950 (order direct).

Herbert Bailey, *Vitamin E: Your Key to a Healthy Heart*. New York, Arc Books, Inc. 1966.

CHAPTERS 28-29
Cancer

Howard Beard, Ph.D., *A New Approach to the Conquest of Cancer, Rheumatic and Heart Diseases*. New York, Pageant Press, 1958.

Alexander Berglas, *Cancer: Nature, Cause and Cure*. Paris, Pasteur Institute, 1957.

Charlotte Carter, R.N., and Dyson Carter, M.Sc., F.C.G.S., M.C.I.C., *Cancer, Smoking, Heart Disease, Drinking in Our Two World Systems*, Toronto, Ontario, Canada, Northern Book House, 1957.

W. D. Chesney, M.D., *A Doctor Is Born*. Milton Junction, Wisc., 1958.

George Crile, Jr., M.D., *Cancer and Common Sense*. New York, Viking Press, 1955.

Max Gerson, M.D., *A Cancer Therapy, Results of Fifty Cases*. New York, Dura Books, 1963.

H. E. Kirschner, M.D. *Nature's Healing Grasses*. Yucaipa, Calif. H. C. White, Publisher, 1960.

Glenn Kittler, Laetrile, *Control for Cancer*. New York, Paperbook Library, 260 Park Ave., South; 1963.

Sir Robert McCarrison, M.D., *Studies in Deficiency Disease*. Milwaukee, Wisc. Lee Foundation for Nutritional Research, 1945.

M. E. Page, D.D.S., and H. Leon Abrams, Jr., *Health Versus Disease*. St. Petersburg, Fla., Page Foundation, Inc., 1960.

D. T. Quigley, M.D., *The National Malnutrition*. Milwaukee, Wisc., Lee Foundation for Nutritional Research, 1943.

Weston A. Price, D.D.S., *Nutrition and Physical Degeneration*. Los Angeles, American Academy of Applied Nutrition, 1950.

Cyril Scott, *Victory Over Cancer*. London, Eng., True Health Publishing Co., 1957. (Available from Health Research, Mokelumne Hill, Calif.).

Boris Sokoloff, *Cancer, New Approach, New Hope*. New York, Devin-Adair, 1952.

Stefansson, V. Cancer, *Disease of Civilization?* New York, Hill and Wang, 1960.

Thomas Sugrue, *There Is a River—The Story of Edgar Cayce*. New York, Henry Holt, 1942.

Andre Voisin, *Soil, Grass and Cancer*. New York, Philosophical Library, 15 E. 40th Street, 1959.

George A. Wilson, D.C., *Things You Should Know About Cancer*. Long Beach, Calif. 6455 Don Julio Street; 1956.

Comfrey plants available from:
Shafers, 238 Sinclair Ave., Glendale 6, Calif.
North Central Comfrey Providers, Box 195e, Glidden, Weisc.
Verne Thomas, Hancock, N.H.
Cristy's Comfrey Gardens, P.O. Box 36, Sandoval, N.M.

CHAPTER 30
Constipation

Adelle Davis, *Let's Eat Right To Keep Fit*. New York, Harcourt, Brace, 1954.

Catharyn Elwood, *Feel Like A Million*. New York, Devin-Adair, 1954.

Boris Sokoloff, M.D., *Middle Age is What You Make It*. New York, Greystone Press, 1938.

CHAPTER 31
Eyes—How to See Better

W. H. Bates, M.D., *Better Eyesight Without Glasses*. New York, Henry Holt, 1940, 1943 (Condensation available at health food stores.)

Clara A. Hackett, with Lawrence Galton, *Relax and See, a Daily Guide to Better Vision*. New York, Harper & Bros. 1955.

R. Brooks Simpkins, *Visible Ray Therapy of the Eyes*. Health Science Press, Rustington Sussex. (Available at Harmony Book Store, New Castle, Pa.

CHAPTER 32
Fall-Out—How to Bypass It

The following periodicals contain valuable information on this general subject:

Reader's Digest, May, 1962.

Jack Harrison Pollack, "World's Greatest Scientist Reports on Fall-Out". *Saga*, April 1962, and Dr. Hermann J. Muller with Jack Harrison Pollack, "Let's Face the Truth about Nuclear Testing."

This Week, June 10, 1962.

"Biological Effects of Atomic Radiation". *Summary Report*, 1956, p. 25, National Academy of Science, Washington, D.C.

Modern Nutrition, Nov. 1962, p. 7.

New York Times, May 11, 1960; Oct. 29, 1961; May 6, 1962.

Ruth and Edward Brecher, "What We Are Not Being Told About Fall-Out Hazards", *Redbook*, Sept., 1962.

South African Medical Journal, July, 1958.

Consumer's Report, Sept., 1962, p. 447.

"These Precious Days," *New Yorker*, Oct. 3, 1959.

Journal of the National Cancer Institute, Aug., 1951.

Modern Nutrition, Nov., 1960; Dec., 1961; Jan. 1962.

Lancet, Sept. 8, 1956.

Journal of the American Medical Association, Nov. 18, 1961; Jan. 20, 1962.

Science News Letter, Jan. 13, 1962; Feb. 3, 1962.

Mira Louise, "Survival In the Atomic Age", 242a Rundle St., Adelaide, South Australia. (Available Harmony Book Shop, New Castle, Pa.)

Hansgeorg Weidner, *E. Sciences, Marschalkenzimmern uber Horb/Schwarzwald*, Germany: Lichthort, No. 45/46, "Millet and Buckwheat as Preventive Medicine Against Radioactive Influences in the Human Organism."

Radiological Health News, 1962, 1963, State of California, Department of Public Health, Bureau of Radiological Health, 2151 Berkeley Way, Berkeley 4, Calif.

CHAPTER 33
Fatigue

Charles De Coti Marsh, *Prescription For Energy*. London, Eng. Thorsons Ltd., 1961. (Available in this country from Mildred Hatch Library, St. Johnsbury, Vermont, or Harmony Book Shop, New Castle, Pa.

Karin Roon's New Way To Relax. New York, Greystone Press, 1949.

CHAPTER 34
Feet

George A. Schroeder, *The Miracle Healing Power of Body Mechanics Therapy*. Englewood Cliffs, Prentice-Hall, 1964.

Simon J. Wikler, D.S.C., *Take Off Your Shoes and Walk: Steps to Better Foot Health*. New York, Devin-Adair, 1961. Murray Space Shoe Corp. 616 Fairfield Ave., Bridgeport 3, Conn.

CHAPTER 35
Migraine Headache

John E. Eichenlaub, M.D., *A Minnesota Doctor's Home Remedies for Common and Uncommon Ailments*. New York, Prentice-Hall, 1960.

Thomas H. Holmes, M.D., Helen Goodall, B.S., Stewart Wolf, M.D., Harold G. Wolf, M.D., *The Nose, An Experimental Study of Reactions Within the Nose in Human Subjects During Various Life Experiences*. Springfield, Ill., Charles C. Thomas, 1950.

Curt S. Wachtel, M.D., *Your Mind Can Make You Sick Or Well*. New York, Prentice-Hall, 1957.

CHAPTER 36
Hearing

Eleanor E. Amend, D.C., *Health Can Be Yours Naturally.* New York, Greenwich Book Publishers, 1958.

Victor L. Browd, M.D., *The New Way To Better Hearing.*

Catharyn Elwood, *Feel Like A Million.* New York, Devin-Adair, 1956.

Lester M. Morrison, M.D., *The Low Fat Way to Health and Longer Life.* New York, Prentice-Hall, 1958.

John A. Victoreen, L.L.D., *Hearing Enhancement.* Springfield, Ill. Charles C. Thomas, 1960.

HEARING SPECIALISTS:

H. J. Israelsen, Consultant, on sound pressure testing. Belmont Custom Hearing Aid Center, 865 Ralston Ave., Belmont, Calif.

Bernard Welt, M.D.F.A.C.S., 135 York Ave., Brooklyn, New York.

Dr. Curtis J. Muncie, Aurist, 150 N.E. 96th St, Miami, Fla.

CHAPTER 37
Heart

Kenneth C. Hutchin, M.D., *Heart Disease and High Blood Pressure.* New York, Arc Books, Inc. 1964.

E. M. Abrahamson and E. W. Pezet, *Body, Mind and Sugar.* New York, Henry Holt Co., 1951.

John X. Loughran, *90 Days To A Better Heart.* New York, Devin-Adair, 1958.

Lester M. Morrison, M.D., *The Low Fat Way to Health and Longer Life,* New York, Prentice-Hall, 1958.

Benjamin P. Sandler, M.D., *How To Prevent Heart Attacks.* Milwaukee, Wis., Lee Foundation for Nutritional Research, 1958.

Hans Selye, M.D., with Fred Kerner, *Strees and Your Heart.* New York, Hawthorne Books, 1961.

Evan Shute, M.D., *Your Heart and Vitamin E.* New York, Devin-Adair, 1956.

Herbert Bailey, *Vitamin E: Your Key to a Healthy Heart.* New York, Arc Books, Inc. 1966.

Max Warmbrand, N.D., *Add Years To Your Heart,* New York, Whittier Books, 1956.

CHAPTER 38
Indigestion—Gallstones—Kidney Stones

R. Swinburne Clymer, M.D., *Nature's Healing Agents.* Philadelphia, Pa., Dorrance and Co., 1963.

John E. Eichenlaub, M.D., *A Minnesota Doctor's Home Remedies For Common and Uncommon Ailments.* New York, Prentice-Hall, 1960.

Claudia V. James, *That Old Green Magic,* Edmonton, Alberta, Canada, Amrita Books, 12114 93rd St., 1952.

H. E. Kirschner, M.D., *Nature's Healing Grasses.* Yucaipa, Calif. H. C. White Publishers, 1960.

Boris Sokoloff, M.D., *Civilized Diseases. You Can Cure Them.* New York, Howell Soskin, 1944.

CHAPTER 39
Infections

Fred R. Klenner, "The Use of Vitamin C as an Antibiotic", *Journal of Applied Nutrition*, VI, 1953, 274; "Massive Doses of Vitamin C and the Virus Diseases", *Southern Medicine and Surgery*, CXIII, 1951, p. 101.

W. J. McCormick, M.D., "Have We Forgotten the Lesson of Scurvy?" *Journal of Applied Nutrition*, Vol. 15, No. 1 & 2, 1962; also, "Studies of the Effects of C", *Medical Record*, Sept. 1947, *Archives of Pediatrics*, N. Y. 69: 151-155, April, 1952; 70: 107-112, April, 1955; 76: 166-171, April, 1959.

"The Key to Good Health—Vitamin C" (booklet of documentation, $1.00) published by Graphic Arts Research Foundation, 112 West Kinzie St., Chicago 10, Ill.

"Vitamin C—Weapon against Disease", *Health Bulletin*, July 20, 1963.

CHAPTER 40
Insomnia

John E. Eichenlaub, M.D., *A Minnesota Doctor's Home Remedies For Common and Uncommon Ailments*, New York, Prentice-Hall, 1960.

William Gutman, M.D., *Prolongation of Life*. Rustington, Essex, Eng. Health Science Press, 1961. (Available Harmony Book Shop, New Castle, Pa.).

Charles P. Kelly, *The Natural Way to Healthful Sleep*. New York, Hawthorne Books, 1961.

Johnnie Lee MacFadden, *Barefoot In Eden*. New York, Prentice-Hall, 1962.

CHAPTER 41
Leg Cramps

Adelle Davis, *Let's Eat Right To Keep Fit*. New York, Harcourt Brace. 1954.

Catharyn Elwood, *Feel Like A Million*. New York, Devin-Adair, 1956.

Benjamin Harrow and Abraham Mazur, *Textbook of Biochemistry*, Philadelphia, Pa. W. B. Saunders, Seventh Edition, 1958.

CHAPTER 42
Overweight and Fasting

Luigi Cornaro, *Discourses on the Sober Life—How to Live 100 Years*. Mokelumne Hill, Calif., Health Research.

Adelle Davis, *Let's Eat Right To Keep Fit*. New York, Harcourt Brace, 1954.

Irving B. Perlstein, M.D. with William Cole, *Diet Is Not Enough*. New York, MacMillan, 1963.

Eric Taylor, *Fitness After Forty*. New York, Arc Books, Inc. 1966.

CHAPTER 43
Ulcers

Eleanor E. Amend, A.B., M.S., D.C. Ph.C. N.D., *Health Can Be Yours Naturally*, New York, Greenwich Books, 1958.

T. L. Cleave, M.D., *Peptic Ulcer, Causation, Prevention and Arrest*. Baltimore, Williams & Williams, 1963.

Captain Frank Roberts, *The Herbal Cure of Duodenal Ulcers*. London, Thorsons, 4th Printing 1960.

Sir Cecil Wakeley, M.D., *Stomach Ulcers*. New York, Arc Books, Inc. 1964.

Index

THESE TWO BOOKS COULD CHANGE YOUR LIFE

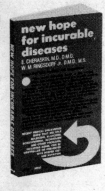

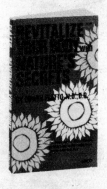

NEW HOPE FOR INCURABLE DISEASES

E. Cheraskin, M.D. and
W.M. Ringsdorf, Jr., M.D.

The revolutionary bestseller that proves in simple, everyday language that the battle against many dread diseases previously considered hopeless is being won—today. Stressing simple organic improvements in diet and nutrition and recent dramatic discoveries in these areas, the authors outline radically new and hopeful treatments for some of the most feared ailments of our time—multiple sclerosis, glaucoma, heart disease, mental retardation, birth defects and others. **"It is likely to become the most valuable guide to good health anyone could posess . . . an historic book, a must for all health seekers. The material on food supplements alone, is worth the price of the book." — Better Nutrition** $1.65

REVITALIZE YOUR BODY WITH NATURE'S SECRETS

Edwin Flatto, N.D., D.O.

A respected homeopathic physician explores every aspect of physical and mental well-being, never losing sight of the fact that health is the natural state of the body while disease is an unnatural state of imbalance. Fasting as a way to cleanse the body of toxic waste, the importance of a diet of wholesome, natural foods and the rewards of right eating are covered, as are exercise as therapy and the health benefits of fresh air and sunshine. Scores of questions on the problems of overweight, ulcers, varicose veins, acne, sinus trouble, constipation, colds and other common ailments are answered. Soundly scientific, easy-to-follow, this simple book promises lasting health, undreamed vigor and the happiness and peace that go with them.

$1.45

"THE MORE NATURAL OUR FOOD THE BETTER OUR HEALTH"

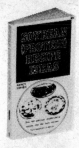 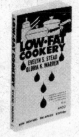 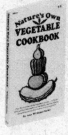

SOYBEAN (PROTEIN) RECIPE IDEAS
Nancy Snider

As a major source of protein soybeans are a nutritious and endlessly versatile food. Here are over 100 unusual and delicious recipes that take the zesty soybean from breakfast to dinner in a fabulous cookbook by a noted home economist and food editor. Scores of diet and dollar stretching recipes—all easy to prepare and serve—and all featuring soy protein—soy stroganoff, meat loaf, soy breakfast items, soups, entrees, side dishes, sandwiches, breads, desserts, much more. Includes menu ideas and tips on cooking with soy.

Illustrated, 95¢

LOW-FAT COOKERY
Evelyn S. Stead and Gloria K. Warren

Here finally is the perfect cookbook for a calorie-conscious, health-happy age. Incorporating more than 250 delicious, easy-to-follow recipes, **Low-Fat Cookery** puts the fun into dietetic cooking—and even more imporant, dietetic eating. Imagine delicious low-fat recipes for baked lasagna, fruitcake, bleu-cheese dressing, butterscotch sauce and lobster newburg. Included are invaluable aids to dietetic cooking with an easy-to-remember summary of the basic points of low-fat cookery, how to modify any recipe to obtain a low-fat content, information about new food products to enrich and diversify a low-fat diet, and a helpful discussion of special diets such as restricted sodium and unsaturated vegetable oil plans.

$1.45

NATURE'S OWN VEGETABLE COOKBOOK
Ann Williams-Heller

Over 350 mouthwatering vegetable recipes—complete with practical information on the buying, storing, cooking, seasoning and nutritional value of each vegetable. With this cookbook, noted nutritionist Ann Williams-Heller has opened the door to an entirely new culinary world. She brings her cooking genius to bear on every available vegetable—in main dishes, casseroles, salads, soups and their countless variations. Also included are recipes for sauces and salad dressings as well as nutrition charts that show the vitamin and mineral content of each vegetable.

$1.45

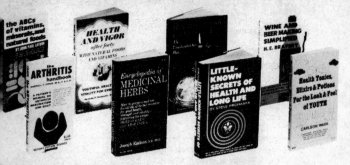

ABC'S OF VITAMINS, MINERALS AND NATURAL FOODS

John Paul Latour

An accurate, up-to-the-minute guide to foods, vitamins, minerals and poisons—their use and abuse. Reveals what to eat and what **not** to eat to achieve radiant good health.   95¢

ENCYCLOPEDIA OF MEDICINAL HERBS

Joseph Kadans, Ph.D.

A practical guide to the medical and cosmetic use of over 600 herbs—with hundreds of simple herbal treatments for all kinds of ailments. Special section on herb and spice cookery. $1.45

LITTLE-KNOWN SECRETS OF HEALTH AND LONG LIFE

Steve Prohaska

How to avoid doctors, dentists, hospitals and medical bills while gaining the blessings of good health and long life through simple, natural means. Features the fabulous Saturation Diet and a proven exercise program. $5.95

THE ARTHRITIS HANDBOOK

Darrell Crain, M.D.

An expert, authoritative guide to alleviating the suffering of arthritis, rheumatism and gout through natural diet and exercise. "A valuable manual."— The Arthritis Foundation
$1.45

WINE AND BEER MAKING SIMPLIFIED

H.E. Bravery

The thinking man's handbook—a lucid and lively guide for the home wine-maker who knows "what to do" but wants to know "why it works." With a section of recipes from apricot wine to light mild ale.   95¢

HEALTH AND VIGOR AFTER 40 WITH NATURAL FOODS AND VITAMINS

Herman Saussele, D.C.

A practicing chiropractic doctor reveals how men and women in the middle years can start the powerful healing forces of nature working for better health, longer life and more joyful living. $1.45

HEALTH TONIC, ELIXIRS AND POTIONS FOR THE LOOK AND FEEL OF YOUTH

Carlson Wade

Scores of easy-to-make, easy-to-use tonics, potions, and elixirs said to bring relief from seemingly hopeless aches and pains and which may help you look and feel years younger than your actual age. $1.45

HEALTHIER JEWISH COOKERY
The Unsaturated Fat Way

June Roth

Hundreds of traditional Jewish recipes, streamlined to remove the saturated fats and retain the old-fashioned tastes. Substitutes vegetable for animal fat, eliminates frying, uses herbs and natural foods.
$4.95

HEALTH and MEDICINE BOOKS

All books are available at your bookseller or directly from ARCO PUBLISHING COMPANY, INC., 219 Park Avenue South, New York, N.Y. 10003. Send price of books plus 25¢ for postage and handling. No. C.O.D.